Handbook of
Geriatric Care
Management
SECOND EDITION

Cathy Cress, MSW
Editor
Instructor
Emphasis in Geriatric/Home Care Management
Master of Arts Degree Program
San Francisco State University

JONES AND BARTLETT PUBLISHERS
Sudbury, Massachusetts
BOSTON   TORONTO   LONDON   SINGAPORE

World Headquarters

Jones and Bartlett Publishers
40 Tall Pine Drive
Sudbury, MA 01776
978-443-5000
info@jbpub.com
www.jbpub.com

Jones and Bartlett Publishers
Canada
6339 Ormindale Way
Mississauga, Ontario L5V 1J2
CANADA

Jones and Bartlett Publishers
International
Barb House, Barb Mews
London W6 7PA
UK

Jones and Bartlett's books and products are available through most bookstores and online booksellers. To contact Jones and Bartlett Publishers directly, call 800-832-0034, fax 978-443-8000, or visit our website www.jbpub.com.

Substantial discounts on bulk quantities of Jones and Bartlett's publications are available to corporations, professional associations, and other qualified organizations. For details and specific discount information, contact the special sales department at Jones and Bartlett via the above contact information or send an email to specialsales@jbpub.com.

The authors, editor, and publisher have made every effort to provide accurate information. However, they are not responsible for errors, omissions, or for any outcomes related to the use of the contents of this book and take no responsibility for the use of the products and procedures described. Treatments and side effects described in this book may not be applicable to all people; likewise, some people may require a dose or experience a side effect that is not described herein. Drugs and medical devices are discussed that may have limited availability controlled by the Food and Drug Administration (FDA) for use only in a research study or clinical trial. Research, clinical practice, and government regulations often change the accepted standard in this field. When consideration is being given to use of any drug in the clinical setting, the health care provider or reader is responsible for determining FDA status of the drug, reading the package insert, and reviewing prescribing information for the most up-to-date recommendations on dose, precautions, and contraindications, and determining the appropriate usage for the product. This is especially important in the case of drugs that are new or seldom used.

6048

Library of Congress Cataloging-in-Publication Data
Handbook of geriatric care management / [edited by] Cathy Cress. --
  2nd ed.
    p. ; cm.
  Includes bibliographical references and index.
  ISBN-13: 978-0-7637-4642-1
  ISBN-10: 0-7637-4642-8
    1. Geriatrics--Handbooks, manuals, etc. 2. Older people--Medical
care--Management--Handbooks, manuals, etc.   I. Cress, Cathy.
  [DNLM: 1. Health Services for the Aged--organization & admini-
stration. 2. Geriatrics. 3. Practice Management--organization &
administration.   WT 31 H236 2007]
RC952.55.C74 2007
362.198'97--dc22
                              2006026600

Production Credits

Executive Editor: Kevin Sullivan
Production Director: Amy Rose
Acquisitions Editor: Emily Ekle
Associate Editor: Amy Sibley
Production Assistant: Jamie Chase
Editorial Assistant: Patricia Donnelly
Manufacturing Buyer: Therese Connell
Marketing Manager: Katrina Gosek

Marketing Associate: Rebecca Wasley
Manufacturing and Inventory Coordinator: Amy Bacus
Composition: Arlene Apone
Cover Design: Kristin E. Ohlin
Cover Image: © Photos.com
Printing and Binding: Malloy, Inc.
Cover Printing: Malloy, Inc.

Printed in the United States of America
11 10 09   10 9 8 7 6 5 4 3

Contents

Contributors

Miriam K. Aronson, EdD
Consulting Gerontologist
Clinical Associate Professor
Albert Einstein College of Medicine
Old Tappan, NJ

Carolyn Barber, MSN, PHN, CMC

Peter S. Belson, MSW LICSW
Program Director, Care Management
Riverside Community Care, Inc.
Needham, MA

Phyllis Mensh Brostoff, CISW, CMC
Co-Founder and President
Stowell Associates SelectStaff Inc.
Milwaukee, WI

Cathy Jo Cress, MSW
Instructor
Emphasis in Geriatric/Home Care
Management
Master of Arts Degree Program
San Francisco State University
San Francisco, CA

Nina Pflumm Herndon, MA, CMC
National Association of Professional
Geriatric Care Managers
Sage Eldercare Solutions
San Francisco and San Mateo Counties, CA

Nancy Hikoyeda, DrPH, MPH
Director, Gerontology Program
San Jose State University
San Jose, CA

Erica Karp, LCSW, CCM
President
GCM Consulting, Inc.
Evanston, IL

Angela Koenig, MA
Freelance writer
Chicago, IL

Stephne Lencioni, MSW, CMC
Certified Geriatric Care Manager
Older Adults Care Management
Palo Alto, CA
A Division of the Institute on Aging
San Francisco, CA

Kathleen McConnell, MSW, LCSW

Christina Miyawaki, MA
Case Manager
Japanese American Services of the East Bay (JASEB)
Berkeley, CA

Barbara Morano, LSCW, CMC
Administrative Officer
GRECC
VA Medical Center
Bronx, NY

Carmen L. Morano, PhD, MSW
Associate Professor
Hunter College School of Social Work
New York, NY

Deborah Newquist, PhD, MSW, CMC
Director of Geriatric Services
ResCare, Inc.
Costa Mesa, CA

Leonie Nowitz, LCSW, BCD
Director
Center for Lifelong Growth
New York, NY

Merrily Orsini, MSSW
Managing Director
Corecubed Communications
Louisville, KY

Robert E. O'Toole, MSW
President
Informed Eldercare Decisions, Inc.
Dedham, MA

Cathie Ramey, MA
President/Gerontologist
Vesta Lifestyles, Inc.
Walnut Creek, CA

Connie Rosenberg, MPS, RN, CCM, CMC
Services and Resources for Seniors, Inc.
Morristown, NJ

Anne Rosenthal, PhD, MFT, CMC
Director of Community Services
Reutlinger Community for Jewish Living
Danville, CA

Emily B. Saltz, LICSW, CMC
Director
Elder Resources
Newton, MA

Victoria Thorpe, MEd
Sage Elder Care Solutions
Millbrae, CA

Monika White, PhD, MSW, CMC
President/CEO
Center for Healthy Aging
Santa Monica, CA
Adjunct Associate Professor of Gerontology
University of Southern California
Los Angeles, CA

Cheryl M. Whitman, BSN, MS, CMC
Director
Care Management Works of Countryside
2010, LLC
Colchester, CT

Foreword

America is definitely going gray as the Baby Boomers (those born between 1946 and 1964) are moving into their 60s. Many Americans are now living into their 80s and 90s and are coping with more age-related challenges than ever before. Health care issues are emerging as we struggle to take care of those afflicted by diseases such as, Alzheimer's, Parkinson's, and dementia. Housing issues are emerging as assisted care living facilities, nursing homes, and continuing care communities are vying for the clientele. Financial issues are becoming increasingly important as our elders are faced with a volatile economy, increasing health care costs, and decreasing insurance and government benefits. Finally, independence issues are in the forefront as our nation's elderly struggle to remain on their own—in their own homes and with a quality of life that they so cherish.

If you are thinking about becoming a geriatric care manager (GCM), are a care manager thinking of starting your own business, or are a family member trying to figure out how to work with a care manager, you have found the right book. Cathy Jo Cress has assembled the nation's premier care managers to write chapters for this book that contain real-life situations and solutions. Care management is not something that you can just "decide to do because you took care of Mom." Care management requires training and supervision. It is a profession that comes with professional liabilities and responsibilities. Caring for our nation's elderly means taking on the problems of a very vulnerable population. It is a position of trust and a valued position in our nation's aging network. Knowledge of health care systems, insurance companies, federal and state benefit programs, housing alternatives, and community resources are vital tools for every GCM.

The first edition of the *Handbook of Geriatric Care Management* was a resounding success that provided guidance on how to build, manage, and market a care management practice. It is recognized by care managers and aging network advocates across the country as a "must-have" reference book. Now, the second edition goes one step further in offering more information in each of these areas, as well as updating and expanding resources for use in a rapidly changing society.

Care, compassion, and concern, coupled with an extensive knowledge of the aging network, are the professional hallmarks of a great GCM. This book explores the training needed, the skills to be obtained, and the traits of a GCM. It takes a special person to make this 24/7 job a career, but it comes with some of the greatest rewards in knowing you are improving the quality of life of each client you touch.

GCMs are taking an increasingly important role with our nation's elderly and with those with disabilities. Many of today's seniors don't have close relatives living within 500 miles. Modern-day families are just making ends meet on two salaries and are dealing with young children of their own. Thus, assisting elderly parents or grandparents during a time of crisis is difficult or nearly impossible. Navigating today's health care system is a challenge for the healthy and nearly impossible for the ill or frail. In addition, many of today's insurance programs, health care systems, and government assistance programs require a strong advocate, if not an attorney, to understand all the nuances and receive maximum results.

GCMs are professionally trained to assist the elderly in a variety of circumstances and to become active advocates for their clients in dealing with housing and transportation issues, health care and insurance issues, financial and benefits issues, and in coordinating and overseeing outside resources. Professional geriatric care managers provide the finesse of a social worker, the medical skills of a nurse, and the tenderness of a family member. GCMs are often in the position to discuss end-of-life issues or transition issues with an elderly person and are seen as "an independent third party" with the best interests of their clients in mind. GCMs also provide communication, advice, and support to family members dealing with their elderly or disabled family members. GCMs become the local extension for the family to identify issues and problem-solve using their knowledge of community and national resources.

Often, GCMs are called in to handle a crisis: Mom has fallen and broken her hip, Dad has Alzheimer's and can no longer live at home, there has been a death in the family, or there are immediate financial problems. GCMs are usually available 24 hours a day, seven days a week. They are the life-savers who are on-site immediately—looking out for the best interests of the elderly. They are the ones with an emergency evacuation plan in place before the hurricane or tornado hits, the ones who can intervene with physicians when there are drug complications, the ones who can discuss documents needed and forms to be filed to ensure that all benefits can be accessed appropriately.

Creating, marketing, building, and maintaining a geriatric care management business has its own unique challenges. This is a business that provides highly personalized care and requires employees who are well trained and supported in working with ill, frail, and often lonely seniors. No aspect of the business is easy, and you will, no doubt, find yourself referring back to this book for answers to your business dilemmas.

Laury Gelardi, MBA
Former Executive Director,
National Association of Professional
Geriatric Care Managers
Tucson, AZ

Linda Aufderhaar, MSW, LCSW, CCM
President, National Association of
Professional Geriatric Care Managers
Tucson, AZ

Acknowledgments

For their assistance with editing, constructive comments, suggestions, and professional perspective, I would like to acknowledge and express sincere thanks to the many individuals who made this book possible.

I would like to thank Phyllis Brostoff for her help in editing. I would like to thank Amy Sibley for initiating this second edition and the Jones and Bartlett team, including Tricia Donnelly, for being such a warm, friendly, and efficient editorial staff.

I would like to thank the authors who contributed to this book: Carmen Morano, Barbara Morano, Deborah Newquist, Connie Rosenberg, Nancy Hikoyeda, Christina Miyawaki, the late B. J. Curry Spitler, Laura Spitler Hansen, Phyllis Mensh Brostoff, Stephne Lencione, Kathleen McConnell, Merrily Orsini, Robert E. O'Toole, Monika White, Cheryl M. Whitman, Erica Karp, Leonie Nowitz, Miriam Aronson, Cathie Ramey, Anne Rosenthal, Emily Saltz, Nina Pflumm Herndom, Victoria Thorpe, Peter S. Belson, and Karen Knutson. Their perseverance, hard work, and vast professional expertise in the field of geriatric care management fills this book. In this still cutting-edge field, these authors are many of the founding mothers and fathers, and I am especially grateful they shared their pioneering work and perspectives in each excellent chapter.

I would like to dedicate this book to Harry Cress, my 86-year-old father. I have his hands, his intelligence, and his writing talents. My ability to finally see all this and accept him in the filially mature here-and-now has made me a better teacher of aging issues, a more knowledgeable geriatric care manager, and, most importantly, a better person.

I would also like to dedicate this to Dr. Anabel Pelham, who invited me to help create and teach in San Francisco State University's master's in gerontology with an emphasis in geriatric care management. This handbook is a direct model of the classes I have developed at SFSU with Anabel's visionary guidance. She has expanded the field of geriatric care management using her educational foresight, and I feel privileged to work with her.

I would also like to dedicate it to Rose Kleiner and B. J. Spitler, who are two of the prime foremothers in the field of geriatric care management. My career as a geriatric care manager began in 1982 when a client brought me a newspaper clipping about Older Adults Care Management, Rose Kleiner's ground-breaking geriatric care management business. I read the story and said, "I want to do that," and doing it changed my life. Rose's pioneering steps in the field of geriatric care management helped launch many GCMs across the country. She also enriched the field of gerontology by endowing a chair in aging at our mutual alma mater, University of California Berkeley School of Social Welfare.

B. J. Spitler was the mentor and friend of many of the authors in this book. She schooled me and countless practitioners in geriatric care management through the brilliant work of her pioneering agency Age Concerns in San Diego. She taught me much about the challenges of juggling work and family. We shared a passionate love of our daughters and a lifetime of learning how to balance family and career. Her ultimate success is her wonderful daughter Laura, also a contributor to this book.

I would also like to offer my love and thanks to my two daughters, Kali Peterson, who recently joined the field of gerontology, and Jill Gallo, a great artist, plus my 13-year-old granddaughter, Julia Gallo. We remain a family of compassionate, smart women who work hard for our beliefs and values and labor assiduously to continue to actualize our vision. I want to thank them for carrying on that tradition.

Finally, let me dedicate this book to my husband Pete Peterson, who every day shares that balance of work and family, making it possible for me to do both. Behind every working woman there should be a guy like Pete.

Cathy Jo Cress

Introduction

Since the first edition of the *Handbook of Geriatric Care Management* came out in 2000, the urgency of families seeking solutions for care of their aging parents has mushroomed like a nuclear event. Every day of the year 2006, 7,918 more people turned 65 years old—that's 330 people an hour. An estimated 44 million family members care for older or disabled relatives in the United States. This backbreaking job assumed by families costs $200 billion in informal care that is not reimbursed by the federal government. Businesses lose between $11 billion and $29 billion a year because family members interrupt, leave, or quit work to uphold their caregiving responsibilities. This loving load of elder care is about to shatter families and make the geriatric care manager a more urgent lifesaver compared to its role in the year 2000 when this book was first published.

Geriatric care management was born at the end of the 20th century to oversee the ballooning, illusive, and many times, unreachable aging continuum of care. This new profession was a beacon of hope for desperate family caregivers. Geriatric care managers (GCMs) are now one of the central points of entry for baby boomers who remain lost in the mystifying maze of aging services. By 2006, GCMs had climbed to the level of national experts. GCMs are friendly helpers, who repair frail elders' safety nets, find needed services, and relieve confounded adult children. GCMs can stare down the convoluted, fractional web of senior services and come up with the correct services and a premium care plan for each older person. GCMs ensure that care is right for the individual, delivered by the right person at the right time. The second edition of the *Handbook of Geriatric Care Management* is being published at a time when geriatric care management is evolving exponentially. Although the field has existed for more than 30 years, it is just coming into its own.

Geriatric care management originated as a cutting-edge addition to case management. But as the profession matured, it mainstreamed and separated from case management. Geriatric care management bridges larger businesses such as elder law, banking, trust departments, accounting, the assisted living industry, senior real estate business, and the ballooning U.S. medical care system that ministers to the chronic care needs of older people. Geriatric care managers are both salient guides to all these senior industries and the gears that help all work better and in tandem, like a well-run machine. The geriatric care management profession's growth is reflected in its increasing inclusion in the portfolios of very large health care businesses and the emergence of large nationwide geriatric care management corporations.

Geriatric care management also bridges several educational domains such as nursing, social work, physical therapy, occupational therapy, and gerontology. The new field synthesizes theory and pedagogical frameworks from all of these disciplines to create a new field, with its own academic degrees and certificates, reflected in the many emerging academic programs at universities all over the country.

Why has this new profession grown so quickly, spread so far, and created an academic place of its own? What created it in the first place? Quite simply, the field evolved out of a genuine gap in aging services that still exists today. It began in the 1980s as a result of astounding demographics—the fastest-growing segment of U.S. population was over age 85. This burgeoning population of middle- and upper-income elders needed community and health care services to remain in their homes. Their needs were not being met. Their adult children, affected since the 1950s by Dad and Mom working and trying to raise a family, were already overpowered by their load. Most adult children had moved long distance from their aging parents. When aging mothers, fathers, aunts, and uncles called out to their adult children for help in the early 1980s, all of these demographic, economic, and family system factors converged to launch the field of geriatric care management, answering the needs of both adult children and their older family members who wished to remain in their homes. What did not evolve was a training program for GCMs, a large gap that this book aims to fill. The *Handbook of Geriatric Care Management, Second Edition* delivers a training program to the growing number of colleges and universities offering geriatric care management programs. This textbook is a great choice for schools that form the front line for geriatric care management education, including those that specialize in social welfare, nursing, gerontology, and physical therapy. It gives educators

throughout the United States and the world a text to add to classes that addresses the multiple needs of aging adults and their families. This book is a critical tool to use in health, social services, and business curricula in undergraduate and graduate courses. This textbook can also be used as an additional reading resource in introductory aging issues classes and can augment courses in related fields, such as physical therapy, occupational therapy, law, insurance, banking, medicine, and real estate, when instructors want to provide a bridge to help their particular profession solve the problems of aging families.

As the vocation of geriatric care management has grown, so has a much-needed GCM credentialing process. This book discusses the many credentialing choices and the credentialing process in general. Why is the credentialing process important? It is a stamp of approval for consumers—families and older people seeking a skilled and professionally trained GCM. The credentialing process is also helpful to GCMs, giving them credibility with the public, thus helping to build their practice. This book can help aspiring and experienced GCMs choose the right credentials to pursue.

The *Handbook of Geriatric Care Management, Second Edition* can help beginning GCMs get their sea legs and seasoned GCMs grow as professionals. Because geriatric care management is a business, whether nonprofit or for-profit, this book covers critical aspects of running, adding to, and operating a geriatric care management practice, including launching the business, promoting the business, running a fiscally sound business, making money, and expanding the business.

This textbook covers critical clinical issues, including the GCM's role in working with dementia clients and their families and giving aid to clients diagnosed with depression. It also pilots GCMs through clinical work such as guiding and problem solving with normal but highly stressed aging families and doing the same for difficult, aging families. It gives readers therapeutic interventions to help families function as a unit to solve the myriad problems of their older parents.

This second edition offers nine substantial new chapters that cover psychosocial assessment, functional assessment, geriatric care management and late-life relocation, working with normal or nearly normal families, working with difficult families, preparing for emergencies, writing a geriatric assessment and care plan, and ethical and cultural considerations in geriatric care management.

New sections, including geriatric assessment and monitoring, are broken down to psychosocial assessment, functional assessment, ethnic and cultural assessment, and writing a geriatric assessment, giving the reader a broad guide to assessment tools that pinpoint an older person's problems.

Because the definition of geriatric care management is still somewhat unclear, marketing geriatric care management services can be difficult. This book offers clear guidance to define geriatric care management as a business product to sell, get new customers, and make a profit. This information is helpful to beginning GCMs, experienced GCMs, nonprofit agencies offering geriatric care management services, health care corporations that already integrate geriatric care management into their menu of services, or law and real estate businesses that want to add GCM to their practices.

This handbook also offers an entire chapter on the ethics of geriatric care management. GCMs try to ensure that senior services are not only highly individualized, appropriate, and coordinated, but also ethical. GCM providers help seniors and their families make very difficult decisions. GCMs have also developed a code of ethics for all practitioners to follow. Consumers should know to choose only GCMs who abide by this code of ethics.

A new chapter on working with clients from different cultural and ethnic backgrounds is a landmark chapter in broadening the scope of practice of GCMs and giving GCMs of multi-ethnic and cultural backgrounds tools to appropriately assess the needs of elders from different cultures.

The *Handbook* will also serve as a tool for the business world. Part 3, *The Business of Geriatric Care Management,* includes information on how to begin or add a geriatric care management business, grow a mature or seasoned geriatric care management business, add a geriatric care management practice to a nonprofit business, and sell GCM services and gain customers thereby critically making money in all of these business arenas. Business owners wishing to integrate geriatric care management into their business or portfolio of businesses (e.g., accountants, elder-law attorneys, persons who work in a trust department or large national health care corporation) will learn all they need to know through this book.

Intended as a practical guide, the *Handbook of Geriatric Care Management, Second Editon* includes sample forms and letters. These tools are meant to both be used as-is and be modified. And because this book is intended as a teaching tool, it contains many case examples. Instructors working with this textbook can use the examples to explain some of the how-to techniques mentioned and give students a good sense of the problems likely to arise and how they can be solved. Some contact information for organizations mentioned in the book is listed in Appendix A. The textbook also offers multiple assessment tools critical to the field, which can assist instructors in helping students learn to appraise the problems of older people and their stressed families.

This textbook is a manual to a stage of life not addressed in the annals of how-to books of the 20th century. Whole series of classes developed for the study of babies and preschoolers. Entire curricula have been developed through schools of nursing and social work to instruct the family facing adolescents and their prospective problems. Yet guidebooks for the difficulties of the midlife family, a distinct new stage of life, are scanty at best. Recently retired baby boomers facing the continued support of their own adult children are now additionally affected by the needs and crises of their aging parents. The textbooks for them are just beginning to be codified and accepted into academia. A flurry of "how to deal with our aging parents" books are just hitting the bookstores in volumes. This textbook is a major contribution to this needed body of literature that addresses this new developmental stage not identified until the last few decades.

Geriatric care management in the not-so-distant year 2025 may be completely differ-

ent from geriatric care management today. This handbook gives a sense of the metamorphosis the field is likely to undergo in the next few decades.

The *Handbook of Geriatric Care Management, Second Edition* is meant as a rich resource discussing this incredibly complex and interesting field. I hope that it will serve you well, helping you become a better GCM , integrate geriatric care management into your business, learn more about aging, and help these midlife families and their aging parents work as successful and loving systems of care.

Cathy Jo Cress

PART 1

Introduction to Geriatric Care Management

Chapter 1

Overview and History of Geriatric Care Management

Cathy Jo Cress

What is geriatric care management? It is a series of steps taken by a professional geriatric care manager (GCM) to help solve older people's problems. A GCM, who may be a social worker, a nurse, a gerontologist, or another human service professional, serves older people and their families. The GCM usually steps in when the older person or family is in crisis. Geriatric care management is also a preventative service rendered on demand, increasing the quality of an older person's life, managing all the players rendering services to the older person, and offering assurance and peace of mind to the adult children of the older individual. How does the GCM solve these problems and render these services? The GCM uses classic social work and nursing tools, including client assessment, care planning, service coordination, and referral and monitoring.

What is a professional GCM? GCMs' jobs are similar to the role of case managers, and GCMs use all the classic tools of case management. But unlike other case managers, GCMs specialize in serving adults aged 65 and older and offer very personalized services. GCMs historically have had much smaller caseloads than case managers have (especially those in public case management settings), giving GCMs great flexibility in delivering highly individualized services to their older clients. Unlike many case managers in public case management settings, GCMs are generally available 24 hours a day, 7 days a week, 365 days a year. They respond to client needs at the convenience of the client, which enables the GCM to cross the line from public sector human services into the for-profit service business. The GCM's product is service, and that product must be available at all times to be useful to older people, their families, and third parties such as trust departments and conservators, who are willing to buy the product if it is offered in this manner.[1]

The GCM is not just the classic anonymous public-sector case manager delivering impersonal services. In fact, the GCM is a kind of surrogate family member with special expertise in the phases and tasks of care management and a long-standing and personal relationship with clients. GCMs deliver the kind of old-fashioned good service that many older clients remember nostalgically. GCMs both respond to clients' demands and are proactive, always maintaining a positive attitude.

In addition, GCMs deliver the level of service that older clients' and adult children expect. These children are usually baby boomers from two-income families who are accustomed to purchasing services (housecleaning, day care, after-school transportation, tax assistance) to help make their busy lives easier. Purchasing geriatric care management services to assist with the problems of their older family members, who frequently live far away, seems logical to these adult children. The GCM is providing time and expertise, neither of which the adult child has. The GCM also sells peace of mind. Most baby boomers do not want to get up in the middle of the night to respond to an older person's crisis, but the GCM will. The adult child may not have enough vacation time to fly to the parent's home to arrange services once the older person gets out of hospital, but the GCM does this. Many adult children want the assurance that the older family member is cared for and safe, without having to solve the problem themselves. So, the personalized services of the GCM, a surrogate family member, appeal to adult children.[2]

In addition to handling client assessment, care planning, service coordination, and referral and monitoring, the GCM keeps track of a giant web of senior services, the continuum of care. GCMs are like Charlotte, the friendly spider in *Charlotte's Web*. They run back and forth across the web, linking services, repairing gaps, spinning new solutions to problems, and coordinating answers. At their root, GCMs are problem solvers.

This chapter offers an overview of what a GCM does and discusses the history of the profession.

■ HISTORY OF GERIATRIC CARE MANAGEMENT

GCMs are now relatively familiar participants in the world of senior services and health care. But what conditions led to the rise of geriatric care management? This section discusses the history of this important profession.

The Origins of Case Management

In a seminal study of geriatric care management, Secord and Parker note that case management itself, the root of geriatric care management, has its foundation in the social services for new immigrants and other poor people that emerged in the late 1800s.[3] At that time, urbanization and industrialization had left so many people poor and homeless that churches and local communities were paralyzed and unable to care for everyone in need. Social service bureaucracies began to arise, which led to the beginning of case management. Secord and Parker hypothesize that the core elements of today's case management were born by "helping the client find the least costly, most appropriate services to meet his or her needs."[3(p4)] Since then, community agencies, social workers, hospital discharge planners, and case coordinators have provided what we now call case management.

No one group or movement was solely responsible for the emergence of case management. In the arena of early social services, in 1833 Joseph Tuckerman organized a group of churches to help needy families. The Settlement House movement at the turn of the 20th century is another example of early case management. The Settlement House movement established institutions called settlement houses that tried to improve living conditions in city neighborhoods. Most settlement houses had social workers on staff. Many charity organizations and societies coordinated assistance for children and families; a case management program was set up by the Massachusetts Board of Charities in the mid-1800s. The roots of case management can also be found in early workers' compensation programs of the 1940s.[4]

In the medical world, case management appeared in the treatment of chronically ill and long-term-care populations, including children, people with disabilities, substance abusers, and people with acquired immune deficiency syndrome. As acute care costs skyrocketed in the United States after World War II, case management techniques developed to lower costs. Case managers appeared in institutional settings and followed patients into the community to coordinate care for high-cost, high-risk individuals. At the same time, private medical case managers appeared to respond to the needs of patients, insurers, and medical providers by helping these constituents make difficult decisions (e.g., is a medical procedure appropriate, is there a less costly alternative, or can a patient spend recovery time at home). Today, the medical case manager makes a path for the patient through the maze of the health care delivery system, coordinates a plan of care, and offers support from family agencies and suppliers of health care or health care entities.[5]

Growth of Case Management for Older People

According to Parker and Secord, case management for older people emerged because of two factors. The first was the rapid growth of the older population in the United States. The second was the increased cost of health care, especially Medicare, in the United States. At the time of their study in 1987, Secord and Parker reported that Medicare expenditures totaled $83 billion in 1981 and were projected to increase to $200 billion in the year 2000.[3] The US Department of Health and Human Services has estimated that Medicare spending in 2006 will be 345.2 billion. So the cost soared exponentially.

When health care costs exploded in the 1950s and 1960s, and the number of older people grew, a national effort was made to stem the fiscal bloodletting. This was true especially with nursing home expenditures, which ate up a large part of public funds, mostly through Medicaid payments for older people. In the 1970s and 1980s, many states developed nursing home preadmission screening programs in an attempt to reduce nursing home placement. In other states, a moratorium was placed on nursing home bed construction. People realized that nursing home placement was not only costly but often unnecessary or inappropriate; many older Americans could be cared for in their own homes.

In addition, services for older people were expanding. This growth was driven (post World War II) by five major federal programs with mandates to finance gerontological services: Title VIII of the Social Security Act (Medicare), Title XIX of the Social Security Act (Medicaid), Title XX of the Social Security Act, the Older Americans Act, and the Department of Veterans Affairs.[6]

As a result of these developments, in the 1960s and 1970s a plethora of senior programs blossomed in the United States. These services included home care, homemaker services, chore services, housing alternatives, transportation services, adult day care, and in-home meals. These senior services, all of which helped keep seniors in their own homes, were not coordinated. Some services emerged from states, some from the federal government, and some from the local community. Because this fragmented system was difficult to navigate, it did not serve older people well.

To help with this fragmentation and lack of a single point of entry into the web of senior programs, many public and private programs developed aspects of case management. In the 1970s, Medicare funded a number of Medicare waiver programs to find out whether older people could remain more independent when provided with community-based coordinated care. Case managers guided older people through the complex web of senior services and decided which services were appropriate for each individual.

A case manager might help in the following way: Suppose an older person who lives alone at home and is very lonely becomes depressed enough to stop eating on a regular basis. The nutritional deficit can lead to confusion, which makes it more likely that the older person will not take needed medications. If these medications, say, are for high blood pressure, the unmedicated older person may have a stroke and need to be hospitalized, and then placed in a nursing home. This eventual nursing home placement could be avoided if the older person had a case manager who knew that depression might lead to this outcome and who understood that a regular friendly visitor could allay the depression. The case manager might also suggest regular visits to a senior center as a way for this person to reenter the world. The case manager might talk to some of the older person's friends and encourage them to visit more frequently or for them to have a weekly meal together so that the older person has company and something to look forward to each week. The case manager might also arrange for the older person to visit his or her physician so medications can be monitored and arrange for prepared meals to be dropped off daily by Meals on Wheels. Thus, the case manager could help avoid an unnecessary nursing home placement by helping the older person navigate the very confusing continuum of care.

The emerging Medicare waiver programs of the 1970s included Connecticut Triage on the East Coast, the Multipurpose Senior Services Project on the West Coast, the National Long Term Care Channeling Project, the 2176 Medicaïd Waiver Programs, and the Community Nursing and Home Health programs. Case management was viewed as central to these Medicare waiver programs. In addition, these programs allowed older people to purchase items they normally would not be able to buy through Medicare, such as medications and eyeglasses. This was done on an experimental basis to see what mix of services would help keep older people out of nursing homes and in the community.

Out of these very experimental programs of the 1970s and 1980s emerged the classic model of case management.[7]

The Emergence of Professional Geriatric Care Management

The frail elderly have historically been the prime consumers of case management services. They experience functional and cognitive impairments that demand a wide array of informal and formal services. Case managers are expert in brokering these services. The publicly funded case management programs of the 1970s and 1980s demonstrated that case management was an ideal tool in brokering these formal and informal services and in helping older people remain in the community. Years of studies showed that older people wanted to stay at home and that they could remain at home with coordinated in-home and community-based services. The key was case management. Many factors came together to encourage the development of geriatric care management, which was at first a specialized form of case management.

One factor that contributed to the rise of geriatric care management was the emergence of a new pool of qualified professional case managers interested in pursuing a slightly different type of work. Many case managers from public case management programs burned themselves out by working in the public system. They wanted more independence in their jobs while still doing good and working with older people. Others from the helping professions (nurses and social workers) had not worked in public case management programs but had experienced burnout and wanted a different, perhaps more exciting career path where they would still be helping others.

At the same time, the voluminous and very fragmented web of senior services continued to expand, tangle, and unravel, with no central point of entry and mind-boggling rules at the federal, state, and local levels. Contemporaneously, the number of older people was increasing. Because long-term care management and chronic care management are not covered by Medicare, these types of care are considered discretionary purchases. In addition, many older people had large enough incomes and amounts of assets to be ineligible for publicly funded and community-based programs. The over-65 cohort is much more affluent than all the age groups under 45 years of age. Seventy percent of the wealth in the United States is controlled by people 50 years old and older. Households headed by persons older than 65 years have considerable purchasing power, controlling one-third of all the discretionary income in the country. Older people in this $800 billion market have at least $115 billion in discretionary income. Therefore, older people needed and could afford geriatric care management services.[6]

Two other factors contributed to the development of geriatric care management. First, more women began working out of the home. Although women remain the principal informal caregivers in the United States today—75% of all relatives who care for elders are women—they have accounted for a significant percentage of the work force since the 1950s. Women entered the work force partly because of societal change, including the women's movement, and families began to need two incomes to stay afloat. Fifty-five percent of all women today work, leaving not only children but older adults in need of care. Despite the crushing emotional, physical, and financial burdens, the U.S. family has not abandoned its elders. A study done in the 1990s by the U.S. House of Representatives showed that the average woman spends 17 years caring for her children and 18 years or more caring for her older parents. Piggybacked on this is another startling statistic: for the first time in U.S. history, Americans today have more living parents than they have children.[8]

Second, most Americans tend to live far from their older family members. The United States is a mobile society. Individuals no longer stay where they grew up. They may work in many different locations while their parents stay in the hometown. According to a study by the American Association of Retired Persons, one-third of all adult children in the United States live at least 30 minutes away from their aging parents.[9] Because the main system of support is still the family, this leaves older people vulnerable if they have a crisis. If the family lives far away, a crisis can turn into a mega-crisis if there is no one to offer assistance.

All of these factors have led to the need for geriatric care management. Public and private case managers as well as nurses and social workers who chose to leave the system saw a wonderful niche to fill. They understood how to provide care professionally. Many understood case management. And they saw the frustration of many older people, who had the money to purchase services but were not sure which services to choose, and of families, usually adult daughters, who were overworked and lived far away. In addition, adult children realized they could do what they already did for housecleaning and other services: they could outsource help for their parents.

■ THE BIRTH OF GERIATRIC CARE MANAGEMENT ORGANIZATIONS

Geriatric care management became a profession gradually. Because the people who started the profession came from diverse fields, in the beginning there was no central meeting ground for them. Social workers belonged to the National Association of Social Workers, whereas nurses belonged to many different associations, including the American Nurses Association. To work on common goals and interests, the new GCMs started several organizations. The most important early ones were the National Association of Professional Geriatric Care Managers and the Case Management Society of America (CMSA).

GCM

The first 12 GCMs, who were scattered across the country, were originally drawn together through a 1984 article in the *New York Times*.[10] GCMs from different areas were surprised to learn that other people were doing what they were doing. Social workers who were interviewed in the article were asked to join a coalition. In January 1985, the first meeting of what would become the National Association of Professional Geriatric Care Managers was held in the home of Adele Elkind, a social worker who was the founding force of the organization.

Professionals who had expertise in this relatively new area began to share information to help each other run better businesses. They agreed that if they could help each other, they could help the public. They put together a brochure to describe their services and moved on to develop criteria to decide who could be a member of the group. They formalized their network into the Greater New York Network on Aging (GNYNA) and began to refer cases to each other. Sarah Cohen, a founding member, suggested the radical idea that the fledgling group have a national conference; in 1985, 100 human service professionals gathered in New York City to take part in the first National Conference of Private Geriatric Care Managers. The gathering was hosted by GNYNA, which was by then a growing group of social workers, psychologists, nurses, and clinical gerontologists. This group had the vision of forming a national association dedicated to private geriatric care management.[11]

In 1986, this vision became a reality when the same group had a conference in Philadelphia, adopted membership standards, and unanimously voted to found the National Association of Private Geriatric Care Managers. In 1992, the association changed its name to the National Association of Professional Geriatric Care Managers, reflecting the fact that members might be from public, private for-profit, or private nonprofit backgrounds.

The association began with 30 members; currently it has 1,800. It has been able to bring unity and consistency to geriatric care management by configuring an information base for aspiring and practicing GCMs. In 22 years of meetings, its members have been able

to gather a body of research about the GCM field. This body of knowledge has been presented in yearly national and regional conferences and in the *GCM Journal*. The journal, in existence for 16 years, publishes research and topical information about the field and addresses points of interest to GCMs, including business practice and clinical issues.

The association includes a resource on the Web site (http://www.caremanager.org) called "Find a Care Manager," where potential GCM clients can locate a GCM anywhere in the United States, and a listserv, which is an electronic bulletin board through which GCMs can communicate with other GCMs from all over the country. The association has committees that benefit individual members and the whole GCM field, including marketing and public relations committees that create national marketing and public relations tools and promote geriatric care management through media stories published across the country. A public policy committee monitors legislation on national and local levels to keep GCMs informed of any significant pending action.

The association has 12 regional chapters that can provide members with peer support and supervision, business and professional development, educational opportunities, clinical information, leadership training, networking, and joint marketing opportunities. Each chapter has a Web site, and many can help members advertise GCM job opportunities.

In the association's store on its Web site, the National Association of Professional Geriatric Care Managers offers many products that are helpful to GCMs who are starting a geriatric care management business. Products include a business start-up kit (GCM Tool Box), several years of workshop tapes and CDs from conferences that cover business issues, a GCM forms book, and many other tools useful for starting, growing, and managing a GCM business. Products can be ordered by contacting the Association (see Appendix A).[12]

CMSA

CMSA is another association that addresses the needs of budding GCMs. CMSA does not specifically focus on geriatric care management but addresses the entire field of case management, including geriatric care management. Many CMSA members work in settings involving geriatric care management. CMSA has workshops and products that meet the needs of GCMs. CMSA also has an Elder Care Special Interest Group that offers an electronic newsletter, Communities of Practice networking, electronic membership directories, roundtable presentations, and specialized education programs.

CMSA was founded in 1990 to support and develop the profession of case management through education, networking, and legislation. CMSA first published *Standards of Practice for Case Managers* in 1995, and then revised these standards in 2002. CMSA merged with the Individual Case Management Association in 1996. It now has 70 affiliated chapters and is associated with CMS UK, CMSAustralia, and OCMA in Canada. The CMSA Web site (http://www.cmsa.org) receives more than 1.4 million hits/month. (See Appendix A.)

CMSA's mission is to advance case management, to promote the growth and value of case management, and to support the evolving needs of the case management professional. CMSA's strategic priorities are education, outcomes, and communications.

Under the education priority, CMSA has produced a large national annual conference and expo, fields more than 40 smaller training sessions nationwide, and is in the process of developing a second main conference. The online Educational Library has an extensive offering of courses in basic, intermediate, and advanced work.

Under the outcomes priority, CMSA has developed the *Case Management Adherence Guidelines*, now in its second phase, to address the issue of patient nonadherence to recommended medication use and treatment. A national study is being conducted to show the impact and value of case management intervention.

Communications is a multifaceted area. CMSA's Health Policy Committee is active, and the CMSA Board makes trips to Capitol Hill in Washington, D.C., to inform legislators about issues like the need for nurse licensure portability from state to state. CMSA has also assembled a Collaborative Practice Advisory Board, which has become the steering committee for crafting appropriate physician–case management partnerships.[13]

Benefits of Membership

For a new GCM, joining an association is a wise step. Like any new professional, new GCMs can learn from those with experience in their chosen field, and associations are a good place to find knowledgeable people who might even become mentors. A rich body of information exists in the field of geriatric care management. Because this profession is relatively new, information is still mainly available through workshops and journals, both of which are produced by associations. However, many courses that offer a certificate and degree in geriatric care management have become available in the past 5 years.

By spending time with other members of professional associations, newcomers to geriatric care management can learn the pitfalls to avoid as they enter the field. GCMs who have practiced for any length of time have opinions in many areas, including whether becoming a GCM is a good idea. They can also provide tips about billing, setting up an office, hiring staff members, conducting geriatric assessments, using prefabricated forms, dealing with the stress of running a small business, and developing a business despite the pressures and stresses.

■ ACADEMIC PROGRAMS IN GERIATRIC CARE MANAGEMENT

In the past few years, several academic courses, certificate programs, and one master's program have emerged in geriatric care management.

These programs offer a career path for students heading into the geriatric care management field or for GCMs who want further education in the business. San Francisco State University's Master of Arts (MA) in Gerontology has made one of the program's three emphases geriatric care management. Geriatric care management is part of the university's master's degree program, and this program is the only MA in gerontology that focuses on geriatric care management. The Web site is http://www.sfsu.edu/ ~sfsugero/programoverview.

The University of Florida offers an online program through which a certificate in geriatric care management can be achieved. University of Florida offers graduate, undergraduate, and continuing education certificates in geriatric care management. The Web site is http://gcm.dce.ufl.edu/.

The Brookdale Center for Aging in New York City offers a Geriatric Care Management Certificate program through which a certificate in professional geriatric care management can be achieved. The Web site is http://www.brookdale.org/pgcm/index.html.

Kaplan University offers an online Geriatric Care Management Certificate program. The student receives a certificate of completion at the end of the program. The Web site is http://www.kaplanonlineprograms.com.

Virginia Commonwealth University is developing a GCM program and has begun offering geriatric care management classes. The Web site is http://www.vchealth.org. Also, GCM classes are offered at the University of Wisconsin.

■ CONCLUSION

The geriatric care management profession developed in response to a societal need: a wide array of fragmented senior services was available, but older people and their adult children were having trouble figuring out which senior services would be helpful. GCMs are caring problem solvers who match older people to the appropriate senior services and monitor their care. Professionals who provide this very personalized service have organized into associations to help define and advance the geriatric care management field.

■ NOTES

1. Parker M. Private care management: how families are served. *J Case Manage*. 1992;1:108–112.

2. Cress C. The business of for-profit case management. *J Case Manage*. 1992;1:113–116.

3. Secord L, Parker M. *Private Case Management for Older Persons and Their Families*. Excelsior, MN: Interstudy; 1987.

4. US Department of Health and Human Services. *A National Agenda for Geriatric Education*. Vol. 1. Rockville, MD: Interdisciplinary Geriatrics and Allied Health Branch, Division of Associated Dental and Public Health Professions, Bureau of Health Professions; 1998.

5. Mullahay CM. *The Case Manager's Handbook*. Gaithersburg, MD: Aspen Publishers; 1998.

6. Kaye LW. The evolution of private care management. *J Case Manage*. 1992;1:103–107.

7. Cress C. Care management news takes hold in long term care. *Aging Int*. September 1992;19.

8. Kilborn B. Eldercare: its impact on the workplace. *Update Aging*. 1990;16.

9. American Association of Retired Persons. *A Profile of Older Americans*. Washington, DC: AARP Fulfillment; 1998.

10. Collins G. Long distance care for the elderly. *New York Times*. January 1984.

11. Elkind A. Development and growth of a regional network. GNYNA: the first two years, joys and growing pains. *Geri Gazette*. 1986;1:1–4.

12. National Association of Professional Geriatric Care Managers. *GCM Directory of Members*. Tucson, AZ: National Association of Professional Geriatric Care Managers; 1999.

13. Case Management Society of America, National Office, 2006.

Chapter 2

Ethics and Geriatric Care Management

Cathy Jo Cress

What is ethics? *Ethics* is a process of studying ourselves and our behavior, according to Nancy Alexander, a geriatric care manager (GCM), social worker, and attorney who has written much on ethics and geriatric care management.[1] According to John Banja, a noted writer on ethics and case management, the word *ethics* derives from the Greek *ethikos*. Banja says that the word *ethikos* means character; for people like Plato and Aristotle, an ethical person had a good character and many virtues.[2]

This idea of virtues had a renaissance in William B. Bennett's best-selling book, *The Book of Virtues: A Treasury of Good Moral Stories.*[2] Banja notes that to the Greeks, being ethical was not difficult. The Greeks simply assumed that a person of good character would make ethical decisions because he or she knew right from wrong. When tough ethical decisions had to be made, Aristotle simply suggested that a group of reasonable and upstanding people decide together. Banja notes that Aristotle believed this process was as good as any decision-making process because deciding what is moral and traversing dilemmas along the way are so complex that there are no simple rules to follow.[2]

Aristotle and the Greeks did not make the process of discovering the ethical choice overly complex. There were no rigid formulas to give one the correct answer. In fact, even today,

knowing the right behavior is relatively easy because this knowledge is so embedded in our societal understanding of the right path. We know the basics: we must pay our debts, be good parents, be honest, be respectful, and so forth. How do we know these basic truths? Some would hold, as Banja points out, that God or another creator imprinted these truths on our souls.[2] Banja then shows us another possible source.

Banja uses Edgar Schein's theories on organizational behavior to explain another way of learning basic truths.[2] Schein says that we first learn moral rules as young people because we are born into a system of ethics. We are taught this system by our parents and the institutions of which we are part (e.g., synagogues, churches, schools, communities). When we become a member of a group, we must then adapt to the external reality the group confronts. Groups then go through a second step, according to Schein's theory. That second step is to integrate their internal operations. This is done through role definition. In the family group, for example, one role is that of mother; in a university, professor; in geriatric care management, GCM.

Here is where morality or the right or wrong of an action comes in. Those who have a certain role within a group (e.g., a mother in the family group, a GCM in the field of geriatric care management) must act consistently in a manner that the group deems acceptable for a person in that role. Persons who have these roles must set aside their own beliefs and be socially responsible to the group and carry out their obligations to the group. Individuals who fail may be penalized by the group.

For instance, consider a young mother who gives in to her need to enjoy herself and leaves her children unattended while she goes out to a bar. She is reprimanded either by society or a group, perhaps by being arrested for child abandonment. She has exposed her children to harm and neglected her obligation as a mother to her family. Even though she has a desire for pleasure and happiness, which is natural and generally acceptable to most people, she does not act morally according to society's concept of harm and duty in the family. So, being a mother means that one has to act in a socially responsible way as defined by the group, setting one's other needs aside if they conflict with the group's expectations.

A GCM must be socially responsible to the group of GCMs and carry out the obligations of the GCM group as defined by the field's professional organizations, the Case Management Society of America (CMSA) and the National Association of Professional Geriatric Care Managers. For example, this means following the association's Pledge of Ethics (Exhibit 2–1).[3] The pledge states, among other things, that GCMs should always make referrals in the client's interest, not in the GCM's own interest. For example, if a GCM has a business relationship with a local physician, the GCM might be tempted to refer all clients to that physician to gain reciprocal business referrals from the physician, despite the facts that the physician may not offer appropriate services for every client and that clients should be offered multiple health care choices. In this situation, by referring all clients to this physician, the GCM has not set aside personal interests and has not put the client's interests first. This GCM also has ignored the obligation to be fair and do no harm to clients, an obliga-

tion codified by CMSA and the National Association of Professional Geriatric Care Managers. This GCM has violated the GCM Pledge of Ethics, which states:

> I will only refer you to services and organizations I believe to be appropriate and of good quality. I will fully explain to you any business relationship I have with any service I propose, and give you information on alternatives, if at all possible, so that you, or a person designated to act for you, can make an informed decision to accept or reject services recommended to you.[1]

Out of this theory of group ethics, we can see how ethical concepts such as goodness, harm, risk, and benefit emerge in a group. All groups develop an understanding of these ideas to help the group survive. We all have our own desires for pleasure or self-gain. However, to act morally in a group, we must go along with the group's understanding of the concepts of harm, benefit, duty, justice, and fairness. These become the rules of the group, and belonging to a group means complying with the group's rules or code of morality. The rules also involve policies, vocabulary, and a system of enforcement within the group. Rules are learned not only when a person joins a group, but also from the time of infancy during the normal socialization process.[2]

Banja points out that the case manager receives a code of moral concepts made up by his or her profession or group.[2] As part of the field of case management, GCMs also follow a professional moral code. For example, as mentioned earlier, GCMs must avoid conflicts of interest. If a conflict exists, the GCM must disclose the conflict to the interested party.[1] GCMs who refer clients to home health agencies in which the GCMs have financial interests violate the GCM code of ethics. The GCM must disclose that interest to the client.

A third step in Schein's theory of learning moral rules then comes up. Banja says that we learn moral rules through basic assumptions taught to us by a group. These basic assump-

Exhibit 2–1   Pledge of Ethics for Members of the National Association of Professional Geriatric Care Managers

Provisions of Service

I will provide ongoing service to you only after I have assessed your needs and you, or a person designated to act for you, understand and agree to a plan of service, the results that may be expected from it, and the cost of service.

Self-Determination

I will base my plan of service on goals you, or a person designated to act for you, have defined, and which enhance the decisions you have made concerning your life.

Cooperation

I will strive to ensure cooperation between all of the individuals involved in providing service and care to you.

Referrals/Disclosure

I will refer you only to services and organizations I believe to be appropriate and of good quality. I will fully explain to you any business relationship I have with any service I propose, and give you information on alternatives, if at all possible, so that you, or a person designated to act for you, can make an informed decision to accept or reject the services I recommend to you.

Termination of Service

I will end service to you only after reasonable notice. I will recommend a plan for you to continue to receive the services as needed.

Confidentiality

I will hold in trust any confidence you give me, disclosing information to others only with your permission, or if I am compelled to do so by a belief that you will be seriously harmed by my silence, or if the laws of this State require me to do so.

Substitute Judgment

I will not substitute my judgment for yours unless I am acting in the role of your guardian, appointed by a Court of Law, or with your approval, or the approval of someone designated to act for you.

Loyalty

My first duty is loyalty to you. I will always provide services based on your best interest, even if this conflicts with my interests or the interests of others.

Qualifications

I am fully qualified in my profession to provide the services I undertake. I continue to improve my skills and knowledge by participating in professional development programs and maintaining certification and licensing in my profession.

Discrimination

I will not promote or sanction any form of discrimination.

Source: Reprinted with permission from Pledge of Ethics for Members of the National Association of Professional Geriatric Care Managers, *GCM Journal*, Vol. 9, No. 4, pp. 4–5, (c) 1999, National Association of Professional Geriatric Care Managers.

tions both drive the system and explain its morality. He reasons that these assumptions tell people when they have to do certain things in a group and what justifies that behavior. Basic assumptions begin to show us the group's policies, beliefs, and practices. These group tenets reveal the group's moral concepts. When we begin to look into this morality, we also look at whether the group's moral system is defensible or acceptable. We then enter the realm of ethics.[2]

Beauchamp and Childress, in their classic *Principles of Biomedical Ethics*, propose that there are four accepted guides to making ethical decisions: beneficence, nonmaleficence, justice, and autonomy (Exhibit 2–2).[4]

The four principles defined by Beauchamp and Childress are the moral principles accepted as guides in the medical field, and they can also be applied to geriatric care management. These are the basic assumptions referred to by Banja. These principles are in balance with each other, and no principle supersedes another. GCMs try to adhere to these principles. They sometimes have difficulty when they are unsure which principle applies or when one principle collides with another.[5] Here we are entering the world of ethical probing and ethical dilemmas.

■ WHAT IS AN ETHICAL DILEMMA?

Banja defines morality as a group's moral code—its policies and its understanding of right and wrong. Ethics, as Banja says, is a major step beyond morals.[2] Ethics considers whether a group's moral beliefs are defensible, coherent, factual, honorable, and fair.

If we are to accept Beauchamp and Childress's four tenets, how do we apply them to a society, where we have limited resources?[2] For instance, if beneficence, or doing the greatest good for all older people, is a goal, why does Medicare not cover home care? We know that one answer given by the federal government is that having Medicare fund home care might damage the federal budget. This is an ethical dilemma. How does one choose between preserving government funds and helping older people?

Another example of an ethical dilemma might be the conflict between a legal mandate and a basic GCM assumption such as the

Exhibit 2–2
Principles of Biomedical Ethics

- Autonomy: Respecting the client's worth
- Nonmaleficence: Refraining from harm
- Beneficence: Advancing an individual's benefit
- Justice: Acting in fairness and equitably giving clients the services they need

autonomy of an older person. An older woman, for instance, might be having memory problems, forgetting to take her medications, burning pots by forgetting to turn off the stove. Such behavior may lead her family members to believe that she can no longer care for herself and that a conservator may need to be appointed. Here an ethical dilemma concerning surrogate decision making might arise. GCMs believe in the basic assumption of autonomy, respecting a person's freedom. However, if the woman's safety or health is compromised by her poor decisions and unsafe actions, should her freedom be curtailed through conservatorship? Is she no longer legally competent—capable of making decisions, understanding, and acting reasonably? The GCM can take a step in solving this dilemma by obtaining the family's and the woman's permission to do a mental competency exam.

In a survey of 251 case managers in 10 states, Rosalie Kane and Arthur Caplan uncovered other ethical dilemmas case managers regularly encounter.[6] Case managers' dilemmas included the following:

- Case managers overwhelmingly agreed that case managers should ensure that clients receive all possible services. But at the same time, the case managers agreed almost as strongly that they should be responsible for seeing that taxpayers' money is well spent. This creates an ongoing ethical dilemma: it is difficult to both restrict costs and provide all the services necessary.
- Case managers believed that family members should care for their older relatives. Yet at the same time, case managers supported the idea that if older people want to keep family members out of their business, they have the right to do so.
- Case managers believed that a client should have the right to die at home. But at the same time, the case managers felt that if the agency could not arrange

enough services for the client to be safe in the home, the agency should withdraw services altogether, perhaps resulting in the client being forced into an institution and not being able to die at home.

Other types of ethical dilemmas described by Kane and Caplan are discussed later in this chapter.

CASE STUDY

Here is a more detailed account of one GCM's ethical dilemma. Mary, a GCM, contracts with a senior housing complex to do geriatric assessments. Her employer, Pleasant Gardens, wants her to do a geriatric assessment on a particular resident. Pleasant Gardens has a rule that if a resident scores a 7 or higher on the mental status quotient (MSQ) exam section of the geriatric assessment, the resident is deemed too confused to live independently and is asked to move. Mary knows this. Mary also knows that when the resident's unit is rented again to another client, Pleasant Gardens receives triple the current rent because housing for older people is in great demand.

Eighty-eight-year-old resident Becca Virden's neighbors state that they have seen her putting silverware in the clothes washing machine, that there is spoiled food in her refrigerator, and that she sometimes wears two dresses at the same time. Mary conducts the geriatric assessment. Becca scores higher than a 7 on the MSQ section. There is some spoiled food in the refrigerator, but Becca has limited vision and may not have been able to see the spoilage. She was not wearing two dresses during the assessment, but her clothes, although clean, are worn and shoddy compared to those of her neighbors, who are obviously more affluent than Becca is. Becca says that she does not want to move out of her apartment where she has lived for 10 years, and she tells Mary that she is terrified to go into a nursing home. She also says that the neighbors who have moved into the complex in the last few years are "hoity-toity," or above her class, and don't like her because she uses common language and was never well-to-do or a "ladies luncheon" person.

Here an ethical dilemma arises. Should Mary tell the Pleasant Gardens staff that Becca has an MSQ score high enough for her to be evicted from her unit, which would almost surely cause her to end up in a nursing home? Mary has contracted with Pleasant Gardens as a consultant, so she is not obligated to report the MSQ score to the Pleasant Gardens staff. Is there anything wrong when a GCM's assessment causes an older person to be forced to move out of her residence, given that the move is certainly in the senior housing facility's fiscal interest? Does the fact that Mary is paid by Pleasant Gardens force her to disclose everything about a resident's assessment? If Pleasant Gardens finds out Mary did not reveal information, could the facility sue her? Before doing the assessment, should Mary have told Becca that she could not promise confidentiality of the results?

If Mary reveals information that results in Becca being moved, will Mary be violating her responsibility as a GCM to always safeguard the best interests of the client? Mary must ask herself who her client is, Becca or Pleasant Gardens? Is Mary inherently unethical if she does not disclose to Becca before the assessment that she works for Pleasant Gardens? Mary now faces the ultimate conundrum. She has been hired, as Banja says, to serve two masters—her employer and her client.[2]

A Collision of Moral Systems

Two different GCMs could easily make totally different decisions about Mary's ethical dilemma. Both individuals might believe that their analysis of the situation is objective and that they have found the ethical answer. Being ethical simply means considering a situation and deciding what response is correct.

This is why, Banja says, we run into ethical dilemmas. If a person's actions are called into question by multiple parties and the ethics of the person's decision is debated, each debating party can reach a different conclusion, with an excellent supporting argument. For example, in ethical dilemmas about such charged issues as physician-assisted suicide and abortion, each side can give fine reasons to justify its position. Each side believes that it has the "most right position," as Banja says.[2(p45)] Each side is calling on its own moral system, which it believes to be superior. These types of unresolved dilemmas usually involve the collision of two moral systems.

For example, a young woman who is unmarried and pregnant might see both a counselor at a women's health clinic and a counselor at a Right to Life clinic to help her decide whether to terminate the pregnancy. Both counselors will give the young woman advice according to their own moral principles. The Right to Life counselor might advise the young woman to carry out the pregnancy, advice based on the counselor's highest religious principles. The woman's health counselor might give the young woman the option of carrying out the pregnancy and the option of a legal abortion, based on the counselor's belief in a woman's freedom of choice. Both counselors would believe that their advice was justified and moral.

■ ETHICAL CONFLICTS BETWEEN THE CLIENT'S NEEDS AND THE CLIENT'S WANTS

As this chapter has already made clear, GCMs encounter many ethical conflicts. Frequently, these revolve around the lack of harmony between what the client needs and what the client wants. In an analysis of the study done on the ethics of home care and case managers, Kane and Caplan refer to this tension.[6] In the study, case managers pointed out the ethical dilemma encountered when the client chooses to do something that the case manager does not feel is healthy, given the client's condition. An example of this is an older woman who is depressed and who is prescribed the drug Zoloft (sertraline), with the specific instruction not to drink alcohol. Despite the warning, the older woman drinks three glasses of wine a day, two before dinner and one with dinner. She never appears drunk or acts inappropriately. Her family hires a GCM to assess her for depression. The GCM knows that the excess alcohol intake might contribute to her depression. The GCM's assessment mentions the need to help the client stop consuming alcohol.

The woman is mentally competent and not under the legal authority of a conservator. She states that she enjoys the wine and is not going to stop drinking it every night. The GCM is then caught between the client's assessed need and the client's right to choose what to do. This kind of tension often frustrates GCMs.

CASE STUDIES

Here are two detailed examples of GCMs facing the conflict between client needs and client wants. John Powers is an 81-year-old colonel and a former aeronautical engineer who worked on many famous U.S. missile systems before retiring because he had Parkinson's disease. He is an attractive, dignified, and mentally competent older man who enjoys the company of his female caregivers, who are there 24 hours a day. He has reached a stage in his Parkinson's where he has several falls a month. Although the private caregivers use transfer belts and do standby assistance at all times, they occasionally must leave him to go to the bathroom or do something else outside his room. When the caregivers are out of the room, John often gets up by himself. He refuses to wear headgear to protect his head from the falls that result from his Parkinson's. He says that he is still in charge of his life and does not want to be restrained in any way or wear anything as unattractive as a helmet.

He is visited weekly by a GCM (who is also a registered nurse [RN]), and she is quite frustrated. She has assessed his need to be protected from falls but is sympathetic to his refusal to wear the headgear. She understands his desire to preserve his dignity and be independent. He is mentally competent and has no appointed conservator, so he has the choice to refuse the restraints and helmet, and his family refuses to force the issue. The GCM is experiencing a dilemma because the client's desires conflict with her assessment of his physical needs.

Alice Manges is a 79-year-old woman who has a gastrointestinal tube inserted in her stomach. She had throat cancer and after the operation could not eat solid foods or drink liquids. She has 24-hour care, and the caregivers are monitored and supervised by both a GCM who is a social worker and a GCM who is an RN. Alice, the GCMs discover, is an alcoholic who had been very protected by her husband, a respected judge in the community. He recently died. The couple have no children, and her nephew is in charge of her care but lives far away. The RN GCM assesses Alice in the beginning of the case and creates a care plan that says to bring no alcohol into the home and to not let Alice drink. Alice is mentally competent, has no conservator and, when given an MSQ, scores perfectly. The care providers start to report

that Alice has a cleaning person bring wine into the house every week. In addition, they report that Alice is drinking the wine through her feeding tube. When the social worker GCM discovers this, she orders the care providers to discard the alcohol. Alice calls her attorney and her trust officer. The attorney reviews the situation and says that Alice is mentally clear, not in need of a conservator, and has the right to drink alcohol even if it may damage her health. The nephew reluctantly agrees, as does the trust officer. Both the RN GCM and the social worker GCM are caught between the client's choice of lifestyle and the client's health needs.

■ THE ETHICAL CONFLICT REGARDING CLIENT EXPLOITATION

Another dilemma mentioned in Kane and Caplan's study is the ethical conflict case managers experience if their clients are associating with individuals who could exploit the clients.[6] Older people who are lonely often end up in new relationships, frequently with members of the opposite sex, because many older people are widowed or divorced. However, these new relationships can alarm case managers and family members if it seems like the new companion might take advantage of the older person by getting cash or having their name added to the older person's will. If the older person is competent, how can the case manager address this dilemma?

CASE STUDY

Emily Jones is a 78-year-old woman who has been married to an alcoholic 82-year-old man for 20 years. This is her second marriage. She is a very attractive older woman who has retained her figure, loves to dress beautifully, and she always looks attractive. Harold Jones, her husband, was well-to-do when they first married, but Emily's extravagant lifestyle and Harold's alcoholism have severely diminished their finances. They have been friends with another couple, Tommy and Heidi Smith, for 15 years. Tommy always flirted with Emily, but it was socially acceptable among the couples and never led to anything more.

Heidi died after a long illness, and Tommy moved 50 miles away but always kept in touch with Emily and Harold because he was very lonely and distraught over the death of his wife of 44 years. Over a 5-year period, a relationship started between Emily and Tommy. They have lunch together frequently, at Emily's instigation and without Harold's knowledge, and are obviously increasingly attracted to each other. Harold's alcoholism causes him to act inappropriately in social situations. Emily has been thinking of leaving Harold for Tommy. One night at a party following a bar mitzvah, Harold acts very inappropriately after drinking. Angry, Emily moves out to a friend's house that evening. However, her real reason for leaving is her attraction to Tommy.

Eventually, Emily moves in with Tommy. She is impoverished because she and Harold had little money, and now she has only her meager Social Security income. Tommy pays all the bills, and his adult children are angry, viewing Emily as a "money grubber." Eventually, Emily talks Tommy into letting her live in his house if he should die, and then when she dies the house will go to his children. Tommy changes his will to this effect. Tommy's children are incensed and tell Tommy they do not approve. Tommy refuses to cooperate,

saying he loves Emily and wants her to have a place to live until she dies. The children believe that Tommy is being exploited and want to force him to make Emily move out and change his will again. They want to move him to the home of one of his children who lives 500 miles away to get him away from Emily. Because Tommy is in his eighties, they feel he will eventually give in to their wishes. They have also talked to Emily's children, who feel bad about the situation and are willing to take her in.

Tommy's children's attorney advises them to get an assessment from a GCM, and the children call in a local GCM. After assessing the situation, the GCM concludes that Emily has influenced Tommy to change his will. The GCM states in her assessment that Emily has been exploitive in this relationship and has influenced Tommy to change his will to her benefit. Tommy's loneliness after his wife's death made him more open to Emily's flirtations. However, the GCM assesses Tommy's mental status and finds him fully competent, with the right to make this choice, even if his children disapprove. The GCM advises the children not to move him at this time. She, however, encourages further assessment if his will is changed again. So, as Kane and Caplan's study points out, the GCM is left with an ethical dilemma between the client's wants and the client's needs.[6] The client is associating with an exploitive person but, in this case at least, has the right to continue the association.

■ CONFLICT BETWEEN THE CLIENT'S SAFETY AND THE CLIENT'S AUTONOMY

Another type of ethical dilemma discussed by Kane and Caplan involves case managers with clients who live a life that involves high risk.[6]

An example of this is older men or women who insist on driving even though they have compromised eyesight, limited response times, or confusion. Does a person's right to be independent supersede his or her safety or the public's safety? If the person has passed a driver's test, what can a case manager do?

■ CONFLICTS AROUND CONFIDENTIALITY AND DISCLOSURE

Kane and Caplan's study also found that case managers experienced ethical conflicts around the issues of confidentiality and disclosure. The largest group of respondents (22%) reported having conflicts over what to disclose to family members. The second-largest group (17%) reported having conflicts over what to disclose to agency providers. More than 50% of those GCMs who reported having conflicts over confidentiality stated that they used their judgment to resolve what to disclose and to whom.[6] The conflict that the GCM Mary experienced with regard to her client Becca, discussed earlier, was partly a conflict involving confidentiality and disclosure. Another example of this type of conflict follows.

CASE STUDY

The White family daughters hired a GCM to do a geriatric assessment of their mother, Blanche. Blanche lived with one son and his wife, whom the other family members suspected of physically abusing, overmedicating, and intimidating their mother. In doing the assessment, the GCM found evidence of potential physical and medication abuse, which warranted turning the situation in to Adult Protective Services (APS). However, the GCM knew that APS was so underfunded and understaffed that it might not do anything about the situation immediately, although by law it would make an investigative visit, which would tip off the son and his wife to the problems uncovered.

The geriatric assessment confirmed the children's fear that the son and his wife were physically abusing the mother and overmedicating her. The other children decided to send their mother to stay with her daughter in Atlanta. One daughter who lived near the son planned to take Blanche out for a supposed day trip and would actually put her on a plane to Atlanta to go live with the sister, who would implement all the GCM's suggestions. These suggestions included a medication review by a geriatric RN, a possible reduction of medication, and attendance at an adult day care program for additional socialization. The family members did not want to tell the brother with whom the mother lived because they feared he would stop them and might harm the mother.

The GCM was in a ethical dilemma. The family members did not want her to report the case to APS until they got their mother on the plane to Atlanta. The GCM worked for the family. However, by law the GCM was obligated to report the case to APS, even though she knew it might stop the plans to get the mother away from the abusive son. The GCM had a conflict about confidentiality involving what to disclose to an agency.

■ ANALYZING ETHICAL DILEMMAS

Patricia Burbank provides one framework for analyzing ethical problems (Exhibit 2–3). Burbank suggests many avenues to help in ethical decision making and states that analysis does not have to be done in isolation. Among her suggestions is using ethics review boards in institutions because they are there to help health professionals resolve ethical dilemmas. If this option is not possible, she suggests team conferences that include all the parties involved

Exhibit 2–3   Analyzing Ethical Problems

1. Review the situation.
   - What health problems exist?
   - What decisions need to be made?
   - Which components are ethical and which are based on scientific knowledge?
2. Gather additional information necessary to make a decision.
3. What are relevant ethical principles?
   - What are the historical, philosophical, and religious bases for each of the principles?
4. What are your values and beliefs?
   - From your family and other personal experience?
   - From your professional code of ethics?
5. What are the values and beliefs of others in the situation?

6. What are the value conflicts in the situation?
7. Who is the best person to make the decision?
8. What is the fullest range of possible decisions and actions?
   - What are the implications/consequences of possible decisions and actions?
   - Do the possible decisions and actions and your professional code of ethics agree?
9. Decide on a course of action and take steps to implement it.
10. Evaluate the outcomes of the decisions and use this information for future decision making.

Source: Reprinted with permission from Legal and Ethical Issues in Health Care of Older Adults, *GCM Journal*, Vol. 9, No. 4, p. 28, (c) 1999, National Association of Professional Geriatric Care Managers.

in the dilemma. She also suggests reaching out to other professionals, while always respecting the confidentiality of the client.[5] GCMs could also use the National Association of Professional Geriatric Care Managers, CMSA, the National Association of Social Workers, or any other professional association with a code of ethics and an ethics committee (see Appendix A for contact information).[5]

E. Haavi Morreim proposes another possible method of ethical dilemma analysis.[7] He suggests that the first step is fact finding. The GCM should seek the primary sources of information, not rely on secondhand information. The GCM should not make unwarranted assumptions or depend on other people's assumptions. Objectively gathering facts to discover basic problems is the first step in routine geriatric assessment. Therefore, it should be familiar to GCMs.

Morreim's second step is to identify all those whose interests and wishes might be affected by the results (e.g., family members, friends, other agencies, other professionals). The client is the GCM's highest responsibility, but Morreim says GCMs must uncover all the other players and then uncover all the values that are at stake (e.g., autonomy, justice, freedom).

The third step involves creative problem solving. Like the other steps in the process, creative problem solving is part of a GCM's basic skill set in geriatric assessment and general geriatric care management. Morreim advises GCMs to respect the important moral values in the problem and to not only consider obvious options but to try to devise creative new options.[7]

■ HOW TO RESOLVE ETHICAL DILEMMAS

Resolving ethical dilemmas is difficult at best. The body of literature on ethics and case or care management—a body of literature that grew considerably in the late 1990s—suggests several different pathways.

In Kane and Caplan's study, case managers who had ethical dilemmas with other case managers or agencies tended to resolve the conflict in various ways. Negotiation and compromise were used by 31% of the case managers responding to the survey. Ten percent mentioned overriding their providers and colleagues. Another 10% said they occasionally appealed to a higher authority and went over the head of the individual who caused difficulty. A strategy of winning the confidence of their providers and colleagues was used by only 6%. Kane and Caplan state that case managers sometimes assisted the client in finding another agency or simply refused to refer again to an organization or professional that caused a conflict. However, Kane and Caplan state that most case managers had a difficult time with the concept of blackballing.[6]

Sixty-eight percent, the largest percentage of case managers in the study, used discussion with their supervisors to solve ethical dilemmas. Because many GCMs operate as entrepreneurs and have no supervisors, GCMs might consider the second most common approach to resolving ethical dilemmas found in Kane and Caplan's study: discussion with colleagues. This method was used by 39% of case managers. Seventeen percent said they used care and case conferences, where professional care managers meet to discuss client problems and resolve ethical dilemmas.[6] If a GCM works for an agency or has many other GCMs in his or her own agency, this is an excellent avenue to consider.

Banja says that the process of resolving ethical dilemmas may reveal not only what to do but also what not to do.[2] He makes another interesting point: when resolving an ethical dilemma, both sides can become very emotional. The average person gets defensive, making all kinds of excuses when there is an allegation of error. A prominent flaw in the majority of the poor reasons used to justify a type of conduct is that the poor reasons rarely address the problems at hand. Instead, these reasons avoid the real issue and involve justifications for disregarding the real issue, causing the ethical dilemma.

■ CONCLUSION

As geriatric care management and case management evolve as professions, GCMs have a great opportunity to learn how to think ethically. GCMs have the codes of ethics of both the National Association of Professional Geriatric Care Managers and CMSA to govern their ethics and help with ethical dilemmas. Both associations also offer ethics committees to help clarify and resolve problems. Both associations have rules, disciplinary procedures, and penalties for breaking these codes. Membership in an association also gives GCMs access to colleagues with whom they can discuss ethical problems—just as the Greeks would have done. As Kane and Caplan's survey shows, professionals find many ways to resolve these interesting but painful ethical dilemmas.

■ NOTES

1. Alexander N. An international code of ethics for care/case managers. *GCM J.* 1999;4:6.

2. Banja J. Ethical decision making: origins, process, and applications to case management. *Case Manager.* 1999;9:41–42.

3. Brostoff PM. A short history of drafting the GCM Pledge of Ethics. *GCM J.* 1999;10:6.

4. Beauchamp T, Childress J. *Principles of Biomedical Ethics*. 4th ed. New York: Oxford University Press; 1994.

5. Burbank PM. Legal and ethical issues in health care of older adults. *GCM J.* 1999;27.

6. Kane R, Caplan AL. *Ethical Conflicts in the Management of Home Care: The Case Manager's Dilemma*. New York: Springer; 1993.

7. Morreim E. Ethical issues in care management: case studies in moral problem solving. *GCM J.* 1999;9.

PART 2

Geriatric Assessment and Care Monitoring

Chapter 3

Psychosocial Assessment

Barbara Morano
Carmen L. Morano

Psychosocial assessment along with the functional assessment (discussed in Chapter 4) provides the foundation for all the care management that follows. Combined, the functional and the psychosocial assessments are not only critical to developing a relevant and appropriate care plan, but in fact they provide an in-depth perspective of the older adult's quality of life.[1] The goals of clinicians and researchers alike have moved from focusing on how long a particular intervention can extend an older adult's life, to a more holistic approach that recognizes the importance of increasing the quality of the older adult's life.[1] (See Chapter 19 for a more complete discussion on quality of life.)

The knowledge gained from a comprehensive psychosocial assessment provides objective measurable information about the cognitive, social, psychological, spiritual, financial, and legal dimensions of the client system, as well as important subjective information about the entire client system's coping mechanisms and relationships. There is no one model or approach to completing a psychosocial assessment, or even a unified consensus on what specific dimensions (cognitive, psychological, financial, social, etc.) make up a comprehensive psychosocial assessment. The care manager must develop a psychosocial assessment that best meets the needs of the clients served, and one that helps to inform, guide, or contribute to making professional judgments about an appropriate care plan.[2] For purposes of this chapter, we have included the cognitive, psychological, economic, and social dimensions, as well as an assessment for potential substance abuse and elder maltreatment. Spiritual assessment is covered in Chapter 14.

"Underlying good care management is good assessment."[3] It is the psychosocial aspects of an assessment that can be labeled the heart and soul of the comprehensive geriatric assessment. It is through this part of the assessment that we determine who the client is, from a systemic, individual, and historical perspective. The care manager will then understand the client's typical behavior, coping capacities, motivations, and the nature of relationships. Once this segment of the assessment is complete, the care manager is able to engage the client more successfully and engage the entire client system in a collaborative working relationship.

Because it is usually a relative who calls initially to refer an older adult for geriatric care management services, it is here where the psychosocial assessment can begin. Our practice model started with a family assessment to obtain reliable information about the family system and to understand the problem more fully from their perspective. This initial time with the family was valuable for developing an approach for the initial engagement of the older adult. Care management is unique in that there are multiple clients, most notably adult children and their parent(s). Any one of this entire client system, but most frequently the older adult, can be resistant to an intervention as a result of denial of the problem, anger at family interference, or fear. By initiating the assessment process with the family, the care manager can understand who this client is to manage this resistance appropriately early on in the relationship and, as important, understand family barriers and supports to developing this crucial relationship.

This chapter delineates the essential elements of the psychosocial assessment. Psychosocial assessment is quite comprehensive and time-consuming, so it is not uncommon to defer certain areas for subsequent visits. Because every care manager must initially assess for safety and risk factors in the client's day-to-day living situation, it is imperative that the cognitive, psychological, and support systems are assessed at the time of the first visit.

The demographic information gathered during the initial family meeting is required to complete an assessment fully. Although a standardized tool does not exist, the following information about the older adult must be obtained:

- Birth date and place
- Nationality/history of immigration
- Religion/affiliation/importance
- Siblings/alive/deceased/relationships/ health
- Childhood
- Education
- Military history
- Marital history/significant others
- Offspring/birth order/relationship to parent(s) and each other/current living arrangement/availability
- Occupation
- Hobbies/interests
- Retirement

As the information about each of the family members is gathered, it can be used to construct a *genogram*. The authors suggest the use of a genogram (see Figure 3-1) to illustrate graphically who is part of the family system and each person's relationship to the identified client. Information about the age, health status, and relationship (good, strained, distant, etc.) to the identified client can be included in the genogram. This enhances the basic genogram that depicts connections members have to each other by providing a richer description of each of the members included.

■ COGNITIVE ASSESSMENT

Cognitive assessment is an integral part of detecting dementia.[4] Because the incidence and prevalence of dementing disorders increases in later life,[4] it is necessary to assess

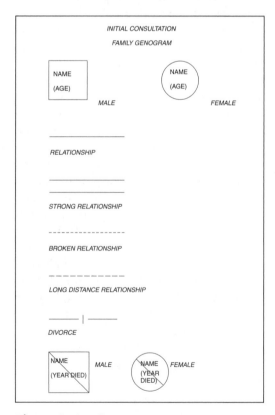

Figure 3-1   Genogram

the older adult's mental status to determine whether the current living arrangement is appropriate and safe. The care manager cannot assume that an older adult has been assessed for mental status by a primary care physician. Research has shown the failure of physicians to perform mental status testing routinely on older patients.[5] Likewise, many of those with cognitive impairment can behave in socially appropriate manners, and are therefore not recognized as having any impairment.

Assessment for mental capacity is accomplished both informally and formally through use of one or more screening tests. An unstructured form of cognitive assessment occurs throughout the entire evaluation process. Because the family has already provided reliable demographic information, the care manager will also ask the older adult many of the same questions as a way to informally gauge memory and recall. Other more informal ways to test memory include these:

- Asking the older adult to perform a multitask function (i.e., getting a glass of water)
- Asking the older adult to identify people in family photos
- Carrying on an informal conversation with the older adult

The care manager should also ask the older adult to assess his or her own cognitive functioning. Understanding the older adult's perception of his or her own functioning is especially informative to the overall assessment and care plan.

Indirect assessment can also be completed by conversing with a family member or other close contact. Family members can provide useful information in this process because they have the historical context of change over time. "The caregiver is able to provide information regarding the mode of onset of cognitive dysfunction (abrupt vs. gradual), progression of symptoms (stepwise vs. continuous), and duration of symptoms."[4]

The most commonly used and most thoroughly researched formal screening test for dementia is the Mini Mental State Examination (MMSE) (Exhibit 3-1) developed by Folstein and colleagues.[6] Concentration, language, orientation, memory, and attention are tested in this short, usually 10-minute, 30-question test. A score of 23 or lower out of a possible 30 has been defined as indicating cognitive impairment. Shortcomings of the test include a wide variation of scoring and test administration styles, as well as inappropriateness for those with physical disability, sensory impairment, and poor command of the English language.

Exhibit 3-1
MMSE Sample Items

Orientation to Time
"What is the date?"

Registration
"Listen carefully. I am going to say three words. You say them back after I stop.

Ready? Here they are . . .

APPLE (pause), PENNY (pause), TABLE (pause). Now repeat those words back to me." [Repeat up to 5 times, but score only the first trial.]

Naming
"What is this?" [Point to a pencil or pen.]

Reading
"Please read this and do what it says." [Show examinee the words on the stimulus form.]

CLOSE YOUR EYES

Source: Reproduced by special permission of the Publisher, Psychological Assessment Resources, Inc., 16204 North Florida Avenue, Lutz, Florida 33549, from the Mini Mental State Examination, by Marshal Folstein and Susan Folstein. Copyright 1975, 1998, 2001 by Mini Mental LLC, Inc. Published 2001 by Psychological Assessment Resources, Inc. Further reproduction is prohibited without permission of PAR, Inc. The MMSE can be purchased from PAR, Inc. by calling (813) 968-3003.

The Short Portable Mental Status Questionnaire (Exhibit 3–2) asks 10 questions with each error scored as 1 point.[7] Intact mental function is indicated by less than 2 errors, and severe mental impairment is indicated by 8 to 10 errors. The scoring is adjusted for educational level.

The Blessed Orientation-Memory-Concentration Test consists of all verbal questions, takes 3 to 6 minutes to administer, counts errors, and has a maximum score of 28, with a score of 10 indicating dementia.[8]

The Clock Drawing Test measures multiple cognitive and motor functions through a clock-drawing task.[9] The individual is given a piece of paper with a 4- to 6-inch circle drawn on it and is asked to write the numbers and draw the hands of the clock to show "10 past 11." Although many clinicians use a qualitative evaluation, there are scales to rank the drawing for completeness and correctness or to rate specific components of the clock drawn and combine the ratings into a score. The clock-drawing interpretation scale recommended by Mendez et al. falls into this latter category.

Although we encourage the use of standardized instruments to assess cognitive status, we suggest that it is important that the findings,

Exhibit 3–2 The Short Portable Mental Status Questionnaire (SPMSQ)

Scoring: Count the number of correct and incorrect responses.		
Question	**Correct Responses**	**Incorrect Responses**
1. What are the date, month, and year?		
2. What is the day of the week?		
3. What is the name of this place?		
4. What is your phone number?		
5. How old are you?		
6. When were you born?		
7. Who is the current president?		
8. Who was the president before him?		
9. What was your mother's maiden name?		
10. Can you count backward from 20 by 3s?		

SCORING

0–2 errors: normal mental functioning
3–4 errors: mild cognitive impairment
5–7 errors: moderate cognitive impairment
8 or more errors: severe cognitive impairment

*One more error is allowed in the scoring if a patient has had a grade school education or less.
*One less error is allowed if the patient has had education beyond the high school level.

Source: Pfeiffer E. A short portable mental status questionnaire for the assessment of organic brain deficit in elderly patients. *Journal of the American Geriatric Society* 1975 Oct. 23(10): 433–441.

regardless of the measure used, are understood within the larger context of older person's ability to process cognitive information. The ability of the older person to function safely within his or her daily routine cannot always be measured by a single cognitive assessment instrument. (See Chapter 20 on dementia.)

■ PSYCHOLOGICAL ASSESSMENT

Older adults are hesitant to discuss psychological problems because of a fear of being labeled as crazy, because it is perceived as a sign of weakness, or because they think it is something to be ashamed of.[5] With numerous somatic or physical complaints, it is not uncommon for both the older adult and family to deny a diagnosis of depression. Frequently, they attribute sadness or anxiety to a normal part of aging and/or illness. The care manager is in a good position to differentially assess psychological compromise from personality traits or cognitive decline.

Through the building of an ongoing and trusting relationship with the geriatric care manager, the older adult may become more comfortable discussing personal problems and fears. Additionally, over time the care manager can assess the older adult's psychological functioning by observing him or her in different circumstances, performing various tasks, and relating to family, friends, and other professionals. Although standardized measures are valuable screening tools, they are not the definitive assessment, but rather are used in conjunction with direct observation and interviews with the older adult and support system.[10]

Depression

Depression is significantly underdiagnosed and undertreated in older adults.[11] It can affect performance on mental status tests and should be considered when cognitive impairment is suspected. As discussed by Gallo and Wittink:

The person with the appearance of cognitive impairment secondary to depression remains oriented and with coaxing can perform cognitive tests. Clues that dementia may be secondary to depression include recent onset and rapid progression, a family history of depressive disorders, a personal history of affective disorders, and onset of the disorder after the age of 60 years.[12(p157)]

The Geriatric Depression Scale (GDS) designed by Yesavage[13] was the first depression assessment scale explicitly for older adults and remains widely used because of its simplicity. The GDS is a 30-question survey that includes yes-or-no questions. A point is given for each answer that matches the answer in parentheses. A score of 10 or more usually suggests depression.

The Beck Depression Inventory is a 21-item self-rating report that assesses symptoms of depression and includes a broad range of questions.[14] Individual questions are scored as 0, 1, 2, or 3. A total score of greater than 11 is indicative of depression. This scale relies heavily on physical symptoms, making it less useful for older adults with physical impairment. It is also difficult to use with those who have cognitive impairment and those with communication and hearing problems.

Anxiety

With community-living older adults, generalized anxiety, more commonly stated as worry, is the most frequently encountered disorder—it is even more prevalent than depression is.[15] Anxiety and depression coexist and can overlap in older adults with symptoms stated as sleeplessness or fatigue. Other symptoms of anxiety can include fear, nervousness, dread, shortness of breath, and rapid heartbeat. All of these symptoms can be misdiagnosed as various medical conditions, such as cardiovascular problems, Parkinson's disease, Alzheimer's disease, or hormonal imbalances.

Anxiety is easily confused with worry, which is an emotional reaction to health and safety concerns rather than a pathological response. Assessing an older adult's concerns during the assessment process is necessary to make this distinction.

The Beck Anxiety Inventory is a 21-item self-report questionnaire of common anxiety symptoms.[16] Respondents rate the intensity of each symptom as 0, 1, 2, or 3, with a score of 22 to 35 indicating moderate anxiety, and a score of more than 36 as severe. It should be noted that there are other anxiety instruments, none of which appear to be used that frequently by care managers.

■ SOCIAL SUPPORT

Social support as presented in the context of this chapter and text refers to both the formal and informal sources of support. Formal supports such as home health care, custodial care, case management, and day care among others, are supportive services that are either purchased by the client or reimbursed through a third-party source (i.e., Medicare, Medicaid) or a local, state, or federal program. Informal support is provided by family members, extended kin, friends, or neighbors. This section focuses exclusively on informal social support.

Both formal and informal support are assessed as part of the psychosocial assessment. The process of conducting an assessment of formal and informal support provides important subjective and objective information that is critical to the development, and ultimately the success, of the care plan.

Approximately 80% of all support to older adults is provided on an informal basis by either an adult child or a spouse.[17] Assessing informal support begins with the very first call to the care manager. Most often, the initial call to the care manager comes from an adult child, frequently the older adult's daughter or daughter-in-law. Understanding why the call to the care manager is being made now as well as why this particular person is making the call initiates the assessment of informal support. In addition to being concerned about a parent(s), this person is often already involved with providing informal support or coordinating formal support. In 2005, family members providing care to someone with a memory impairment provided on average 30 hours per week of care.[18] Many of the family systems working with a care manager will have both primary and secondary caregivers involved with providing varying levels of support. Thus, it is not surprising that those involved with providing support, especially to someone with cognitive impairment, can experience significant strain.[19,20]

Identifying all primary and secondary informal caregivers, perhaps starting with those represented in the genogram and then expanding to include other family, extended kin, friends, or neighbors who might be involved or have the potential to become involved, can be the starting point for assessment of social support. As discussed previously, the genogram is a useful tool that will depict not only the relationship each family member has to the identified patient, but it can also be useful when assigning roles and responsibilities for the care plan.

Because the entire informal support system may not be present during the initial assessment, it is important to establish an accurate assessment of the motivation of both those present and involved as well as those who are not present but who might be involved. The assessment of social support should ultimately reflect an accurate picture of who the informal supports are and the nature of the relationship they have with the older person. Frequently, some of those who are most involved are also reported to have the most strained relationship with the older person.[21]

Some care managers use an informal, semistructured interviewing process to assess social support, whereas others, the authors included, use a combination of a semistructured interview along with one of the many standardized instruments that can measure informal support. The semistructured interview process can provide the care manager with valuable information about how individuals relate to each other as well as to the care manager, whereas a standardized instrument reports quantified information that can be used as an objective outcome to evaluate the effects of the intervention. Whatever format the care manager uses, the size of the network and the availability of assistance for the client, as well as the caregiver, should be assessed by the conclusion of the social support assessment.

A number of standardized instruments measure social support, but not in a uniform way. Some focus only on family members, some focus on both family and friends,[21] and yet others focus only on the older person's perception of support.[19] The Lubben Social Support Scale uses a series of nine questions to assess the client's social support system, including family and friends.[22] This instrument can be used equally well with the client and the caregiver to provide a broad-based picture about the size of the support network and its availability to assist with care and decision making. Another formal assessment instrument is the Norbeck Social Support Questionnaire.[23] This scale has also been shown to have strong validity, and it has demonstrated utility for measuring social support not only with caregivers, but also for the clients themselves. The Norbeck subscales permit some determination of the areas in which a person perceives adequate social support and those areas in which the person perceives social support as lacking. As previously mentioned, in addition to assessing the availability of support, it is important to then measure the level of strain or burden that those involved with providing support might be experiencing.

Not all supportive relationships are positive relationships. In fact, overwhelming evidence shows that being a caregiver, especially a primary caregiver, can result in feelings of strain or burden,[24-26] and a growing body of evidence shows that some caregivers also report feelings of gain.[26,27] If there is evidence, or if the care manager has an intuitive feeling that a particular caregiver is at risk of becoming overwhelmed, it is advisable to assess the caregiver's level of burden. As with social support, a number of instruments can be used to assess the caregiver's burden and satisfaction. The Lawton Scale of Appraised Burden and Appraised Satisfaction,[28] the Caregiver Burden Inventory,[29] and the Caregiver Strain Index (CSI)[30] are just some of the multidimensional scales that can be used to measure strain. The CSI has 13 items that assess five dimensions or sources of strain (financial, physical, time, social, and employment). A positive response to more than seven indicates a need for a more focused assessment to determine the most appropriate intervention.

■ ELDER MISTREATMENT

The actual rate of elder mistreatment is probably much higher than is reported because secrecy and isolation, common in all forms of intimate abuse, prevent an accurate count. The National Elder Abuse Incidence Study calculated that for every case reported to Adult Protective Services (APS), five additional cases were known to community agencies.[31] Furthermore, less than one-half of reported cases are substantiated.[32] Elders are vulnerable to abuse and neglect because of a greater likelihood of their suffering from physical and cognitive impairments and their need to rely on caregivers and family members for basic physical care.[1]

For purposes of the psychosocial assessment, elder mistreatment is defined as physical, psychological or emotional, financial, or sexual abuse, as well as financial exploitation, use of undue influence, neglect, and self-neglect inflicted actively, passively, or unintentionally. All states have some form of protection and services for vulnerable older adults, yet seven states rely only on voluntary reporting (Colorado, Illinois, New Jersey, New York, North Dakota, Pennsylvania, and Wisconsin).

As with other areas of psychosocial assessment, elder mistreatment can be assessed both formally and informally. The care manager is directly involved with the older adult and his or her caregiver and can assess mistreatment by direct observation, interview, or by report from others. An unexplainable sudden decline in the older adult's functional, cognitive, or psychological status can be an indicator of mistreatment. "The assessment of elder mistreatment begins when there is a suspicion that the elders' relationships are contributing to unnecessary suffering, or when elders hint at or directly report relationship problems."[31]

The instruments used to assess elder mistreatment are designed to assess the risk for abuse, cognitive ability, and functional status. The Elder Assessment Instrument developed by Fulmer, Street, and Carr is a 46-item instrument that reviews signs, symptoms, and subjective complaints of elder abuse, neglect, exploitation, and abandonment.[33] There is no score, but this instrument is used as a guide for referral to APS if the following conditions exist:

1. If there is any evidence of mistreatment without sufficient clinical explanation
2. Whenever there is a subjective complaint by the elder of mistreatment
3. Whenever the clinician believes there is a high risk of or probable abuse, neglect, exploitation, or abandonment

■ ECONOMIC AND LEGAL ASSESSMENT

Developing an appropriate care plan requires an accurate picture of the older adult's economic status. If the care plan is not affordable, or a particular community-based service is not accessible or available, the plan is inappropriate. A thorough financial assessment helps to screen for risk of financial exploitation, the unintentional and perhaps inappropriate dissipation of assets, as well as to facilitate the access to future community-based or long-term-care services. Unfortunately, many older adults are uncomfortable or hesitant to disclose the particulars of their finances to their own children or to the care manager. It is not uncommon that the adult child or children will not have a clear picture of the older adult's financial status and are uncomfortable in broaching the subject.

A complete financial assessment needs to include an evaluation of income and assets, as well as health insurance and long-term-care insurance. If the care manager senses any discomfort or resistance in this area, assessing the older adult's financial resources can be initiated by asking a few indirect questions to assess their openness to discussing this especially sensitive area. Questions such as, "Do you worry about your finances?" "Have you ever delayed getting a prescription filled?" "Do you have sufficient healthy foods?" can help initiate discussion about finances. Because many older adults are living on a fixed income, unexpected expenses, such as for additional medications, special nutritional supplements, or home care or day care, can be difficult to manage.

Although social security frequently represents a significant percentage of monthly income, income from retirement pensions, annuities, interest income, employment, and/or income from real estate must be accounted for. Information about the source of the income, as well as conditions attached to the income (taxable or tax free, time limited or for life, etc.), should also be obtained.

In addition to obtaining reliable information about income, it is important to include the older adult's assets as part of the financial assessment. Given the increased lifespan and years spent in retirement, what was once considered as adequate income and savings for retirement might turn out to be inadequate for meeting the older adult's future health and care needs. Additionally, most entitlement programs have specific income and asset qualifying limits. Therefore, just as with income, a complete and accurate assessment of assets must be obtained to determine the affordability of a care plan and also to determine eligibility for various entitlement programs. Accurate information about all assets (i.e., home, stocks, bonds, life insurance, property, etc.) must be accounted for. A referral to an elder law attorney or estate planner can be considered when there are considerable, or even reasonable, assets to plan for future care needs and/or to protect assets for a well spouse.

Many older adults, as well as their adult children, do not understand eligibility requirements for community-based entitlement programs and long-term care. False assumptions about what older adults are entitled to or not entitled to must be addressed. And although not every care management client will need to access an entitlement program, it is important that the care manager provides current and accurate information about any relevant entitlement programs and services. Care managers can use their knowledge of the various local programs and their expertise in navigating the bureaucracy to access these programs to increase the older adult's willingness to provide accurate information about finances.

In addition to income and assets, a comprehensive economic assessment should include an assessment of the older adult's insurance policies, including health, life, pharmaceutical, home, and long-term-care insurance. It is especially important that the care manager confirm that all insurance policies are current and in effect, and that they represent adequate and practical coverage. For example, some long-term-care policies have long waiting periods (elimination days), some as long as 90 days, before benefits can be accessed. Also, other restrictions can limit the policy-holder's choice of provider, eligible diagnoses, or type of care.

A final dimension of the economic assessment includes an assessment of the older adult's legal affairs, or what is known as *advance directives* (i.e., health care proxy, power of attorney, living will, etc.). This is another area in which the care manager is advised to confirm and verify the status of these documents. Although many older adults have some, or even all, of these documents, the documents may be outdated, not compliant with current law, executed in a state other than where the older adult is currently residing, or inappropriate as a result of the death or cognitive decline of the appointed agent. The care manager must be knowledgeable of the state's laws with respect to advance directives and must make an immediate referral to an appropriate elder law attorney to initiate or update these documents.

■ SUBSTANCE ABUSE

Substance abuse or dependence, including alcohol use, drug misuse, and nicotine use, can have severe negative physical, cognitive, and psychological consequences for the older adult. Screening for this is essential, not only to detect the problem, but to identify potentially harmful interactions with other physical and mental conditions that could lead to high blood pressure, falls, or memory loss. Improper substance use can increase comorbidities and interfere in the treatment process, and therefore increase medical complexity.[34]

"Heavy drinking, even in the absence of abuse and dependence, can be detrimental to the care of older adults; however moderate drinking may be associated with certain health benefits."[34(p176)] Having a clear definition of what constitutes problem drinking in the elderly is difficult, though. With younger adults, clear criteria are defined in the *Diagnostic and Statistical Manual of Mental Disorders*, including disruption of role function, financial instability, and decreasing social networks.[35] These criteria can be present in the older adult population at large without a substance abuse problem. Additionally, substance abuse problems are masked by other problems associated with aging, including falls, injury, confusion, self-neglect, depression, emotional lability, memory loss, sleep disturbance, and adverse drug interactions. Furthermore, an elder's tendency to use alcohol frequently or heavily is dismissed as "the only vice she has left" or "something to help him sleep."[1]

Even though the frequency of drinking and the amount consumed declines with age, it is estimated that 49.4% of persons over the age of 65 drink alcohol at least on a semiregular basis, compared to 73.1% of persons between the ages of 18 and 29 years. Approximately 10% of elders are defined as problem drinkers.[1] Of significance is the acceptance and casual attitude of alcohol consumption and drug use in the younger population, including the baby boomers, suggesting a dramatic increase in substance abuse in the elderly in coming decades.

Formally assessing alcohol abuse in older adults is difficult because most screening instruments are not age specific and rely on self-report. The Short Michigan Alcoholism Screening Instrument—Geriatric Version was developed as the first short-form screening instrument for the elderly.[36] A score of two or more "Yes" responses suggests an alcohol problem. The goal of the screening is to identify an at-risk population of older adults who use alcohol on a regular basis.

More commonly used is the following CAGE screening questionnaire, a simple-to-administer, four-question instrument.[37] A positive response to any question indicates the need for further evaluation. The major drawback to the validity of this instrument is the reliance on self-report. The older adult may deny any problem when confronted with these questions.

CAGE Screening Questionnaire

1. Have you ever felt you should *cut down* on your drinking?
2. Have people *annoyed* you by criticizing your drinking?
3. Have you ever felt bad or *guilty* about your drinking?
4. Have you ever had a drink first thing in the morning to steady your nerves or get rid of a hangover (*eye-opener*)?

The care manager must also rely on observation to detect alcohol use or abuse. Such indicators as deteriorating hygiene, increased number of falls, slurred speech, the smell of alcohol, and moodiness may indicate a potential problem with alcohol. As mentioned earlier, other physical and cognitive impairments must be ruled out first.

Drug dependency and misuse in the elderly population entails both the use of illicit drugs and the misuse of prescription medications. Drug dependency develops faster in this population because of an older adult's slower metabolic process. The kidneys and liver are not as efficient in removing these substances from the body in older adults. Currently, a very small number of older adults have a life-long history of illegal drug use. However, this number will rise dramatically as a result of the longer life expectancies and the widespread acceptance of recreational drug use among more recent generations.[1]

The most common drug misuse among older adults is with psychoactive medications for the treatment of depression, anxiety, and pain. These medications can cause both physical and psychological dependency. Women are more at risk for drug dependency because they are more likely to seek treatment for somatic complaints and other emotional problems. The care manager must pay close attention to all medications currently prescribed by the older adult's physicians and must be aware of multiple pharmacies to prevent duplication that could potentially lead to lethal dosages.

■ CONCLUSION

Psychosocial assessment is important for both what it can accomplish and what can happen if it is not completed thoroughly and correctly. A comprehensive and accurate psychosocial assessment can better ensure the development of an appropriate intervention and successful care plan. The accurate and timely use of psychosocial assessment tools must be combined with good interviewing skills. The ability to develop and maintain relationships, knowledge of human behavior, understanding of family and caregiver dynamics, knowledge of the effects of aging and disability, and the awareness of community resources and services are critical to all that follows.[2] An assessment that either is incomplete or ignores good clinical and professional judgment can result in the failure to develop a healthy relationship between the care manager and older adult, which can only result in eventual failure of even the best care plan.

The National Association of Professional Geriatric Care Managers has developed a forms book as a benefit for its members. Included in this comprehensive manual are many assessment forms a new care manager can use, as well as a number of the assessment tools mentioned in this chapter (e.g., MMSE, GDS). As stated earlier, the care manager must adapt the psychosocial assessment to the population served to ensure appropriate and relevant information is obtained to develop the care plan. Care must be taken to use only those forms, or those sections of forms, found in the manual that are reflective of the needs of the individual practice population.

■ NOTES

1. McInnis-Dittrich K. *Social Work with Elders: A Biopsychosocial Approach.* 2nd ed. Boston, MA: Allyn & Bacon; 2005.

2. Geron D. Guidelines for case management practice across the long-term care continuum. *Report of the National Advisory Committee on Long-Term Care Case Management.* Bristol, CT: Connecticut Community Care, Inc; 1994.

3. Aronson J. Assessment: the linchpin of geriatric care management. *Geriatric Care Management.* 1998;8(1):11–14.

4. Langley LK. Cognitive assessment of older adults. In: Kane RLKRA, ed. *Assessing Older Persons.* New York: Oxford University Press; 2002.

5. Gallo JJW. Cognitive assessment. In: Gallo JJ, Fulmer T, Paveza GJ, eds. *Handbook of Geriatric Assessment.* 4th ed. Sudbury, MA: Jones and Bartlett Publishers; 2006:46.

6. Folstein MF, Folstein SE, McHugh PR. Mini-Mental State: a practical method for grading the cognitive state of patients for the clinician. *J Psychiat Res.* 1975;12(3):189–198.

7. Pfeiffer E.. A short portable mental status questionnaire for the assessment of organic brain deficit in elder patients. *J Am Geriatr Soc.* 1975;23:433–441.

8. Katzman R, Brown T, Fuld P, Peck A, Schechter R, Schimmel H. Validation of a short Orientation-Memory-Concentration Test of cognitive impairment. *Am J Psychiatry.* 1983;140:734–739.

9. Mendez MF, Ala T, Underwood KL. Development of scoring criteria for the clock drawing task in Alzheimer's disease. *J Am Geriatr Soc.* 1992;40:1095–1099.

10. Berkman BJ, Maramaldi P, Breon EA, Howe JL. Social Work Gerontological Assessment revisited. *Gerontological Social Work.* 2002;40(1/2).

11. Grann JD. Assessment of emotions in older adults: mood disorders, anxiety, psychological well-being, and hope. In: Kane IRLKRA, ed. *Assessing Older Persons.* New York: Oxford University Press; 2000:129–169.

12. Gallo JW. Depression assessment. In: Gallo JJ, Fulmer T, Paveza GJ, eds. *Handbook of Geriatric Assessment.* Sudbury, MA: Jones and Bartlett Publishers; 2006: 20.

13. Yesavage TL. Development and validation of a geriatric depression scale: a preliminary report. *J Psychiatr Res.* 1983;17:37–49.

14. Beck AT, Ward CH, Mendelson M, Mock J, Erbaugh J. An inventory for measuring depression. *Arch Gen Psychiatry.* 1961;4:561–571.

15. Gellis Z. Older adults with mental and emotional problems. In: Berkman B, ed. *Handbook of Social Work and Health in Aging.* New York: Oxford University Press; 2006:10.

16. Beck AT, Epstein N, Brown G, Steer R. An inventory for measuring clinical anxiety: psychometric properties. *J Consult Clin Psychol.* 1988;56:893–897.

17. Albert S. *Public Health and Aging.* New York: Springer; 2004.

18. Albert SM, Sano M, Bell K, Merchant C, Small S, Stern Y. Hourly care received by people with Alzheimer's disease: results from an urban, community-based survey. *Gerontologist.* 1998;38(6):704–714.

19. Pearlin LI, Mullan JT, Semple SJ, Skaff MM. Caregiving and the stress process: an overview of concepts and their measures. *Gerontologist.* 1990;30:583–594.

20. Schulz R, O'Brien, A. T., Bookwala, J., et al. Psychiatric and physical morbidity effects of dementia caregiving: prevalence, correlates, and causes. *Gerontologist.* 1995;35(6):771–791.

21. Antonucci TC, Sherman AM, Vanderwater EA. Measures of social support and caregiver burden. *Generations.* 1997;XXI(1):48–51.

22. Lubben, J. Assessing social networks among elderly populations. *Family and Community Health.* 1988;11:42–52.

23. Norbeck JS, Lindsey AM, Carrieri VL. The development of an instrument to measure social support. *Nursing Res.* 1981;30:264–269.

24. Aneshensel CS, Pearlin LI, Schuler RH. Stress, role captivity, and the cessation of caregiving. *J Health Soc Bhvr.* 1993;34:54–70.

25. Schulz R. Caregiving as a risk factor for mortality: the caregiver health effects study. *JAMA.* 1999;282:2215–2219.

26. Morano C. Appraisal and coping: moderators or mediators of stress in Alzheimer's disease caregivers? *J Soc Work Res.* 2003;27:116–128.

27. Kramer BJ. Gain in the caregiving experience: where are we? What next? *Gerontologist.* 1997;37(2):218–232.

28. Lawton MP, Kleban MH, Moss M, Rovine M, Glicksman A. Measuring caregiving appraisal. *J Gerontol.* 1989;44(3):P61–P71.

29. Novak M, Guest C. Application of a Multidimensional Caregiver Burden Inventory. *Gerontologist.* 1989;29:798–803.

30. Robinson BC. Validation of a Caregiver Strain Index. *J Gerontol.* 1983;38(3):344–348.

31. Tomita S. Mistreated and neglected elders. In: Berkman IB, ed. *Handbook of Social Work and Health in Aging.* New York: Oxford University Press; 2006:219–230.

32. National Center on Elder Abuse. NCEA National Incidence Study. 1998. Available at: http://www.elderabusecenter.org/. Accessed March 2006.

33. Fulmer T, Street S, Carr K. Abuse of the elderly: screening and detection. *J Emerg Nurs.* 1984;10(3):131–140.

34. Zanjani D. Substance use and abuse assessment In: Gallo JJ, Fulmer T, Paveza GJ, eds. *Handbook of Geriatric Assessment.* Sudbury, MA: Jones and Bartlett Publishers; 2006:175–192.

35. American Psychiatric Association. *Diagnostic and Statistical Manual—Text Revision (DSM-TR).* Washington, DC: American Psychiatric Association; 2000.

36. Blow FC, Gillespie BW, Barry KL, et al. Brief screening for alcohol problems in elder populations using the short Michigan Alcoholism Screening Test—Geriatric Version (SMAST-G). *Alcohol Clin Exp Res.* 1998;22:13A.

37. Ewing, J.A. Detecting alcoholism: the CAGE Questionnaire. *JAMA.* 1984;252:1905–1907.

Chapter 4

Functional Assessment

Deborah Newquist, Connie Rosenberg, and Carolyn Barber

■ INTRODUCTION

One maxim of geriatric care management is to promote the autonomy of older individuals to the greatest extent possible. A careful and competent functional assessment of the older person provides information that is critical to ascertaining how that person's autonomy can be maximized through medical, social, mechanical, and/or environmental manipulations.[1] For this reason the ability to function is a central focus of all geriatric care management evaluations. It is not enough to know about a person's diagnoses because this information alone is insufficient to predict the impact of health problems on a person's daily life. The ability to live as one chooses and to perform basic activities throughout the day is affected by a multitude of factors—health problems, attitude, environmental features, social roles, resources, to name a few. Evaluation of an older person's functional status is key to helping that person maintain his or her autonomy and quality of life because functional abilities are of paramount importance to overall health, well-being, and potential need for services.

The functional assessment should be done by a professional, certified geriatric care manager (GCM). Functional ability is assessed through the measurement of the basic skills of role function. This includes measurement of the performance of basic activities of daily living (ADLs), such as bathing, grooming, dressing, eating, transferring, toileting, and more advanced instrumental activities of daily living (IADLs), including handling financial matters appropriately, finding one's way away from home and back, and managing medication regimens. Evaluation of the older person's functional abilities is a critical component of the geriatric assessment. "One of the goals of a responsive health care system is to assist clients in maintaining their functional well-being. Functional status in the older person is characterized by the gradual decreases in organ function that accompany normal aging and the more rapid declines associated with acute and chronic illness."[2] Medical review of symptoms and diagnosis does not by itself predict an individual's functional impairments. These impairments may be the determining factor in deciding on the living situation that person will require. Together, the medical diagnosis and a description and appraisal of the client's function provide the most accurate assessment. Impairments in ADLs have been identified as risk factors for falls, injuries, and institutionalization.

As stated by Gallo, functional assessment helps set priorities around which the available medical, social, and economic resources can be rallied.[3] Changes in function signal a problem whose source should be addressed and whose solution may be not in a medical response but in a realignment of the social situation.[4] In older persons, functional assessment is critical for use with ongoing clients as well as at the time of initial assessment because functional assessment is a barometer of health status in this age group. Loss of functional ability is the most sensitive indicator for identifying new disease and monitoring the progress of treatment.[3] According to Fretwell, most older persons have one "most vulnerable function" (e.g., cognition, memory, continence, ability to walk).[5] Disorders such as pneumonia, urinary tract infection, myocardial infarction, and heart failure may present initially as confusion, incontinence, and other function-related symptoms in certain older adults. Having knowledge of a person's baseline functional status allows early detection of disease, and the subsequent improvement of that functional impairment is a sensitive indicator of recovery.

Some impairments can be identified by interview or observation of the older person performing common everyday functions. Others require the use of screening tools and methods to differentiate them from other impairments and conditions and to determine their severity. Functional impairment of ADLs and IADLs can often be identified by history taking and by demonstration and observation. When questioning the older person, it is more effective to ask about recent activities such as, "Did you drive here today?" rather than "Are you still driving?" and, "Did you dress yourself this morning?" rather than "Do you dress yourself?" Asking questions in this manner helps focus the older person on what is possible right now and minimizes the reporting of inaccurate information. If the older person is cognitively impaired, responses should be confirmed with a caregiver. Observation of the client's behavior and abilities at the time of the assessment meeting, such as ability to rise from a chair, ambulate, and respond appropriately when speaking, can provide much valuable infor-

mation. It is also critical to note whether any activities performed are done slowly, with difficulty, unsafely, or only partially.[6]

If deficits in ADLs are identified, it is important to try to determine the underlying cause of the loss of function and how long ago it occurred. This information will help the GCM determine whether the condition is permanent or is potentially reversible, perhaps a symptom of an illness that can be treated, restoring function. Many factors affect the ability to perform ADLs safely and completely. No matter what the determination, it is usually wise to involve the client in treatment to alter the dysfunction because, with the proper treatment, many clients have the ability to regain at least partial function. Living with a growing loss of function has a major impact on the quality of life of older people and their caregivers.[6]

■ MEASURING ACTIVITIES OF DAILY LIVING

A variety of tools are available to assist the care manager in evaluating the needs of the client. Below are a sample of some of the formal tools that are available.

The Tools[6(pp187–194)]

The instrument most familiar to researchers and clinicians for performing functional assessment is the Katz Index of ADL (Exhibit 4–1). This instrument measures independence of function in bathing, dressing, toileting, transfers, continence, and feeding. It is widely used for assessing treatment outcomes of older persons and the chronically ill. It provides a standardized measure of biological and psychological function and a framework for assessing the ability to live independently. When deficiencies are found, it provides guidelines for care planning for correction of those deficiencies. The client is ideally witnessed by the GCM while performing the ADLs and rated either *independent* or *dependent*

Exhibit 4–1   Katz Index of ADL

Independence means without supervision, direction, or active personal assistance, except as specifically noted below. This is based on actual status and not ability. A patient who refuses to perform a function is considered as not performing the function, even though he or she is deemed able.

Bathing (Sponge, shower, or tub)

Independent: assistance only in bathing a single part (back or disabled extremity) or bathes self completely

Dependent: assistance in bathing more than one part of body; assistance in getting in or out of tub; does not bathe self

Dressing

Independent: gets clothes from closets and drawers; puts on clothes, outer garments, braces; manages fasteners; act of tying shoes is excluded

Dependent: does not dress self or remains partly undressed

Going to Toilet

Independent: gets to toilet; gets on and off toilet; arranges clothes; cleans organs of excretion (may manage own bedpan used at night only and may or may not be using mechanical supports)

Dependent: uses bedpan or commode or receives assistance in getting to and using toilet

Transfer

Independent: moves in and out of bed and in and out of chair independently (may or may not be using mechanical supports)

Dependent: assistance in moving in or out of bed and/or chair; does not perform one or more transfers

Continence

Independent: urination and defecation entirely self-controlled

Dependent: partial or total incontinence in urination or defecation; partial or total control by enemas, catheters, or regulated use of urinals and/or bedpans

Feeding

Independent: gets food from plate or its equivalent into mouth (precutting of meat and preparation of food, as buttering bread, are excluded from evaluation)

Dependent: assistance in act of feeding (see above); does not eat at all or parenteral feeding

Evaluation Form

Name _____

Date of Evaluation _____

For each area of functioning listed below, circle description that applies (the word "assistance" means supervision, direction, or personal assistance).

Bathing—either sponge bath, tub bath, or shower

Receives no assistance (gets in and out of tub by self if tub is usual means of bathing)
Receives assistance in bathing only one part of body (such as back or a leg)
Receives assistance in bathing more than one part of body (or does not bathe self)

Dressing—gets clothes from closets and drawers; puts on clothes, including underclothes, outer garments; manages fasteners (including braces, if worn)

Gets clothes and gets completely dressed without assistance
Gets clothes and gets dressed without assistance except for tying shoes
Receives assistance in getting clothes or in getting dressed or stays partly or
    completely undressed

continues

Exhibit 4–1   Katz Index of ADL (continued)

Toileting—going to the "toilet room" for bowel and urine elimination; cleaning self after elimination and arranging clothes

Goes to "toilet room," cleans self, and arranges clothes without assistance (may use object for support such as cane, walker, or wheelchair and may manage night bedpan or commode, emptying same in morning)

Receives assistance in going to "toilet room" or in cleansing self or in arranging clothes after elimination or in use of night bedpan or commode

Does not go to room termed "toilet" for the elimination process

Transfer

Moves in and out of bed and in and out of chair without assistance (may use object for support such as cane or walker)

Moves in or out of bed or chair with assistance

Does not get out of bed

Continence

Controls urination and bowel movement completely by self

Has occasional "accidents"

Supervision helps keep urine or bowel control; catheter is used or is incontinent

Feeding

Feeds self without assistance

Feeds self except for getting assistance in cutting meat or buttering bread

Receives assistance in feeding or is fed partly or completely by tubes or intravenous fluids

Source: Republished with permission of the Gerontological Society of America, 1030 15th Street, NW, Suite 250, Washington, DC 20005. *Progress in the Development of the Index of ADL* (Tool), S. Katz, T.D. Downs, H.R. Cash, et al., *Gerontologist*, 1970, Vol. 1. Reproduced by permission of the publisher via Copyright Clearance Center, Inc.

---

based on the definitions for performance of each ADL as established by Katz.[7] Caregiver report is often used in situations where it is not practical for the GCM to witness ADL activities. The need for assistance is further broken down into categories for supervision, direction, or personal assistance so that subjectivity of the clinician is minimized. A client refusing to perform any function is categorized as not performing the function even though it might be obvious to the tester that, based on the overall functional abilities, the client is capable of performing the particular ADL. A combined measure of the six ADL functions can be used to quantify changes over time. Although this instrument is easy to use in a home or facility environment, it is somewhat time-consuming to administer and might be of more use to the GCM who is assessing the client on an ongoing basis rather than one performing a one-time assessment.

The Rapid Disability Rating Scale-2 (Exhibit 4–2) rates individuals' performance of ADLs and their degree of disability on a four-point scale from "None" (needing no assistance) to "Total" (needing total assistance). It includes a selection of both ADL and IADL tasks and has sections for "degree of disability" and "degree of special problems." As with other scales, it is important to rate the client on what the client does, not what the client says he or she does. This scale is useful for monitoring changes in clients' conditions over time.

Exhibit 4–2   Rapid Disability Rating Scale (RDRS-2)

Directions: Rate what the person does to reflect current behavior. Circle one of the four choices for each item. Consider rating with any aids or prostheses normally used. None = completely independent or normal behavior. Total = that person cannot, will not, or may not (because of medical restriction) perform a behavior or has the most severe form of disability or problem.

Assistance with Activities of Daily Living

Eating	None	A little	A lot	Spoon-fed; intravenous tube
Walking (with cane or walker if used)	None	A little	A lot	Does not walk
Mobility (going outside and getting about with wheelchair, etc., if used)	None	A little	A lot	Is housebound
Bathing (include getting supplies, supervising)	None	A little	A lot	Must be bathed
Dressing (include help in selecting clothes)	None	A little	A lot	Must be dressed
Toileting (include help with clothes, cleaning, or help with ostomy/catheter)	None	A little	A lot	Uses bedpan or unable to care for ostomy/catheter
Grooming (shaving for men, hairdressing for women, nails, teeth)	None	A little	A lot	Must be groomed
Adaptive tasks (managing money/ possessions; telephoning; buying newspaper, toilet articles, snacks)	None	A little	A lot	Cannot manage

Degree of Disability

Communication (expressing self)	None	A little	A lot	Does not communicate
Hearing (with aid, if used)	None	A little	A lot	Does not seem to hear
Sight (with glasses, if used)	None	A little	A lot	Does not see
Diet (deviation from normal)	None	A little	A lot	Fed by intravenous tube
In bed during day (ordered or self-initiated)	None	A little (<3 hr)	A lot	Most/all of the time
Incontinence (urine/feces, with catheter or prosthesis, if used)	None	Some-times	Frequently (weekly +)	Does not control
Medication	None	Some-times	Daily, taken orally	Daily; injection (+oral if used)

Degree of Special Problems

Mental confusion	None	A little	A lot	Extreme
Uncooperativeness (combats efforts to help with care)	None	A little	A lot	Extreme
Depression	None	A little	A lot	Extreme

Source: Reprinted with permission from *Journal of the American Geriatric Society*, Vol. 20, pp. 318–382, (c) 1982, Lippincott, Williams & Wilkins.

Other comprehensive assessment tools that include the functional domain along with other components identified as determining factors of ability to live independently are useful in assessment and care planning. The most widely mentioned in the literature are the Barthel Index, which rates 10 different items[8]; the Older American Rehabilitation Services (OARS), which includes within its extensive format of many health parameters the same items as the Katz Index but relies on self-reports of clients[9]; and the PULSES (Physical, Upper Limbs, Lower Limbs, Sensory, and Social Factors) Profile, which measures wider dimensions of functions but includes ADLs.[10]

One of the most widely used instruments, mainly used in nursing homes, is the Minimum Data Set (MDS). The MDS is based on direct observations made by professionals and a review of clinical records.[11] The Minimum Data Set for Home Care is now a tool required by several states to assess the needs of persons living at home. It is a multidimensional assessment instrument similar to the long-term-care MDS and is used in combination with the Clinical Assessment Protocols (CAPs) to form the Resident Assessment Instrument–Home Care. CAPs provide guidelines for individualized care planning of triggered problems.[12]

Disease-related assessment scales are available for some conditions, such as gait and balance dysfunction. The Tinetti Balance and Gait Evaluation (Exhibit 4–3) is a 28-point assessment tool that is performed by a trained evaluator.[13]

A condensed version of the Tinetti is also available. This test, the Get Up and Go Test, is simple to administer, requires no special equipment, and can be conducted in a brief amount of time.[14] The test begins with the client sitting up straight in a high-seat chair, which allows the person to sit with hips at a 90-degree angle to knees. The client is then instructed to (1) get up (without using arm-rests if possible), (2) stand still, (3) walk forward 10 feet, (4) turn around and walk back to the chair, and (5) turn and be seated. The evaluator notes sitting balance, transfers from sitting to standing, pace and stability of walking, and ability to turn without staggering. Statistical verification of the test by the developers showed good correlation between test scores and other measures of gait, which in some cases involved more sophisticated laboratory-based measures of balance and gait.

The Activities of Daily Living

Below are the activities of daily living assessed by the care manager during an evaluation.

Bathing

Determining the exact amount of assistance that a person needs in each ADL is necessary to make the best recommendations in a plan of care. For example, in bathing, if we find that the person needs only standby assistance in getting into and out of the tub or shower, the person might only need the assistance of a companion (or family member) who can provide this service rather than assistance by a certified home health aide. Each state has its own laws regarding who can legally provide what service in a home care setting. If the person indicates that he or she isn't showering because of a fear of falling, the person might only need to have the security of a shower chair and handheld shower spray. If the person has dementia and the family reports that he or she is not bathing, the person might only need reminders to bathe.

More specific knowledge of joint function is also helpful in determining the amount and type of assistance that a person might need. For example, if the person has limited range of motion in one or both shoulders, will that person be able to bathe him- or herself? Will physical therapy improve shoulder function?

Exhibit 4–3   Tinetti Balance and Gait Evaluation

Balance

Instructions: Subject is seated in hard, armless chair. The following maneuvers are tested.

1. Sitting balance

Leans or slides in chair	=	0
Steady, safe	=	1 _____

2. Arises

Unable without help	=	0
Able but uses arms to help	=	1
Able without use of arms	=	2 _____

3. Attempts to arise

Unable without help	=	0
Able but requires more than 1 attempt	=	1
Able to arise with 1 attempt	=	2 _____

4. Immediate standing balance (first 5 sec)

Unsteady (staggers, moves feet, marked trunk sway)	=	0
Steady but uses walker or cane or grabs other objects for support	=	1
Steady without walker or cane or other support	=	2 _____

5. Standing balance

Unsteady	=	0
Steady but wide stance (medial heels more than 4 in. apart) or uses cane, walker, or other support	=	1
Narrow stance without support	=	2 _____

6. Nudged (subject at maximum position with feet as close together as possible, examiner pushes lightly on subject's sternum with palm of hand 3 times)

Begins to fall	=	0
Staggers, grabs, but catches self	=	1
Steady	=	2 _____

7. Eyes closed (at maximum position No. 6)

Unsteady	=	0
Steady	=	1 _____

8. Turning 360°

Discontinuous steps	=	0
Continuous	=	1
Unsteady (grabs, staggers)	=	0
Steady	=	1 _____

9. Sitting down

Unsafe (misjudged distance, falls into chair)	=	0
Uses arms or not a smooth motion	=	1
Safe, smooth motion	=	2 _____

Balance score: _____/16

continues

Exhibit 4–3   Tinetti Balance and Gait Evaluation (continued)

Gait

Instructions: Subject stands with examiner; walks down hallway or across room, first at his "usual" pace, then back at "rapid, but safe" pace (using usual walking aid such as cane, walker).

10. Initiation of gait (immediately after told to "go")

Any hesitancy or multiple attempts to start	=	0
No hesitancy	=	1 ____

11. Step length and height

a. Right swing foot

Does not pass left stance foot with step	=	0
Passes left stance foot	=	1
Right foot does not clear floor completely with step	=	0
Right foot completely clears floor	=	1 ____

b. Left swing foot

Does not pass right stance foot with step	=	0
Passes right stance foot	=	1
Left foot does not clear floor completely with step	=	0
Left foot completely clears floor	=	1 ____

12. Step symmetry

Right and left step length not equal (estimate)	=	0
Right and left step appear equal	=	1 ____

13. Step continuity

Stopping or discontinuity between steps	=	0
Steps appear continuous	=	1 ____

14. Path (estimated in relation to floor tiles, 12-in. diameter; observe excursion of 1 foot over about 10 ft of the course)

Marked deviation	=	0
Mild/moderate deviation or uses walking aid	=	1
Straight without walking aid	=	2 ____

15. Trunk

Marked sway or uses walking aid	=	0
No sway but flexion of knees or back or spreads arms out while walking	=	1
No sway, no flexion, no use of arms, and no use of walking aid	=	2 ____

16. Walking stance

Heels apart	=	0
Heels almost touching while walking	=	1 ____

Gait score: ____/12

Total score: ____/28

Source: Reprinted with permission from Tinetti Balance and Gait Evolution, *Journal of the American Geriatric Society,* Vol. 34, pp. 119–126, (c) 1986, Lippincott, Williams & Wilkins.

Grooming

Oftentimes, a care manager can make recommendations that will improve a person's grooming and allow for continued independence. For example, switching from a regular razor to an electric razor can make shaving easier and safer for a person who may have hand tremors or arthritis. Encouraging a woman to go to the assisted-living beauty salon for manicures and hair washes can provide her with the feeling of "treating" herself plus improve hygiene. Cueing for clients with dementia to brush their teeth or comb their hair can give them a continued sense of accomplishment and independence.

Dressing

Again, detailed questioning can assist the care manager in making the most appropriate recommendations. If the family reports that the client is wearing soiled clothes, it may be that the person has a visual impairment that is preventing him or her from seeing that the soiled clothes should be changed. However, it may also be that, if the person has dementia, he or she is forgetting to change clothes and might just need reminders or need to have a caregiver lay out the appropriate clothes to wear. If a person can get dressed unassisted except for shoes and socks, recommending that the person use adaptive devices such as a long shoehorn will enable the person to continue to be independent. Persons who need hands-on assistance because they are unable to dress themselves because of physical problems, such as Parkinson's disease or cognitive loss, will need a referral to a home health aide if family members are not available.

Pain is an often-overlooked problem. Frequently, pain can be great enough to inhibit a person from functioning independently. Pain can definitely be a problem that affects a person's ability to dress him- or herself. The care manager needs to be aware of whether pain is decreasing a person's function and recom-mend a pain evaluation. In addition, a referral for physical therapy for range-of-motion exercises or other therapeutic interventions may assist with improving function in dressing as well as accomplishing other ADLs and IADLs.

Toileting

A person who needs assistance getting on and off the toilet because of physical problems may also need a referral for a home health aide. However, installing a raised toilet seat or adding a grab bar next to the toilet may help to keep this person independent. If a person has difficulty getting to the toilet, for example, at night, having a commode next to the bed may allow him or her to toilet safely alone without awaking a caregiver. In addition, if in a review of medications the care manager notes that the person is taking a diuretic in the afternoon and getting up frequently to toilet at night, a change to a morning dosage can be suggested to the person's physician.

Transfers

Is the person having difficulty getting in or out of bed? The care manager can recommend that the bed be lowered so that it is closer to the floor or that the person rent a hospital bed so that he or she can use the side rails to assist with the transfer. Also, check to see whether a pillow-top mattress is making the bed too high.

Does the person have difficulty getting in or out of a chair? A chairlift can ease the transfer, or perhaps the person can even use a walker for added support. If physical assistance is needed, the care manager should always ask whether a person needs assistance from one or two people. This can make the difference between a person being able to stay at home with one caregiver or needing to be placed in a nursing home. In some instances, the care manager may recommend a hoyer lift to be used at home so that a transfer is safe for the person and the caregiver.

Continence

Fifteen percent to 30% of adults living in the community and almost 50% of nursing home residents are affected by urinary incontinence.[15] The prevalence in older women is twice that of prevalence in older men. Despite the fact that incontinence is common in aging, it should never be considered a normal condition of aging. Various methods of managing and reducing incontinence have been developed, and many older persons have been assisted with incontinence so that the quality of their life is not so greatly affected.

Because of embarrassment and worry about appearance and odor, clients may not report incontinence unless asked directly. Incontinence increases the risk of falls in older persons. It is isolating and has a major impact on quality of life. Often, the development of incontinence is the final factor influencing family caregivers to institutionalize those they care for. Few older people realize that incontinence often is treatable. Oftentimes, they will self-treat by decreasing fluid intake, which in turn can lead to dehydration, which in turn can lead to falls. The care manager should refer the person to the primary care physician or a urologist for a workup before assuming that the incontinence is untreatable. Many times, this condition can be caused by an acute urinary tract infection.

Also, other strategies can be recommended to increase continence such as frequent reminders to toilet or developing the habit of sitting on the toilet to have a bowel movement at the same time every day. Using disposable undergarments that pull up and down easily may also allow a person with incontinence to be more independent in managing his or her incontinence.

Eating

This is not to be confused with meal preparation. This is totally a person's ability to get food from the plate to the mouth. A referral to an occupational therapist by the care manager may improve the person's independence in this area. For example, the therapist may suggest adaptive utensils for a person with arthritis who is unable to grasp a common fork. For persons who are blind, having a dish with a straight rim allows them to feel when they have touched the edge of the plate. Cups that have lids with spouts prevent spills for persons with tremors from Parkinson's, for example. Think adaptive to keep a person independent.

Also, for a person with dementia, providing finger foods or cueing to continue eating may improve nutrition and allow for more independence. Having the caregiver cut food into bite-size pieces and setting up drinks so they can be more easily reached are other useful strategies for persons with cognitive or physical impairments.

The care manager needs to be alert to the fact that problems in this area can seriously affect the client's nutritional status. Asking questions about weight loss will provide added information. If the client is in a nursing home setting, it is important to look at the monthly weight chart. If there is weight loss, the client may not be finishing meals as a result of dementia or the physical inability to continue feeding him- or herself. The nursing home physician may need to order nutritional supplements, and the staff may need to provide more oversight at mealtimes. Visiting a client at mealtime in a nursing home or assisted living facility can provide invaluable information for the care plan.

■ AMBULATION AND MOBILITY

One factor influencing ADL performance is mobility. Direct observation can identify problems in gait and balance. Early detection of deficits in mobility can identify those clients at risk of injury. Whenever possible, rehabilitation can then assist in restoring functional losses and reduce the risk of falls.

For those deficits that cannot be rehabilitated, assistive equipment such as a cane or walker can be provided.

Immobility and inactivity can lead to the older person becoming chair- or bed-bound. These older persons often go on to develop edema, contractures, incontinence, or pressure sores. These complications place them at increased risk of falls and nursing home placement. It is important to inquire about recent falls and the circumstances under which they occurred and to test gait performance in all older adults. One tool, as noted earlier, is the Tinetti Balance and Gait Evaluation tool. Those at high risk can be identified so that preventive measures can be taken as part of care planning. Factors increasing risk include confusion, incontinence, impaired mobility, generalized weakness, use of sedating medications and alcohol, postural hypotension, and history of previous falls.[6(p183)]

To note the character of the gait it is best for the care manager to observe the person ambulating. Is the gait slow and shuffling or too fast and without concern for the environment? Note the person's balance. Did the person need to grab onto the furniture to prevent a fall? Can he or she walk up the flight of steps to get to the bedroom or even up the two steps from the living room to the kitchen? Would a stairlift provide improved safety? It is important to observe footwear. Is the stylish older woman still wearing a shoe with a raised heel? Is the stylish older man still wearing a slip-on shoe that does not provide proper support? Recommending proper footwear can be the first step in preventing falls. Asking the person for a tour of the home is an excellent way to observe how he or she gets around and to make observations regarding home safety.

What about ambulating outside? Does the person need adaptive equipment outside because of uneven surfaces even if he or she is fine when ambulating on a smooth floor inside? Is the person able to get up the outside stairs? Are there railings to keep the person safe? Does the person need a ramp? Is the person cognitively intact enough to use a scooter for longer distances traveled in the nursing home? Does the person need a prescription for a wheelchair because he or she is unable to walk the long distance to the doctor's office?

Falls

Every year, approximately 30% of older persons living at home fall. As stated earlier, getting more information about where falls occur is vital. A practical mnemonic for reviewing the actual fall is as follows[16]:

S	Symptoms experienced at the time of fall
P	Previous number of falls or near-falls
L	Location of falls
A	Activity engaged in or attempted at time of fall
T	Time (hour) of fall
T	Trauma (e.g., physical or psychological) associated with falls

Prevention of falls is of utmost importance because after a fall the fear of another fall can become a vicious cycle. Fear leads to inactivity that then results in decreased strength that then leads to increased risk of another fall.[17] Many falls by older persons occur in the bathroom. Adaptations in the environment can decrease the risk. If your client is falling at night, ask about the use of sedating medications at bedtime. Or perhaps does the person fall because he or she ambulates slowly and needs to rush to answer the only phone in the home, which is located on the kitchen wall? Getting a portable telephone may decrease the risk of another fall. Was the person experiencing specific symptoms secondary to medical problems, for example, dizziness or postural hypotension? Reviewing these symptoms with the physician can result in treatment or change in medications that will reduce the risk of a repeat fall.[18]

Changes in the environment, attention to adaptations, and medical evaluation will make it safer for a person with impaired mobility to get around the home. In addition, with the goal of improved mobility and balance, the care manager should think about the possibility of physical therapy for strength training, personal trainers who can come to the home or the assisted living facility to do light exercise, or even a membership at a local senior-friendly gym that offers tai chi classes, which are known to improve balance. In addition, for clients in nursing homes the care manager needs to advocate for needed therapies and medical evaluations to improve mobility and decrease falls.

■ MEASURING INSTRUMENTAL ACTIVITIES OF DAILY LIVING

The wide range of abilities involved in IADLs (not only physical but mental and social variables) and the complexity and variation of interpretations of the test results mean that there are more problems with IADL instruments than there are with ADL instruments. IADL scales sometimes result in falsely low scores for men and women who have not performed certain food preparation or financial tasks during their lifetime but who are perfectly capable of performing other IADL functions. The scale most widely used and with well-documented reliability and validity in the older population is the IADL Scale developed in the 1960s by Lawton and Brody (Exhibit 4–4).[19] The scale measures eight aspects of living that are critical to those living independently.[6]

The Lawton IADL Scale was the first tool to measure more complex activities related to a person's ability to adapt and function in the environment. It was designed for use as a guide in determining appropriate living environments for older persons. It measures performance rather than ability and therefore is subject to sex role biases that need to be accounted for during use. Originally, it was intended that eight items would be used for women and five items for men, but common use has blurred this approach. The items are ordered in a Guttman scale form with the first item, ability to use a phone, being the lowest level, and handling finances the highest functional activity.

Exhibit 4–4   IADL Scale

Male Score		Female Score
	A. Ability to use telephone	
1	1. Operates telephone on own initiative; looks up and dials numbers, etc.	1
1	2. Dials a few well-known numbers	1
1	3. Answers telephone but does not dial	1
0	4. Does not use telephone at all	0
	B. Shopping	
1	1. Takes care of all shopping needs independently	1
0	2. Shops independently for small purchases	0
0	3. Needs to be accompanied on any shopping trip	0
0	4. Completely unable to shop	0

Exhibit 4–4   IADL Scale (continued)

Male Score		Female Score
	C. Food preparation	
	1. Plans, prepares, and serves adequate meals independently	1
	2. Prepares adequate meals if supplied with ingredients	0
	3. Heats and serves prepared meals, or prepares meals but does not maintain adequate diet	0
	4. Needs to have meals prepared and served	0
	D. Housekeeping	
	1. Maintains house alone or with occasional assistance (e.g., heavy-work domestic help)	1
	2. Performs light daily tasks such as dish washing and bed making	1
	3. Performs light daily tasks but cannot maintain acceptable level of cleanliness	1
	4. Needs help with all home maintenance tasks	1
	5. Does not participate in any housekeeping tasks	0
	E. Laundry	
	1. Does personal laundry completely	1
	2. Launders small items; rinses socks, stockings, etc.	1
	3. All laundry must be done by others	0
	F. Mode of transportation	
1	1. Travels independently on public transportation or drives own car	1
1	2. Arranges own travel via taxi, but does not otherwise use public transportation	1
0	3. Travels on public transportation when assisted or accompanied by another	1
0	4. Travel limited to taxi or automobile, with assistance of another	0
0	5. Does not travel at all	0
	G. Responsibility for own medication	
1	1. Is responsible for taking medication in correct dosages at correct time	1
0	2. Takes responsibility if medication is prepared in advance in separate dosages	0
0	3. Is not capable of dispensing own medication	0
	H. Ability to handle finances	
1	1. Manages financial matters independently (budgets, writes checks, pays rent and bills, goes to bank); collects and keeps track of income	1
1	2. Manages day-to-day purchases, but needs help with bank for managing purchases, etc.	1
0	3. Incapable of handling money	0

Source: Republished with permission of the Gerontological Society of America, 1030 15th Street, NW, Suite 250, Washington, DC 20005. *Assessment of Older People: Self-monitoring and Instrumental Activities of Daily Living* (Scale), M.P. Lawton and E.M. Brody, *Gerontologist*, 1969, Vol. 9. Reproduced by permission of the publisher via Copyright Clearance Center, Inc.

Another tool for IADL assessment is the instrument called the Older Americans Resources and Services Multidimensional Functional Assessment Questionnaire (OARS-IADL), which was developed in the 1970s.[20] The OARS questionnaire assesses five domains of functioning: social, economic, mental health, physical health, and self-care capacity and service utilization. The IADL component has been developed into a separate, seven-item tool that uses a self-reporting approach.[21] (See Exhibit 4–5.) Unlike the Lawton instrument, all items are to be used with both men and women. The tool is useful as a screen for determining the need for more in-depth evaluation and for service planning.

IADL tools generally are viewed as concentrating on activities necessary for independent living in the community. They incorporate an inherent emphasis on cognitive functioning with items such as financial and medication management. Cultural and sex role issues need to be considered in their use so as to avoid unreliable results.

Dementia and Function

Incipient or more pronounced dementia by definition impairs functional performance.

Indeed, the diagnosis of dementia requires that a cognitive condition be severe enough to interfere with the performance of daily activities. It is through functional problems that dementia is often first noticed by patients and their families. IADL instruments, which measure higher-level functioning, are particularly helpful in detecting incipient dementias. Changes in habits indicating difficulty paying bills and managing finances or troubles with medication regimens are often telltale signs that cognitive changes are afoot. These, in fact, may be clues to care managers that other problems less apparent superficially are present.

Dementia can also pose challenges to the care manager in conducting an assessment of IADLs. This is because the reliability of self-reports may be eroded in dementia patients. It is important, therefore, that care managers probe to learn what the person is actually doing, not just what the person says he or she can do, and also for the care manager to gather information about past patterns to determine whether recent changes have occurred. Sorting out capacity from behavior—what the person can do but chooses not to do versus what he or she can no longer do

Exhibit 4–5   OARS-IADL Scale

	Response Option
	Without help (2) With help (1) Unable (0)
Question	
Can you use the telephone?	
Can you get to places out of walking distance?	
Can you go shopping (groceries/clothing)?	
Can you prepare your own meals?	
Can you do your own housework?	
Can you take your own medications?	
Can you handle your own money?	

Source: Reprinted with permission of the American Geriatric Society, c/o Blackwell Publishing, 9600 Garsington Road, Oxford OX4 2DQ, UK. "Components of the Older Americans Resources and Services Instrumental Activities of Daily Living." (Scale), G.G. Fillenbaum, *Journal of the American Geriatrics Society,* 1985, Vol. 33(10), 698–706. Reproduced by permission of the publisher.

but makes the excuse of preferring not to do—takes experience and judgment on the part of the care manager.

Gathering information from various sources—the older persons themselves, their caregivers (ideally in private conversations), observation of the person in the environment, and keen observation of the environment itself—all provide clues about functioning. For example, are medication bottles or systems organized, or are bottles of current and past medications scattered throughout the house? Are random pills left on countertops or tables? Can the person show you which medications he or she takes and tell you his or her routines? Does the person evidence difficulty remembering which medications are taken and when, and if so, can the person problem solve to tell you the routine accurately?

If appropriate (i.e., if needed and with permission of the patient), count the medications in the bottle and calculate the number that should be there based on the prescription instructions and date the prescription was filled. Check the cupboards and refrigerator to see if they are well stocked and kept current. Are there numerous spoiled and/or expired foods in the refrigerator? Are there abundant numbers of the same item in the cupboard, which can indicate the person forgets what is in the cupboards and buys foods repeatedly out of habit, is not able to make a shopping list, or is unable to remember what supplies are needed. (Of course, everyone does these things to some extent, but the care manager must look at degrees of problems and whether any patterns are present.)

Are bills and papers organized, or is the house heavily cluttered with stacks of papers? Have there been reports that utilities or other services have been discontinued or threatened to be shut off because of nonpayment? Are there signs of mail "contests" and other solicitations for "charities" present and in abundance? If the person will let you see his or her checkbook, is it in order or does it show signs of frequent errors, double payments, transposed numbers, and the like?

Dementia interferes with many higher-level functions and, in its more advanced stages, with basic ADLs. Assessing the older person's functional performance can help guide the care manager's plan of care, direct communication with other professionals when further diagnostic tests might be needed, or tailor appropriate supports when independence is no longer possible.

IADL Tasks

Several core functional activities form the bases of IADL assessments. How an older person performs on these activities gives important information about that person's ability to live independently with safety and quality of life.

Telephone Use

Determining a person's ability to make and receive phone calls can help identify home safety issues. From higher-level activities, such as locating or remembering a phone number or looking up a number, to following through to place a call and completing a call all give clues to a person's ability to manage independently and safely at home. If there was a fire, could or would the person be able to call for help? Can the person call the doctor's office and make an appointment? If there was a water leak, could the older person locate and call a plumber, or would the person need to call a family member or friend to get that person to locate help?

Determining capacity in this regard can be tricky. First, determine whether the person has the physical capacity to use the phone: can the person reach the phone, hold it, hear well enough to use it? Asking the person to place a call to the doctor to reconfirm an appointment is one method of evaluating behavior. Another is to ask what the person would do in an emergency. Then ask the person to give the numbers of the persons he or she would need to call. Document the person's responses. When conducting assessments for IADLs, there is the risk that people will give false-positive responses—stating they can perform a function when in fact they may have difficulty performing it. Observation and gathering information from several sources help the care manager pinpoint areas of strength and limitations.

Shopping

Is the older person able to assess needs for supplies and plan and execute shopping excursions independently? What type and level of help are needed if the older person cannot do these tasks alone? Asking the person questions about who does the shopping and having the person describe his or her last shopping trip can give information useful for care planning. Some persons may have difficulty carrying grocery bags but be able to make a shopping list and drive to the store. Others may have cognitive problems that interfere with the ability to survey needs, make a list, find the items in the store, and pay accurate amounts at the checkout counter. Other persons may have ambulation difficulties or low stamina as a result of a heart condition, for example, which precludes the person from walking up and down grocery aisles or going to the mall to buy clothing.

Food Preparation

This task is subject to classic sex role influences. The care manager needs to ascertain past and current role behaviors and integrate that information into the assessment evaluation.

Food preparation involves cognitive functions, including memory, executive function, forecasting, sequencing, and visual-spatial abilities. In addition, physical abilities involving manual dexterity; stamina; ability to reach, stoop, lift, and carry; and balance and gait are involved as a person moves about the kitchen cooking. Deciding what to eat, obtaining the foods to eat, preparing the foods, and storing and cleaning up after meal preparation are all involved. The level of complexity of the meals

and their nutritional value are important considerations for the care manager to note. Safety issues are also involved in remembering to turn off the stove or to regulate cooking temperatures, deciding whether a food is safe to eat or past its expiration date, and storing foods at appropriate temperatures.

It is helpful for the care manager both to ask questions and to observe for telltale signs of trouble. Is the refrigerator stocked with fresh, healthy foods? Is the cupboard or pantry bare, or are there adequate staples on hand? Are there any signs of burnt pans? Are there signs that the meal described was prepared? Are breakfast dishes in the sink? It is very helpful if a visit is close to a time when the care manager has been told the older person normally eats. It gives the care manager a chance to see whether meal preparations are underway. Asking for a tour of the home or for a drink of cold water is an easy way to observe the kitchen unobtrusively if an older person is not forthcoming with information in this area.

Housekeeping

Again, sex role differences can influence responses on this item, and the care manager needs to take account of these issues. Also, some people use the services of a housekeeper and may have for years, so their nonperformance in this area needs to reflect long-established patterns. Finally, individual standards of cleanliness vary, and these need to be acknowledged.

A tour of the house of the older person, in addition to asking direct questions about housekeeping habits, provides information for the care manager to consider. In addition, information about past practices helps the care manager to ascertain whether functioning has changed and when. The care manager should look for signs of neglect. Also signs of hoarding should be noted. Safety issues in the home are also important to record for future follow-up.

Laundry

Like housekeeping, laundry tasks are subject to sex role and support (housekeeping) staff practices. It is important to note actual behavior and health issues or disabilities that interfere with the behavior, if any. Any changes in habits should be followed to learn what triggered and/or caused the behavior change. Also note the person's general appearance. Is the person wearing soiled clothing? Is the person reported to wear the same clothes day in and day out? When touring the house, note whether there are signs of neglect, heavily soiled towels in the bathroom, for example. Where is the laundry room? Is it down a flight of stairs in the basement? Does that pose a risk or difficulty if the person must carry laundry baskets back and forth? Is the laundry in another building or outside in the garage? In the winter, are there environmental difficulties or risks involved in doing the laundry? For example, does a person with unsteady gait or arthritis in the knees need to go down snow- or ice-covered steps to get to the laundry facilities?

Mode of Transportation

In our automobile-oriented society, many people drive as their normal mode of transportation. Age-related changes can threaten driving ability, however. Health problems can interfere with functioning in this area in obvious and less obvious ways. Problems with vision, reaction time, information processing, concentration, and visual-spatial abilities all interplay to influence driving capacity. Motor skills and coordination also affect performance.

Determine through discussion the older person's usual mode of transportation. Then integrate that with information about the person's lifelong habits. Did the person ever drive? How much? It is also important to screen for any concerns about whether the person should be driving and to probe and gather information from various sources to ascertain whether the self-reported behavior can be corroborated. Observing the car itself can also be helpful to see whether there are dents or scratches present and, if so, to learn about their origin.

For many men and women, driving is both a symbolic and a functional basic necessity. It affords freedom to come and go when and where one chooses, even for persons who no longer venture far, and thus is the hallmark of independence and full personhood. The idea that one can go when, where, and whether one chooses is key to many people's sense of autonomy. It is not surprising, then, that many people hold fast to driving as a basic right. Not surprisingly, too, many people continue to drive even when age or infirmity or even the removal of their driver's license dictate that they should not.

It is not within the GCM scope of practice to evaluate a person's driving capacity. The care manager should, however, screen for problems and concerns in this area, note transportation modes being used, and note any need for intervention or evaluation or assistance to afford the older client continued opportunities for freedom of movement.

Older drivers have a higher risk of traffic fatalities because they are involved in more accidents per mile driven than middle-aged drivers are and because they are more fragile and therefore more likely to suffer more serious injuries should an accident occur.[22] For their safety and the safety of others, it is important that concerns about driving ability be addressed. The American Medical Association (AMA) has an Older Drivers Project designed to educate physicians about the public health issues related to older driver safety. It has developed a Physician's Guide to Assessing and Counseling Older Drivers to aid in addressing issues surrounding fitness to drive. Driver rehabilitation and older driver safety training initiatives are available in many communities. Occupational therapists and driver evaluation programs at universities, state motor vehicle departments, or specialty clinics can aid older persons and their families with driving concerns as well.

Medication Management

The ability to procure, organize, and follow medication regimens is vitally important. Medication mismanagement is widely prevalent in the elderly population. Its consequences can be profound, leading to preventable health declines, hospitalization, and sometimes even death. Moreover, physicians are often unable to ascertain whether or not their patient is compliant with the prescribed medications. Hence, medical management can become misguided inadvertently as a result of noncompliance behaviors. The GCM can play a critical role in evaluating this vital component of functioning among older clients.

In assessing functioning in this area, it is important to combine information gathered from self-reports, reports of others close to the patient, and direct observation. Incipient dementia can interfere with abilities to manage medications, as noted earlier. This is compounded when a person's medication regimen is complicated, for example, take this pill 1 hour before meals, this one with meals, this one 2 hours after eating; sit up for 30 minutes after taking this medication, and so forth. Early-stage dementia patients may forget that they forget to take their medications and may give you false reports about their behavior. Or they may try to cover their deficits and minimize or fail to reveal difficulties. It is therefore important to observe, count medications if possible, and gather information from others as well as the older person. Suggest the use of a pillbox if one is not present. Other more targeted pill organizers and reminders may also be needed and can be recommended as part of the care plan.

Handling Financial Affairs

Can the older person plan, budget, manage investments, pay bills, balance a checkbook, and manage day-to-day purchases without assistance? Is the person at risk for scams, undue influence, credit problems, or other financial difficulties because of functional limitations? Does the person show good judgment in regard to finances? Has the person changed lifelong habits in how he or she manages money?

On first meeting someone, often it is difficult to gain enough trust to fully assess functioning in this area. As a first step, direct questions about who pays the bills and manages investments opens up the topic. Based on responses to earlier less threatening questions, the care manager may detect some clues that can shed light on functional capacity here. For example, if someone has difficulty shopping because Alzheimer's disease has affected his or her ability to make a shopping list and go through the market independently to shop, it is expected that this person will need assistance with bookkeeping and money matters. Because the Lawton scale is ordered, it is important to recall that the less demanding tasks are presented first and those requiring higher cognitive functioning are presented later. Thus, difficulties performing the easier tasks indicate the likelihood of difficulties performing the higher-order functions.

When the GCM tours the house, he or she can discreetly and with permission look for unpaid bills lying about or piles of mail that need attention. Stacks of solicitations for charities and/or contests should be noted. Enlisting information from key informants, such as adult children, is important to round out the evaluation of this area. Adult children may be able to review the older person's checkbook to make sure things are in order. They may be aware of utilities or insurances that have threatened termination for nonpayment. They may know whether the older adult participates in "contests" or gives more money than ever before to charities. Financial advisors for the older person may also be a source of information for assistance in evaluating functional performance. Because finances are a very private topic in many families, this subject needs to be handled with delicacy and discretion.

■ SENSORY LOSS

Hearing

Hearing loss affects one-third of 65-year-olds, two-thirds of those over age 70, and three-fourths of those 80 years of age and older.[23] Loss of the senses, for example, hearing and vision, can impact function. Hearing loss affects one's ability to drive or use the telephone or perhaps hear a smoke alarm sound. This in turn affects the client's safety. It is important for the care manager to ask about the client's perception of his or her own hearing. If there is a question, just doing a simple test of whispering so that the lips cannot be read or asking the person whether he or she can hear a ticking watch can be a quick screening tool.

Oftentimes, clients just assume that experiencing a sensory loss is a normal part of aging when, in fact, their ears may be filled with wax. Thus, it is important for the care manager to recommend that the person first see the primary care physician if this has not already been done. Then a referral for an evaluation for treatable causes and for testing is appropriate. Many clients are very resistant to getting hearing aids that will correct their hearing problem. They don't always realize the extent of their loss and what they are not hearing until they have the aids in place. Many are too embarrassed to ask people to repeat themselves and thus may simply nod and smile when they have not heard what has been said. Asking the client to repeat what you have just said is helpful in making sure that the person has heard you.

In addition to an evaluation for a hearing aid, other adaptations are useful. One example is a handheld assistive device that amplifies sound and can be used on an as-needed basis. Other adaptations include doorbells or telephones that trigger a light to go on when they ring. Telephones made especially to be used with hearing aids can make hearing on the phone easier. In addition, adapters for televisions are available that will enable a spouse without loss to listen to the TV at normal sound and the person with the hearing impairment to wear headphones that amplify the volume.

Hearing loss can lead to social isolation and depression,[24] which can in turn lead to other complications that affect function. It is important for the care manager to recommend a plan of care that decreases the likelihood of this occurring and improves the person's quality of life, for example, eating out in restaurants that are not noisy or going in off-hours when it may be the most quiet. Informing others in the person's social circle that the person has hearing loss helps ensure that the person is included in conversations. The care manager can see whether area theaters and performing arts centers have devices available that amplify sound for those with hearing impairment. For clients in a nursing home or an assisted living facility, the staff need to be alerted to the person's need to be wearing a hearing aid. It is important to keep the client with hearing impairment involved as a part of his or her community.

Vision

Visual impairment is very common in older persons and has a major impact on performance of daily activities. More than 90% of older persons wear glasses. Sixteen percent of those between ages 75 to 84 years and 27% of those older than age 85 are blind in both eyes.[23] Age-related illnesses resulting in progressive vision loss include macular degeneration, cataracts, glaucoma, and diabetic retinopathy. Acute vision loss can be caused by stroke or giant-cell arteritis. Many older people are unaware of losses in peripheral vision and central acuity.

Visual acuity information pertaining to the ability to function in the environment can be gathered by observing the client walking, shaking hands, and completing forms. The client can be asked by the care manager to read a headline and a sentence from the newspaper. Ability to read both denotes normal visual acuity. Ability to read only the headline signifies moderate impairment, and inability to read either indicates severe impairment.[6(p186)]

Vision loss can affect a person's ability to perform many ADLs and IADLs. Older persons with vision loss may have problems with ambulation because they do not see obstacles in their path or changes in the ground surfaces outside; problems with dressing because they do not see that their clothes are soiled or do not match; problems with feeding because they do not see the food clearly on their plate; problems with the telephone because they don't see the numbers; problems with food preparation because they can't read directions; problems with transportation because of the inability to drive; problems with medication use because they can't identify the pills or see that they have dropped them on the floor; problems with finances because they can't see to write checks. The list of potential problems can go on and on.

To begin, the care manager should ask whether the person wears glasses and ascertain that the glasses are being worn, especially in a nursing home or assisted living facility where the glasses may be kept in a drawer. Next, the care manager should know when the last ophthalmology exam was performed. Frequently, older persons forget to have their eyes examined, especially if they perceive that they are seeing well enough. However, checks for glaucoma and other eye disease should be done annually. Other clients may require a referral to a low vision center that can offer adaptations, such as specialty magnifiers, to improve

vision.[25] In addition, the care manager can recommend changes in the home to prevent falls such as applying brightly colored tape on the last step, using color contrast when the floor surface changes, or improving contrast in the environment such as not using a red chair on a red carpet.[23] Improved lighting and removing clutter also reduce the risk of falls, which can lead to nursing home placement. In addition, large clocks, calendars, and telephone dials can improve independence in function. An excellent source for strategies on dealing with vision loss is The Lighthouse (1-800-829-0500), which also provides a Web site for purchasing products that improve independence.

■ SLEEP

Lack of sleep can have a definite impact on clients' quality of life and their ability to participate in their ADLs and IADLs. Thus, part of every care manager's assessment should include questions about the client's sleep pattern, such as, "What time do you fall asleep at night?" "Do you get up in the middle of the night?" "Do you fall back to sleep without problems?" "What time do you wake up in the morning?" If there are indications of problems with sleep, a follow-up question should be asked about whether the client naps during the day to see if this is why the person cannot sleep at night.

Oftentimes, a person with dementia can have marked sleep problems that include a reversal of sleeping and awake hours. This has a major effect on family caregivers and may result in placement into an assisted living or nursing home because the client may not have the funds to pay for a caregiver or home health aide who can be awake at night.

Inadequate amounts of sleep can affect the amount of energy the person has to dress in the morning, make breakfast, or go grocery shopping. It is important to attempt to find out the reasons for the poor sleep. Is arthritic pain keeping the person awake at night? Is the person drinking alcohol, which affects the ability to stay awake, or caffeinated soft drinks, which may impair sleep? Would increased exercise during the day improve sleep at night? Is the person depressed? Is the person getting up to toilet too frequently because of a urological problem that can be improved with medication? Is the person taking medications that have side effects that disturb sleep such as cause nightmares or leg movements?[23] For clients in a facility, the problem may be staff checkups at night or early in the morning that may awaken them. Attempts to address the root of the problem are important before prescribing medications for sleep that may then have the added problematic effect of increasing the risk of falls or causing oversedation in the morning. The care manager may consider having an evaluation at a sleep center conducted, which can diagnose problems such as sleep apnea. Changes in bedtime routine such as taking a bath, drinking warm milk, having a snack, listening to soothing music, or removing the television from the bedroom may have a positive effect on the ability to fall and stay asleep.

■ HOME ENVIRONMENT ASSESSMENT[6(PP196–200)]

One-fifth of all households are maintained by a person or persons aged 65 and over. Many older persons choose to live alone if health and finances permit. With advancing age, solitary living increases. In 1990, 47% of those aged 85 and over lived alone. Forty-five percent of those over 85 years are projected to be living alone by 2020. The majority of those over 75 years living alone are women.[26]

The living situations of this group are diverse. Older persons are more vulnerable to the problems of inadequate, unsafe housing as a result of other problems such as poverty, lack of social support, reduced physical reserves or disabilities, and cognitive impairment. The three most common hous-ing-related problems of older persons are adequacy of housing for the individual's needs, suitability of the neighborhood, and cost.[5] The majority of older persons own their own homes, but the homes may not be adequate or in good repair. In a study done in 1979, it was found that 53% of homes owned by older persons were built 40 or more years earlier.[27] These homes are more likely to have physical defects because of age than do the homes lived in by younger persons. Some of these defects, such as inadequate insulation, may actually increase the costs of day-to-day living for older persons, who often live on fixed incomes.

Other vital components of the home (e.g., wiring, roofing) may need repairs and upgrades that the older person cannot afford. As a result of the factors listed earlier and the reluctance of some older persons to consider making any changes to accommodate physical disabilities, such as the installation of grab bars in bathrooms, relocation to a downstairs area for sleeping, and the addition of ramps for safe entry and exit, some older persons are living in unsafe conditions. This group is at increased risk for falls and fractures and the institutionalization that frequently follows such events.

It is very important and necessary to perform a home assessment as part of the geriatric assessment process. The assessment should include the evaluation of safety factors (e.g., functioning smoke alarms, adequate wiring) and how effectively the older person is able to function within the floor plan and room arrangement of his or her home. While the home might be safe for a person without disabilities or cognitive impairments, if there are features (e.g., a second story, sunken rooms or hallways, tiny bathrooms) that are obstacles or potential dangers to a person needing assistive devices or forgetful of steps, that home is not safe for that person. Observation of the client as he or she performs ADLs is invaluable for assessment of the client's home safety and environmental needs as well as functional abilities.

Using a checklist is a time-efficient and comprehensive method for ascertaining the safety of a home. The Home Safety Checklist (Exhibit 4-6) is one tool that can be used to identify fall hazards in the home.[28] Its detailed questions provide some education to the older person in practices that can be initiated to minimize the likelihood of falling. As part of the assessment, caregivers can be educated to be alert for hazards and to evaluate the need for added safety features (e.g., alarms on outside doors, grab bars, raised toilet seats) that the older person may need as his or her condition progresses.

Once safety hazards have been identified and necessary changes have been listed and explained to the client, the GCM has to make sure that changes will be made by addressing hazards as problems in the care plan and writing an intervention for their solution. Often, older persons are unable or unwilling to make changes. Suggested changes should be addressed with the older person, and every attempt should be made to get the person to agree and plan for the prompt implementation needed. If the older person resists, family or other support persons should be notified of the risk to the older person in remaining in the unchanged environment. These persons often can influence the older person and assist with the practical matters of implementation of changes.

■ CONCLUSION

As noted earlier, the evaluation of an older person's functional status is key to helping that person maintain his or her autonomy and quality of life. Functional abilities are of paramount importance to overall health, well-being, and potential need for services. The functional assessment helps set priorities around which the available medical, social, and economic resources can be rallied. Once the functional assessment along with the psychosocial and cognitive assessments (see Chapter 3) are completed, the care manager can develop a plan of care (see Chapter 5).

Exhibit 4-6   Consumer Product Safety Commission Safety for Older Consumers Home Safety Checklist

Each year, many older Americans are injured in and around their homes. The U.S. Consumer Product Safety Commission (CPSC) estimates that in 1981, over 622,000 people over age 65 were treated in hospital emergency rooms for injuries associated with products they live with and use every day.

CPSC believes that many of these injuries result from hazards that are easy to overlook, but also easy to fix. By spotting these hazards and taking some simple steps to correct them, many injuries might be prevented.

Use this checklist to spot possible safety problems that may be present in your home. Check YES or NO to answer each question. Then go back over the list and take action to correct those items that may need attention.

Keep this checklist as a reminder of safe practices, and use it periodically to re-check your home.

This checklist is organized by areas in the home. However, there are some potential hazards that need to be checked in more than just one area of your home.

These are highlighted at the beginning of the checklist, and short reminders are included in each other section of the checklist.

Exhibit 4–6   Consumer Product Safety Commission Safety for Older Consumers Home Safety Checklist (continued)

ALL AREAS OF THE HOME

In all areas of your home, check all electrical and telephone cords; rugs, runners, and mats; telephone areas; smoke detectors; electrical outlets and switches; light bulbs; space heaters; wood-burning stoves; and your emergency exit plan.

CHECK ALL CORDS

QUESTION: Are lamp, extension, and telephone cords placed out of the flow of traffic?
YES ＿＿   NO ＿＿

RECOMMENDATION: Cords stretched across walkways may cause someone to trip.
- Arrange furniture so that outlets are available for lamps and appliances without the use of extension cords.
- If you must use an extension cord, place it on the floor against a wall where people can not trip over it.
- Move the phone so that telephone cords will not lie where people walk.

QUESTION: Are cords out from beneath furniture and rugs or carpeting?
YES ＿＿   NO ＿＿

RECOMMENDATION: Furniture resting on cords can damage them, creating fire and shock hazards. Electric cords that run under carpeting may cause a fire.
- Remove cords from under furniture or carpeting.
- Replace damaged or frayed cords.

QUESTION: Are cords attached to the walls, baseboards, etc., with nails or staples?
YES ＿＿   NO ＿＿

Nails or staples can damage cords, presenting fire and shock hazards.
- Remove nails, staples, etc.
- Check wiring for damage.
- Use tape to attach cords to walls or floors.

QUESTION: Are electrical cords in good condition, not frayed or cracked?
YES ＿＿   NO ＿＿

Damaged cords may cause a shock or fire.
- Replace frayed or cracked cords.

QUESTION: Do extension cords carry more than their proper load, as indicated by the ratings labeled on the cord and the appliance?
YES ＿＿   NO ＿＿

Overloaded extension cords may cause fires. Standard 18 gauge extension cords can carry 1250 watts.
- If the rating on the cord is exceeded because of the power requirements of one or more appliances being used on the cord, change the cord to a higher rated one or unplug some appliances.
- If an extension cord is needed, use one having a sufficient amp or wattage rating.

continues

Exhibit 4–6 Consumer Product Safety Commission Safety for Older Consumers Home Safety Checklist (continued)

CHECK ALL RUGS, RUNNERS, AND MATS

QUESTION: Are all small rugs and runners slip-resistant?
YES ____ NO ____

CPSC estimates that in 1982, over 2,500 people 65 and over were treated in hospital emergency rooms for injuries that resulted from tripping over rugs and runners. Falls are also the most common cause of fatal injury for older people.
- Remove rugs and runners that tend to slide.
- Apply double-faced adhesive carpet tape or rubber matting to the backs of rugs and runners.
- Purchase rugs with slip-resistant backing.
- Check rugs and mats periodically to see if backing needs to be replaced.
- Place rubber matting under rugs. (Rubber matting that can be cut to size is available.)
- Purchase new rugs with slip-resistant backing.

NOTE: Over time, adhesive on tape can wear away. Rugs with slip-resistant backing also become less effective as they are washed. Periodically, check rugs and mats to see if new tape or backing is needed.

QUESTION: Are emergency numbers posted on or near the telephone?
YES ____ NO ____

RECOMMENDATION: In case of emergency, telephone numbers for the Police, Fire Department, and local Poison Control Center, along with a neighbor's number, should be readily available.
- Write the numbers in large print and tape them to the phone, or place them near the phone where they can be seen easily.

QUESTION: Do you have access to a telephone if you fall (or experience some other emergency which prevents you from standing and reaching a wall phone)?
YES ____ NO ____
- Have at least one telephone located where it would be accessible in the event of an accident that leaves you unable to stand.

CHECK SMOKE DETECTORS

QUESTION: Are smoke detectors properly located?
YES ____ NO ____

RECOMMENDATION: At least one smoke detector should be placed on every floor of your home.
- Read the instructions that come with the smoke detector for advice on the best place to install it.
- Make sure detectors are placed near bedrooms, either on the ceiling or 6-12 inches below the ceiling on the wall.
- Locate smoke detectors away from air vents.

QUESTION: Do you have properly working smoke detectors?
YES ____ NO ____

RECOMMENDATION: Many home fire injuries and deaths are caused by smoke and toxic gases, rather than the fire itself. Smoke detectors provide an early warning and can wake you in the event of a fire.

Exhibit 4–6   Consumer Product Safety Commission Safety for Older Consumers
Home Safety Checklist (continued)

- Purchase a smoke detector if you do not have one.
- Check and replace batteries and bulbs according to the manufacturer's instructions.
- Vacuum the grillwork of your smoke detector.
- Replace any smoke detectors that cannot be repaired.

NOTE: Some fire departments or local governments will provide assistance in acquiring or installing smoke detectors.

CHECK ELECTRICAL OUTLETS AND SWITCHES

QUESTION: Are any outlets and switches unusually warm or hot to the touch?
    YES ____   NO ____

Unusually warm or hot outlets or switches may indicate that an unsafe wiring condition exists.
- Unplug cords from outlets and do not use the switches.
- Have an electrician check the wiring as soon as possible.

QUESTION: Do all outlets and switches have cover plates, so that no wiring is exposed?
    YES ____   NO ____

RECOMMENDATION: Exposed wiring presents a shock hazard.
- Add a cover plate.

QUESTION: Are light bulbs the appropriate size and type for the lamp or fixture?
    YES ____   NO ____

RECOMMENDATION: A bulb of too high wattage or the wrong type may lead to fire through overheating. Ceiling fixtures, recessed lights, and "hooded" lamps will trap heat.
- Replace with a bulb of the correct type and wattage. (If you do not know the correct wattage, use a bulb no larger than 60 watts.)

CHECK SPACE HEATERS

QUESTION: Are heaters that come with a 3-prong plug being used in a 3-hole outlet or with a properly attached adapter?
    YES ____   NO ____

RECOMMENDATION: The grounding feature provided by a 3-hole receptacle or an adapter for a 2-hole receptacle is a safety feature designed to lessen the risk of shock.
- Never defeat the grounding feature.
- If you do not have a 3-hole outlet, use an adapter to connect the heater's 3-prong plug. Make sure the adapter ground wire or tab is attached to the outlet.

QUESTION: Are small stoves and heaters placed where they cannot be knocked over, and away from furnishings and flammable materials, such as curtains or rugs?
    YES ____   NO ____

RECOMMENDATION: Heaters can cause fires or serious burns if they cause you to trip or if they are knocked over.
- Relocate heaters away from passageways and flammable materials such as curtains, rugs, furniture, etc.

continues

Exhibit 4–6 Consumer Product Safety Commission Safety for Older Consumers Home Safety Checklist (continued)

QUESTION: If your home has space heating equipment, such as a kerosene heater, a gas heater, or an LP gas heater, do you understand the installation and operating instructions thoroughly?
YES ____ NO ____

RECOMMENDATION: Unvented heaters should be used with room doors open or window slightly open to provide ventilation. The correct fuel, as recommended by the manufacturer, should always be used. Vented heaters should have proper venting, and the venting system should be checked frequently. Improper venting is the most frequent cause of carbon monoxide poisoning, and older consumers are at special risk.
- Review the installation and operating instructions.
- Call your local fire department if you have additional questions.

CHECK WOODBURNING HEATING EQUIPMENT

QUESTION: Is woodburning equipment installed properly?
YES ____ NO ____

RECOMMENDATION: Woodburning stoves should be installed by a qualified person according to local building codes.
- Local building code officials or fire marshals can provide requirements and recommendations for installation.

NOTE: Some insurance companies will not cover fire losses if wood stoves are not installed according to local codes.

CHECK THE EMERGENCY EXIT PLAN

QUESTION: Do you have an emergency exit plan and an alternate emergency exit plan in case of a fire?
YES ____ NO ____

RECOMMENDATION: Once a fire starts, it spreads rapidly. Since you may not have much time to get out and there may be a lot of confusion, it is important that everyone knows what to do.
- Develop an emergency exit plan.
- Choose a meeting place outside your home so you can be sure that everyone is accounted for.
- Practice the plan from time to time to make sure everyone is capable of escape quickly and safely.

Remember periodically to re-check your home.

KITCHEN

In the kitchen, check the range area, all electrical cords, lighting, the stool, all throw rugs and mats, and the telephone area.

CHECK THE RANGE AREA

QUESTION: Are towels, curtains, and other things that might catch fire located away from the range?
YES ____ NO ____

Exhibit 4–6   Consumer Product Safety Commission Safety for Older Consumers Home Safety Checklist (continued)

RECOMMENDATION: Placing or storing non-cooking equipment like potholders, dish towels, or plastic utensils on or near the range may result in fires or burns.
- Store flammable and combustible items away from range and oven.
- Remove any towels hanging on oven handles. If towels hang close to a burner, change the location of the towel rack.
- If necessary, shorten or remove curtains that could brush against heat sources.

QUESTION: Do you wear clothing with short or close-fitting sleeves while you are cooking?
YES ____   NO ____

RECOMMENDATION: CPSC estimates that 70% of all people who die from clothing fires are over 65 years of age. Long sleeves are more likely to catch fire than are short sleeves. Long sleeves are also more apt to catch on pot handles, overturning pots and pans and causing scalds.
- Roll back long, loose sleeves or fasten them with pins or elastic bands while you are cooking.

QUESTION: Are kitchen ventilation systems or range exhausts functioning properly and are they in use while you are cooking?
YES ____   NO ____

RECOMMENDATION: Indoor air pollutants may accumulate to unhealthful levels in a kitchen where gas or kerosene-fire appliances are in use.
- Use ventilation systems or open windows to clear air of vapors and smoke.

QUESTION: Are all extension cords and appliance cords located away from the sink or range areas?
YES ____   NO ____

RECOMMENDATION: Electrical appliances and power cords can cause shock or electrocution if they come in contact with water. Cords can also be damaged by excess heat.
- Move cords and appliances away from sink areas and hot surfaces.
- Move appliances closer to wall outlets or to different outlets so you won't need extension cords.
- If extension cords must be used, install wiring guides so that cords will not hang near sink, range, or working areas.
- Consider adding new outlets for convenience and safety; ask your electrician to install outlets equipped with ground fault circuit interrupters (GFCIs) to protect against electric shock. A GFCI is a shock-protection device that will detect electrical fault and shut off electricity before serious injury or death occurs.

For more information on cords, refer to the beginning of the checklist (pages 1 and 2).

QUESTION: Does good, even lighting exist over the stove, sink, and countertop work areas, especially where food is sliced or cut?
YES ____   NO ____

RECOMMENDATION: Low lighting and glare can contribute to burns or cuts. Improve lighting by:
- Opening curtains and blinds (unless this causes too much glare).
- Using the maximum wattage bulb allowed by the fixture. (If you do not know the correct wattage for the fixture, use a bulb no larger than 60 watts.)
- Reducing glare by using frosted bulbs, indirect lighting, shades or globes on light fixtures, or partially closing the blinds or curtains.
- Installing additional light fixtures, e.g., under cabinet/over countertop lighting.

(Make sure that the bulbs you use are the right type and wattage for the light fixture.)

continues

Exhibit 4–6   Consumer Product Safety Commission Safety for Older Consumers Home Safety Checklist (continued)

QUESTION: Do you have a step stool which is stable and in good repair?
  YES ____   NO ____

RECOMMENDATION: Standing on chairs, boxes, or other makeshift items to reach high shelves can result in falls. CPSC estimates that in 1982, 1500 people over 65 were treated in hospital emergency rooms when they fell from chairs on which they were standing.
  • If you don't have a step stool, consider buying one. Choose one with a handrail that you can hold onto while standing on the top step.
  • Before climbing on any step stool, make sure it is fully opened and stable.
  • Tighten screws and braces on the step stool.
  • Discard step stools with broken parts.

Remember: Check all of the product areas mentioned at the beginning of the checklist.

LIVING ROOM/FAMILY ROOM

In the living room/family room, check all rugs and runners, electrical and telephone cords, lighting, the fireplace and chimney, the telephone area, and all passageways.

QUESTION: Are chimneys clear from accumulations of leaves, and other debris that can clog them?
  YES ____   NO ____

RECOMMENDATION: A clogged chimney can cause a poorly-burning fire to result in poisonous fumes and smoke coming back into the house.
  • Do not use the chimney until the blockage has been removed.
  • Have the chimney checked and cleaned by a registered or licensed professional.

QUESTION: Has the chimney been cleaned within the past year?
  YES ____   NO ____

RECOMMENDATION: Burning wood can cause a buildup of a tarry substance (creosote) inside the chimney. This material can ignite and result in a serious chimney fire.
  • Have the chimney checked and cleaned by a registered or licensed professional.

CHECK THE TELEPHONE AREA

For information on the telephone area, refer to the beginning of the checklist.

CHECK PASSAGEWAYS

QUESTION: Are hallways, passageways between rooms, and other heavy traffic areas well lit?
  YES ____   NO ____

RECOMMENDATION: Shadowed or dark areas can hide tripping hazards.
  • Use the maximum wattage bulb allowed by the fixture. (If you do not know the correct wattage, use a bulb no larger than 60 watts.)
  • Install night lights.
  • Reduce glare by using frosted bulbs, indirect lighting, shades or globes on light fixtures, or partially closing blinds or curtains.
  • Consider using additional lamps or light fixtures. Make sure that the bulbs you use are the right type and wattage for the light fixture.

Exhibit 4–6   Consumer Product Safety Commission Safety for Older Consumers Home Safety Checklist (continued)

QUESTION: Are exits and passageways kept clear?
  YES ____   NO ____

Furniture, boxes, or other items could be an obstruction or tripping hazard, especially in the event of an emergency or fire.
  • Rearrange furniture to open passageways and walkways.
  • Remove boxes and clutter.

Remember: Check all of the product areas mentioned at the beginning of the checklist.

BATHROOM

In the bathroom, check bathtub and shower areas, water temperature, rugs and mats, lighting, small electrical appliances, and storage areas for medications.

CHECK BATHTUB AND SHOWER AREAS

QUESTION: Are bathtubs and showers equipped with non-skid mats, abrasive strips, or surfaces that are not slippery?
  YES ____   NO ____

RECOMMENDATION: Wet soapy tile or porcelain surfaces are especially slippery and may contribute to falls.
  • Apply textured strips or appliques on the floors of tubs and showers.
  • Use non-skid mats in the tub and shower, and on the bathroom floor.

QUESTION: Do bathtubs and showers have at least one (preferably two) grab bars?
  YES ____   NO ____

RECOMMENDATION: Grab bars can help you get into and out of your tub or shower, and can help prevent falls.
  • Check existing bars for strength and stability, and repair if necessary.
  • Attach grab bars, through the tile, to structural supports in the wall, or install bars specifically designed to attach to the sides of the bathtub. If you are not sure how it is done, get someone who is qualified to assist you.

QUESTION: Is the temperature 120 degrees or lower?
  YES ____   NO ____

Water temperature above 120 degrees can cause tap water scalds.
  • Lower the setting on your hot water heater to "Low" or 120 degrees. If you are unfamiliar with the controls of your water heater, ask a qualified person to adjust them for you. If your hot water system is controlled by the landlord, ask the landlord to consider lowering the setting.

NOTE: If the water heater does not have a temperature setting, you can use a thermometer to check the temperature of the water at the tap.
  • Always check water temperature by hand before entering bath or shower.
  • Taking baths, rather than showers, reduces the risk of a scald from suddenly changing water temperatures.

continues

Exhibit 4–6 Consumer Product Safety Commission Safety for Older Consumers Home Safety Checklist (continued)

CHECK LIGHTING

QUESTION: Is a light switch located near the entrance to the bathroom?
YES ⎯⎯ NO ⎯⎯

RECOMMENDATION: A light switch near the door will prevent you from walking through a dark area.
- Install a night light. Inexpensive lights that plug into outlets are available.
- Consider replacing the existing switch with a "glow switch" that can be seen in the dark.

CHECK SMALL ELECTRICAL APPLIANCES

QUESTION: Are small electrical appliances such as hair dryers, shavers, curling irons, etc., unplugged when not in use?
YES ⎯⎯ NO ⎯⎯

RECOMMENDATION: Even an appliance that is not turned on, such as a hairdryer, can be potentially hazardous if it is left plugged in. If it falls into water in a sink or bathtub while plugged in, it could cause a lethal shock.
- Unplug all small appliances when not in use.
- Never reach into water to retrieve an appliance that has fallen in without being sure the appliance is unplugged.
- Install a GFCI in your bathroom outlet to protect against electric shock.

CHECK MEDICATIONS

QUESTION: Are all medicines stored in the containers that they came in and are they clearly marked?
YES ⎯⎯ NO ⎯⎯

RECOMMENDATION: Medications that are not clearly and accurately labeled can be easily mixed up. Taking the wrong medicine or missing a dosage of medicine you need can be dangerous.
- Be sure that all containers are clearly marked with the contents, doctor's instructions, expiration date, and patient's name.
- Dispose of outdated medicines properly.
- Request non-child-resistant closures from your pharmacist only when you cannot use child-resistant closures.

NOTE: Many poisonings occur when children visiting grandparents go through the medicine cabinet or grandmother's purse. In homes where grandchildren or other youngsters are frequent visitors, medicines should be purchased in containers with child-resistant caps, and the caps properly closed after each use. Store medicines beyond the reach of children.

Remember: Check all of the product areas mentioned at the beginning of the checklist.

BEDROOMS

In the bedroom, check all rugs and runners, electrical and telephone cords, and areas around beds.

Exhibit 4–6   Consumer Product Safety Commission Safety for Older Consumers
Home Safety Checklist (continued)

CHECK AREAS AROUND BEDS

QUESTION: Are lamps or light switches within reach of each bed?
    YES ____   NO ____

RECOMMENDATION: Lamps or switches located close to each bed will enable people getting
up at night to see where they are going.
  • Rearrange furniture closer to switches or move lamps closer to beds.
  • Install night lights.

QUESTION: Are ash trays, smoking materials, or other fire sources (heaters, hot plates,
teapots, etc.) located away from beds or bedding?
    YES ____   NO ____

RECOMMENDATION: Burns are a leading cause of accidental death among seniors. Smoking
in bed is a major contributor to this problem. Among mattress and bedding fire related deaths
in a recent year, 42% were to persons 65 or older.
  • Remove sources of heat or flame from areas around beds.
  • Don't smoke in bed.

QUESTION: Is anything covering your electric blanket when in use?
    YES ____   NO ____

RECOMMENDATION: "Tucking in" electric blankets, or placing additional coverings on top of
them can cause excessive heat buildup that can start a fire.

QUESTION: Do you avoid "tucking in" the sides or ends of your electric blanket?
    YES ____   NO ____

RECOMMENDATION:
  • Use electric blankets according to the manufacturer's instructions.
  • Don't allow anything on top of the blanket while it is in use. (This includes other blan-
    kets or comforters, even pets sleeping on top of the blanket.)
  • Don't set electric blankets so high that they could burn someone who falls asleep while
    they are on.

QUESTION: Do you ever go to sleep with a heating pad that is turned on?
    YES ____   NO ____

RECOMMENDATION: Never go to sleep with a heating pad if it is turned on because it can
cause serious burns even at relatively low settings.

QUESTION: Is there a telephone close to your bed?
    YES ____   NO ____

RECOMMENDATION: In case of an emergency, it is important to be able to reach the telephone without getting out of bed.
Remember: Check all of the product areas mentioned at the beginning of the checklist.

BASEMENT/GARAGE/WORKSHOP/STORAGE AREAS

In the basement, garage, workshop, and storage areas, check lighting, fuse boxes or circuit
breakers, appliances and power tools, electrical cords, and flammable liquids.

continues

Exhibit 4–6   Consumer Product Safety Commission Safety for Older Consumers Home Safety Checklist (continued)

CHECK LIGHTING

QUESTION: Are work areas, especially areas where power tools are used, well lit?
    YES _____   NO _____

RECOMMENDATION: Power tools were involved in over 5,200 injuries treated in hospital emergency rooms to people 65 and over in 1982. Three-fourths of these were finger injuries. Good lighting can reduce the chance that you will accidentally cut your finger.
    • Either install additional light, or avoid working with power tools in the area.

QUESTION: Can you turn on the lights without first having to walk through a dark area?
    YES _____   NO _____

RECOMMENDATION: Basement, garages, and storage areas can contain many tripping hazards and sharp or pointed tools that can make a fall even more hazardous.
    • Keep an operating flashlight handy.
    • Have an electrician install switches at each entrance to a dark area.

CHECK THE FUSE BOX OR CIRCUIT BREAKERS

QUESTION: If fuses are used, are they the correct size for the circuit?
    YES _____   NO _____

RECOMMENDATION: Replacing a correct size fuse with a larger size fuse can present a serious fire hazard. If the fuse in the box is rated higher than that intended for the circuit, excessive current will be allowed to flow and possibly overload the outlet and house wiring to the point that a fire can begin.
    • Be certain that correct-size fuses are used. (If you do not know the correct sizes, consider having an electrician identify and label the sizes to be used.)
NOTE: If all, or nearly all, fuses used are 30-amp fuses, there is a chance that some of the fuses are rated too high for the circuit.

CHECK APPLIANCES AND POWER TOOLS

QUESTION: Are power tools equipped with a 3-prong plug or marked to show that they are double insulated?
    YES _____   NO _____

RECOMMENDATION: These safety features reduce the risk of an electric shock.
    • Use a properly connected 3-prong adapter for connecting a 3-prong plug to a 2-hole receptacle.
    • Consider replacing old tools that have neither a 3-prong plug nor are double insulated.

QUESTION: Are power tools guards in place?
    YES _____   NO _____

RECOMMENDATION: Power tools used with guards removed pose a serious risk of injury from sharp edges or moving parts.
    • Replace guards that have been removed from power tools.

Exhibit 4–6   Consumer Product Safety Commission Safety for Older Consumers Home Safety Checklist (continued)

QUESTION: Has the grounding feature on any 3-prong plug been defeated by removal of the grounding pin or by improperly using an adapter?

YES ____   NO ____

RECOMMENDATION: Improperly grounded appliances can lead to electric shock.

• Check with your service person or an electrician if you are in doubt.

CHECK FLAMMABLE AND VOLATILE LIQUIDS

QUESTION: Are containers of volatile liquids tightly capped?

YES ____   NO ____

RECOMMENDATION: If not tightly closed, vapors may escape that may be toxic when inhaled.

• Check containers periodically to make sure they are tightly closed.

NOTE: CPSC has reports of several cases in which gasoline, stored as much as 10 feet from a gas water heater, exploded. Many people are unaware that gas fumes can travel that far.

QUESTION: Are gasoline, paints, solvents, or other products that give off vapors or fumes stored away from ignition sources?

YES ____   NO ____

RECOMMENDATION: Gasoline, kerosene, and other flammable liquids should be stored out of living areas in properly labeled, non-glass safety containers.

• Remove these products from the areas near heat or flame such as heaters, furnaces, water heaters, ranges, and other gas appliances.

STAIRS

For all stairways, check lighting, handrails, and the condition of the steps and coverings.

CHECK LIGHTING

QUESTION: Are stairs well lighted?

YES ____   NO ____

RECOMMENDATION: Stairs should be lighted so that each step, particularly the step edges, can be clearly seen while going up and down stairs. The lighting should not produce glare or shadows along the stairway.

• Use the maximum wattage bulb allowed by the light fixture. (If you do not know the correct wattage, use a bulb no larger than 60 watts.)
• Reduce glare by using frosted bulbs, indirect lighting, shades or globes on light fixtures, or partially closing blinds and curtains.
• Have a qualified person add additional light fixtures. Make sure that the bulbs you use are the right type and wattage for the light fixture.

QUESTION: Are light switches located at both the top and bottom of the stairs.

YES ____   NO ____

RECOMMENDATION: Even if you are very familiar with the stairs, lighting is an important factor in preventing falls. You should be able to turn on the lights before you use the stairway from either end.

continues

Exhibit 4–6   Consumer Product Safety Commission Safety for Older Consumers Home Safety Checklist (continued)

- If no other light is available, keep an operating flashlight in a convenient location at the top and bottom of the stairs.
- Install night lights at nearby outlets.
- Consider installing switches at the top and bottom of the stairs.

QUESTION: Do the steps allow secure footing?
     YES ____   NO ____

RECOMMENDATION: Worn treads or worn or loose carpeting can lead to insecure footing, resulting in slips or falls.
- Try to avoid wearing only socks or smooth-soled shoes or slippers when using stairs.
- Make certain the carpet is firmly attached to the steps all along the stairs.
- Consider refinishing or replacing worn treads, or replacing worn carpeting.
- Paint outside steps with paint that has a rough texture, or use abrasive strips.

QUESTION: Are steps even and of the same size and height?
     YES ____   NO ____

RECOMMENDATION: Even a small difference in step surfaces or riser heights can lead to falls.
- Mark any steps that are especially narrow or have risers that are higher or lower than the others. Be especially careful of these steps when using the stairs.

QUESTION: Are the coverings on the steps in good condition?
     YES ____   NO ____

RECOMMENDATION: Worn or torn coverings or nails sticking out from coverings could snag your foot or cause you to trip.
- Repair coverings.
- Remove coverings.
- Replace coverings.

QUESTION: Can you clearly see the edges of the steps?
     YES ____   NO ____

RECOMMENDATION: Falls may occur if the edges of the steps are blurred or hard to see.
- Paint edges of outdoor steps white to see them better at night.
- Add extra lighting.
- If you plan to carpet your stairs, avoid deep pile carpeting or patterned or dark-colored carpeting that can make it difficult to see the edges of the steps clearly.

QUESTION: Is anything stored on the stairway, even temporarily?
     YES ____   NO ____

RECOMMENDATION: People can trip over objects left on stairs, particularly in the event of an emergency or fire.
- Remove all objects from the stairway.

REMEMBER PERIODICALLY TO RE-CHECK YOUR HOME.

Source: Consumer Product Safety Commission. *Safety for Older Consumers Home Safety Checklist.* CPSC Document #701. Available at: http://www.cpsc.gov/cpscpub/pubs/701.html. Accessed August 21, 2006.

■ NOTES

1. Kane RL, Ouslander JG, Abrass IB. *Essentials of Clinical Geriatrics*. New York: McGraw-Hill, Health Professions Division; 1999.

2. Newcomer R, Harrington C, Kane R. Implications of managed care for older persons. In: Katz P, Kane R, Mezey M, eds. *Emerging Systems in Long-Term Care*. New York: Springer Publishers; 1999:118-148.

3. Gallo J. *Handbook of Geriatric Assessment*. 3rd ed. Gaithersburg, MD: Aspen Publishers; 1999.

4. American Geriatrics Society. Comprehensive Geriatric Assessment Position Statement. October 1996. Available at: http://www.american geriatrics.org. Accessed March 15, 1999.

5. Fretwell M. Comprehensive functional assessment. In: Abrams W, Berkow R, eds. *The Merck Manual of Geriatrics*. Rathway, NJ: Merck & Co.; 1990:170-174.

6. Barber C. Geriatric assessment. In: Cress C, ed. *Handbook of Geriatric Care Management*. Gaithersburg, MD: Aspen Publishers; 2001:187-194.

7. Katz S, Downs T, Cash H. Progress in the development of the index of ADL. *Gerontologist*. 1970;10:20-30.

8. Mahoney F, Barthel D. Functional evaluation: the Barthel Index. *Md State Med J*. 1965;14:61-65.

9. Fillenbaum G, Smyer M. The development, validity and reliability of the OARS multidimensional functional assessment questionnaire. *J Gerontol*. 1981;36:428-434.

10. Moskowitz E, McCann C. Classification of disability in the chronically ill and aging. *J Chronic Dis*. 1957;5:342-346.

11. Morris J, Harues C, Murphy K. Designing the National Resident Assessment Instrument for Nursing Homes. *Gerontologist*. 1990;30:293-307.

12. Heeren T, Lagaay A, vonBeck W, Rooymans H, Hijman W. Reference values for the Mini-Mental State Examination in octo- and nonagenarians. *J Am Geriatr Soc*. 1990;38:1093-1096.

13. Tinetti M. Performance oriented assessment of mobility: problems in elderly patients. *J Am Geriatr Soc*. 1986;34:119-126.

14. Mathias S, Nayak U, Issacs B. Balance in elderly patients: the Get Up and Go Test. *Arch Phys Med Rehab*. 1986;67:387-389.

15. Resnick N, Wells T. Maintaining and restoring continence. In: Funk S, Tornquist M, Champagne M, Weise R, eds. *Key Aspects of Elder Care*. New York: Springer Publishers; 1992:135-154.

16. Tideiksaar R. *Falls in Older Persons, Prevention and Management*. 2nd ed. Baltimore, MD: Health Professions Press; 1998.

17. Davies G, Scully F. *Fall Prevention: Stay on Your Own Two Feet*. West Conshohocken, PA: Infinity Publishing; 2006.

18. Castle S, Opava-Rutter D. Practical fall risk assessment in older adults with multiple medical problems and/or chronic disease. *Geriatric Care Manage J*. Summer-Fall 2003;13(2):17-23.

19. Lawton M, Brody E. Assessment of older people: self-maintaining and instrumental activities of daily living. *Gerontologist*. 1969;9:179-186.

20. Pearson VI. Assessment of function in older adults. In: Kane R, Kane R, eds. *Assessing Older Persons*. New York: Oxford University Press; 2000:17-48.

21. Fillenbaum GG. Screening the elderly. A brief instrumental activities of daily living measure. *J Am Geriatr Soc*. 1985;33(10):698-706.

22. American Medical Association. Safety and the Older Driver, Physician's Guide to Assessing and Counseling Older Drivers. 2006. Available at: http://www.ama-assn.org. Accessed May 7, 2006.

23. Matteson M, McConnell E. *Gerontological Nursing*. Philadelphia: Saunders; 1988.

24. Weinstein BE. Hearing loss and hearing aides. *Geriatric Care Manage J*. Summer 2002;12(2):7.

25. Strand CH. Vision loss—a focus on function. *Geriatric Care Manage J*. Summer 2002;12(2):3.

26. National Safety Council and American Association of Retired Persons. *Falling—The Unexpected Trip*. Chicago, IL: National Safety Council and American Association of Retired Persons; 1982.

27. Campbell A, Converse P. *Quality of Life in America*. New York: Russell Sage; 1976.

28. U.S. Consumer Product Safety Commission, Safety for Older Consumers Home Safety Checklist. CPSC Document #701. Available at: http://www.cpsc.gov/cpscpub/pubs/701.html. Accessed August 21, 2006.

Chapter 5

Care Planning and Geriatric Assessment

Cathy Jo Cress and Carolyn Barber

■ INTRODUCTION

The process of geriatric assessment is like the method detectives use to solve a crime. Just as detectives meticulously sift through clues, leave no stone unturned, ensure all evidence is taken into account before reaching conclusions, so must geriatric care managers (GCMs). Like Sherlock Holmes, GCMs conducting a geriatric assessment must strive to make sure all facts have been gathered and examined, both individually and in combination with one another, before writing a report and developing a care plan. However, unlike Sherlock Holmes, GCMs often have to first meet a client because of an immediate crisis, and they sometimes have to begin to assist that client without being able to gather all of the information they might like.

Comprehensive geriatric assessment has been defined as a "multidisciplinary evaluation in which the multiple problems of older people are uncovered, described, and explained, if possible, and in which the resources and strengths of the person are catalogued, need for services assessed, and a coordinated care plan developed to focus on interventions of the person's problems."[1] Additionally, the resources and strengths of the older person must be ascertained and evaluated so that they can be part of the development of a care plan, in recognition of the uniqueness and individuality of that per-

son. Assessment of the impact of illnesses and the aging process on an older person's physical, emotional, spiritual, and social functioning is a critical component of the provision of appropriate health care. Doing comprehensive geriatric assessment and care planning is a challenge for GCMs.

The Comprehensive Geriatric Assessment Position Statement of the American Geriatrics Society includes the following statements: "Comprehensive geriatric assessment has demonstrated usefulness in improving the health status of frail, older patients. Therefore, elements of Comprehensive Geriatric Assessment should be incorporated into the acute and long-term care provided to these elderly individuals" and "Medicare and other insurers should recognize as a reimbursable service or procedure: (1) periodic assessment of patients and (2) the support services required for effective application on Comprehensive Geriatric Assessment."[2]

A comprehensive assessment is essential to provide the right services at the right time. Older people often have complex health problems with atypical presentations. Elders have cognitive and affective problems that make history taking difficult. They react strongly to medication and are frequently socially isolated and can be economically compromised. If a comprehensive assessment is not done, older people may be at risk for premature or inappropriate institutionalization. Problems often involve more than one domain of the assessment. Treatment of a medical problem or living condition can sometimes affect cognitive or functional status. On the other hand, the client's cognitive and functional status and values must often be taken into account before deciding how aggressively medical problems should be approached.

The geriatric assessment should be carried out by an experienced GCM. This person is usually either a registered nurse (RN) or human services professional such as a gerontologist or social worker. As more classes, certificates, and concentrations in geriatric care management evolve throughout the United States, GCMs can actually have specific educational backgrounds in geriatric care management. Many have passed a certification exam in geriatric care management. A team approach involving an RN and a social worker can be very effective, but a non-RN GCM using a functional assessment tool can gather both the health and psychosocial information needed for a comprehensive assessment.

The assessment process begins with a case-finding approach and employs screening instruments and techniques, unless this information is already available from the client's medical record. Based on the initial interview, more detailed assessments may be recommended. This may mean referrals to a number of professional disciplines, such as audiology, psychology, nutrition, physical therapy, occupational therapy, pharmacy, and speech therapy. The assessment should take account of the older person's physical and emotional health. It should reflect his or her ethnic and spiritual background and preferences, finances, and support systems so realistic plans for long-term care can be made if necessary. The older person's own goals and wishes should be taken into account in the planning as much as possible.

The initial assessment is also the GCM's first contact with the client and family. First impressions are important, so the GCM should present him- or herself in a professional manner by being on time, being well dressed, and being thorough. The GCM must be the quality professional the client and family want to work with on an ongoing basis. This assessment is also the basis for getting paid a fee, so making an excellent initial impression is essential if you want to do further work with the client and family.

■ GOALS OF A WRITTEN GERIATRIC ASSESSMENT

The GCM does a geriatric assessment to create a care plan, which proposes recommendations to repair the holes in the older client's personal safety net using the family system and the continuum of care. The recommendations suggest services at the right time for the right amount of money.

The first GCM goal of a written geriatric assessment is to convey in an organized and thorough manner the information gathered and recorded with the assessment tools, interviews, and observations. These pieces of information are all the clues. The second goal is to draw conclusions from that information or clues and present them in a persuasive manner. The final goal is for the GCM to prepare recommendations based on the conclusions. These conclusions are presented to the client, family, or third party who requested the assessment. Hopefully they are convincing enough that the family or third party will agree with those needed solutions to the documented problems. By preparing a thorough, well-reasoned geriatric care assessment, the GCM has begun the process of developing an ongoing relationship with that client and family.

■ ELEMENTS OF THE ASSESSMENT

The first step the GCM takes in a basic geriatric assessment is looking at the client's physical and mental health and social, spiritual, economic, functional, and environmental status. Much like Sherlock Holmes or his new sleuthing wife, Mary Russell, you observe the clients through the lens of a magnifying glass, which is the GCM's assessment tools.

You measure change in an assessment—change in the client's present problems; change in the client's present functioning; change in the support system that might necessitate need for different solutions. As an example of this process, consider a client we will call Mamie Nixon, who lives in Santa Cruz, California. Her son calls you and asks you to assess his Mom because she drove to the grocery store, got lost, and was picked up by the highway patrol, disoriented and confused. Mamie has actually had difficulty driving for 20 years, first ameliorated by eye-glasses and, then, 10 years later, she agreed not to drive at night. But now a new problem has developed. Her original vision problem is now complicated by mental confusion. A client could have a change in functional ability: she can't remember well enough to drive from home to the supermarket.

Mamie also experienced a change in appearance. She dressed appropriately a year ago, and now is always dressed in dirty, unmatched clothes. A year ago Mamie walked around unaided, and now she needs to use a cane. Twelve months ago she was mentally clear enough to execute a will, but now her mental status has declined to the point where she may not have the capacity to change her will. She could pay her bills a year ago but now can't. Twelve months ago she regularly attended the Live Oak Senior Center, but last month she stopped going to the classes in current affairs she has always loved. During the course of the geriatric care assessment, you discovered and reported all these changes in Mamie.

The next step is to recommend ways to repair the holes in Mamie's safety net: a secure way to shop, get to church, and attend to her activities of daily living (ADLs) such as bathing, grooming, and washing her clothes. In preparing your recommendations, you will consider her strengths and what resources she has to fill these holes. For example, Mamie's resources include her son Pete Nixon, the geriatric psychiatrist at Dominican Mental Health Center, the home care aides available through Senior Network Services, and adequate financial resources from Mamie's income and assets to pay for these services.

Physical Health

The first element of a geriatric assessment is a physical assessment that identifies specific diseases or symptoms for which curative, restorative, palliative, or preventive treatment may be available. Special attention is directed toward visual or hearing impairment, nutritional status, incontinence, and conditions that may contribute to falling or difficulty in ambulation. Of course, any actual physical examination should be done by a nurse practitioner or a physician. Gathering health information about the client and reporting it to the physician, through assessment tools, can be done by the GCM who has a background in gerontology, the health sciences, or social work or psychology.

Psychosocial Status

The GCM evaluates the cognitive, behavioral, and emotional status of a client. Identification of signs of dementia, delirium, and depression is particularly important. A range of assessment instruments is available for screening and differentiating among these conditions. Following screening, the care manager may refer clients for a thorough psychiatric or neurological consultation. (See Chapter 3 on dementia and Chapter 20 on depression and psychosocial issues.)

Caregiving and Ethnic, Social, Spiritual, and Economic Status

Identification of present and potential caregivers and assessment of their willingness, competence, and acceptability to the older person is determined through interviews with the client's family and the social network. An evaluation of caregiver stress and the support network of the client are also evaluated. (See Chapter 17 on the family and Chapter 15 on caregivers.) Assessment of the older person's cultural, ethnic, and spiritual values should also be included in a geriatric assessment. The older person's concept of what constitutes quality of life should be assessed. End-of-life decisions and verification of written advance directives should be included as well, although this information may not be appropriate to gather in an initial interview. (See Chapter 6 on ethnic asssessment, Chapter 14 on spiritual assessment, Chapter 17 on family assessment, Chapter 3 on psychosocial assessment, and Chapter 19 on quality of life.)

Economic resources also need to be evaluated because they are crucial for planning for the provision of personal care and the living arrangements of the client and can be a factor in compliance with medical treatment. (See Chapter 3 on psychosocial assessment.)

Functional Status

A functional assessment is a measure of the person's ability to perform adequately and safely basic ADLs, including bathing, dressing, toileting, transferring, and feeding. Instrumental activities of daily living (IADLs), such as meal preparation, shopping, housework, financial management, medication management, use of the telephone, and driving, are evaluated by direct observation in the home, interviews with the client and family, and administration of standardized questionnaires. (See Chapter 4 on functional assessment.)

Environment

Evaluation of the client's physical environment is essential. Home safety must be evaluated. Problem areas must be identified and corrected if the client is to remain in the home environment. (See Chapter 4 on functional assessment and Chapter 16 on Late Life Relocation.) Evaluating the physical environment in combination with an understanding of the client's ability to perform the ADLs enables the care manager to understand the level of care the client needs. This is the basis for recommending when a client should consider a move to another setting.

Goals of Geriatric Assessment

In 1987, the Consensus Development Conference on Geriatric Assessment Methods for Clinical Decision Making established the following goals of comprehensive geriatric assessment: (1) to improve diagnostic accuracy, (2) to guide the selection of interventions to restore or preserve health, (3) to recommend an optimal environment for care, (4) to predict outcomes, and (5) to monitor clinical change over time.[3] The effectiveness of geriatric assessment has been demonstrated most convincingly with clients in geriatric and rehabilitation units and inpatient geriatric units. Less evidence is available regarding home and ambulatory settings.[3] Outcomes demonstrated include improved diagnostic accuracy, prolonged survival, reduced medical care costs, reduced use of acute hospitals, and reduced use of nursing.

■ CARE PLAN

After the initial assessment information is gathered, a comprehensive list of the client's problems and interventions should be generated at a multidisciplinary team conference with other GCMs on staff. This list is called a *care plan*. If you practice alone, having an agreement with a more experienced GCM, mentor, or a consultant to review your care plans is a really good idea.

A care plan is a strategy to repair the holes in your clients' web or safety net. Your client is experiencing problems because the web of support or his or her own functioning has deficits or holes. The care plan suggests a way to repair those holes by recommending the right services at the right time for the right amount of money. Again, you are Charlotte, the crafty spider from *Charlotte's Web*, using the large continuum of care in your community to recommend ways to repair holes in the older person's personal web.

The care plan is also like a prescribed remedy. The GCM identifies each problem the client is experiencing in the problem section and gives an intervention for each problem in the intervention section of the care plan. You, the GCM, are like a health practitioner. You examine your patient—using your psychosocial and functional assessment tools plus any other needed assessments (spiritual, dementia, etc.). You then make a diagnosis based on your assessments—the problem list in the care plan. Then, you prescribe the solution to the client's problems—the interventions or solution in the care plan. (See Exhibit 5–1.)

How do you create a care plan or your professional opinion of what the family ought to do to solve its problems? You begin by gathering all of the data with your assessment tools: your functional assessment data (see Chapter 4 on functional assessment) and your psychosocial assessment data (see Chapter 3 on psychosocial assessment). You then add additional data you have gleaned from any specialized assessment you have done, such as depression, spiritual, or quality of life.

The next step is to sort through these data, like Holmes.

Exhibit 5–1 Care Plan

1. Examine the client = Assessment
2. Come up with a diagnosis = problems list
3. Prescribe the solution to the problems
   = Intervention list

   2 + 3 = Care Plan

This is where you sift through clues, leaving no stone upturned, to ensure that all evidence has been taken into account before reaching conclusions. You must examine the clues closely. Talk to each person in the formal or informal support system and make sure all evidence is taken into account. Everyone has a different version of what happened. Analyze the client's problems from all perspectives and then synthesize all the opinions into one truth, which will form your professional opinion. Collect all the data, and then look at each person's point of view to come up with your own professional GCM point of view.

As a GCM, you should start your care plan with the problem you were asked to solve initially. Why was your agency called in? For example, was the client very dirty and unable to shower alone when the out-of-town son visited? Start there. This becomes your first problem in your care plan. Always start with the initial presenting problem.

How do you find the remaining problems in the care plan? After addressing the first problem, continue by listing the client's functional problems. What are the deficits you discovered in your functional assessment? A few examples might be the following: unable to prepare meals, unable to walk without a cane, unable to bathe, in pain, poor diet.

Next, list problems you have found in the psychosocial assessments. Some examples are as follows: unable to handle finances, unable to drive to store because driver's license was taken away, unable to participate in activities as a result of depression.

Frequently, many older clients have similar deficits as they age. See Exhibit 5–2 for a sample problem list that lists problems older people often develop when they become more frail and vulnerable. Most care plans will include one or more of these problems, and it is good to incorporate this list into your assessment tools.

Exhibit 5-2   Sample Care Plan Problem Checklist

Below is a list of the most frequent problems older people experience. If these problems are not addressed by an assessment tool, keep this list handy to draw from when you create a care plan.

❑ Self-care deficit
❑ Impaired home management
❑ Alternation in nutrition
❑ Impaired mobility
❑ Knowledge deficit
❑ Alteration in bowel elimination
❑ Alteration in urinary elimination
❑ Impaired skin integrity
❑ Loneliness
❑ Depression
❑ Pain
❑ Caregiver burnout

■ INTERVENTIONS IN THE CARE PLAN

Where do you get the interventions or solutions for the problems listed in your care plan? In part, you take them from the continuum of care. In Chapter 17 on the family, GCM Anne Rosenthall wisely states, "Just as no man is an island—no GCM stands alone."

Every GCM must know a staggering array of other experts who make up the web of senior services in the community. These experts practice in areas to which GCM skills do not extend (attorneys, trust officers, moving companies, plumbers). It is the care manager's expert knowledge of the continuum of care in the community that is the heart of the care management role. As stated in the Chapter 1, a GCM is like Charlotte, the friendly spider. The GCM runs across the web of senior services (continuum of care), linking services, repairing gaps, spinning new solutions, and coordinating answers. You need to know how to locate all those services to implement your care plan and find interventions to the problems you have uncovered.

Finding Interventions for the Care Plan

How do you find this continuum? As a GCM, you should already have significant experience in this continuum before you open your GCM door for business. In Chapter 7, this is what is meant by your core competence to open a geriatric care management business. You need to know your community's continuum of care from day one.

However, because the web billows, expands, compresses, and changes constantly, you need the real Web to help you keep up. You can access most areas of the continuum of care and all its changes (new businesses, new senior services offered) through the World Wide Web and Internet. You can access your county's or Area Agency on Aging Web site, which will usually list all the current senior services available in your town. You can review your business plan and find all the sources you listed there such as the National Association of Elder Law Attorneys Web site for elder law attorneys. In 2006, most organizations serving seniors maintained a Web site. Of course, you should only recommend services that you know to be competent and able to solve the particular problem you are seeking to ameliorate. For example, if you recommend a local conservator or guardian, there should be an organization in your county of guardians with a Web site.

You can expand your knowledge beyond your local continuum of care nationally by using the Eldercare Locator, which is available at http://www.eldercare.gov.

Crafting Interventions

Interventions in a care plan to be placed in the home and followed by care providers are less complex at times than interventions in a written geriatric assessment sent to a judge.

The judge and attornies are not health care providers and may need less jargon-free interventions.

Once you know where to find the interventions for your care plan, tailor these interventions to the client. For example, consider another of Mamie Nixon's problems in her care plan—her self-care deficit, namely, that she is apparently unable to bathe without supervision. The intervention to this problem might be hiring a paid care provider to come for 2 hours, 3 days a week to bathe Mamie. Each intervention must have a clear plan. You must state in your intervention who will carry out the intervention, how it will be carried out, the number of times it will be carried out, and how you will measure that it was carried out.

Make Interventions Doable

In the example of recommending an aide to bathe Mamie 3 days a week, you could suggest that the family call a home care agency in the community that provides bonded care providers for 2-hour blocks of time. Also, someone has to carry out the intervention or you risk that it will not be done. Who will carry it out? Your intervention could specify that the family will locate care providers by calling three home care agencies as recommended by the GCM. But before you recommend this, check with the family and confirm they will do this. It may be that the family wants you to interview the care providers and recommend which one they should hire. So, remember to create a solution based on facts. This makes the solution doable.

Make Interventions Measurable

Your recommended interventions should be measurable. This means you should specify the number of times an intervention will be carried out. For example, the agency will send an aide 3 times a week, for 2 hours each time.

You need to show the family exactly how to measure whether the intervention was completed. For example the care provider might fill out and sign a charting page for his shift. This also provides the GCM who monitors the care of the older person a basis to review both status of the older person and whether the care provider was present. If the care provider has come only once a week, you know you need to follow up. If the family wants to monitor the care, this approach also tells them how to measure the care.

Make Interventions Understandable

Each intervention must be written in straightforward and objective language so that the person carrying out the plan can understand it. It is important to communicate clearly to families, who need jargon-free language. Unskilled caregivers, who may think in another language, need you to use simple, straightforward sentences. The care providers should read the care plan and understand it completely because they are the people who will carry it out in many cases.

Make Interventions with a Timeline

Your intervention should have measurable goals based on a timeline. For example, the problem of loneliness: Mrs. Virden recently lost her husband of 50 years, and she is not socializing and resists outside help. Intervention: The GCM will visit weekly for 1 month to help Mrs. Virden accept community services to relieve some of her loneliness and ongoing grief.

■ MULTIPLE INTERVENTIONS

The GCM can recommend more than one intervention to solve a single problem. For example, an additional intervention to assist Mrs. Virden could be as follows: Intervention: GCM will arrange a Friendly Visitor to visit

Mrs. Virden weekly for 6 months; and Intervention: GCM to call the Blessed Christian Church to ask whether a minister could visit Mrs. Virden weekly for a month and offer spiritual comfort and encouragement to attend church on Sundays after that month; and Intervention: GCM to encourage Mrs. Virden to attend weekly adult exercise class at local senior center within one month.

Because older clients often have chronic disease, the absence of disease or cure for problem or return to normal is rarely a goal. Mrs. Virden may not really fully recover from the death of her husband, but the GCM can fashion interventions that will help her better accept his death over time, and these interventions can be written in a way that you, the client, and her family can measure.

Care Plan Is Subject to Change

Everyone who follows the care plan must understand that it is subject to change. Mrs. Virden may start to attend her church on Sundays, make a male friend at the Blessed Christian Church, and decide to remarry, or she may refuse to accept the friendly visitor you have arranged.

Care Plan Needs to Be Acceptable: Dealing with Rejected Interventions

Sometimes the family or third party may not accept your intervention. For example, you discover that Mrs. C is pouring wine brought in by the cleaning lady down her gastrointestinal tube. Intervention: Trust officer is to replace the cleaning lady within 24 hours, and all alcohol is to be removed from the home by the GCM.

However, the GCM may find that a planned intervention cannot be carried out. For example, Mrs. C may call her attorney, who may insist that a geriatrician hired by the court has tested Mrs. C's competency and concluded that she is competent and has the

right to drink alcohol if she wishes. The GCM has developed an intervention that the client rejects and will not carry out. When care plans are rejected, the GCM may have to wait until the client or the family will accept the solution. If they do not, the GCM will have to accept the wishes of the legally competent client and family. If the GCM feels that not carrying out the solution will seriously endanger the client's health and safety, the GCM can report the situation to Adult Protective Services. The GCM should consult with Adult Protective Services and an attorney about mandatory reporting state laws.

Care Plan Needs to Be Affordable

The care plan must be something that the older person's assets and income can afford or that the family is willing to pay for. If your client has a self-care deficit, cannot bathe or groom without assistance, and requires ongoing oversight to remain safely in her home, you may recommend 24-hour care. However, if the client cannot afford 24-hour care, you must offer other, cost-effective solutions, such as having the client move in with a family member. This is why a financial assessment is needed before you can prepare your care plan. Financial resources should be investigated on the psychosocial intake form.

Consider this example: Mrs. Scott is unable to get to Happy Trails assisted living dining room every night. Solution: Daughter will hire a care provider from a home health agency to take Mrs. Scott to the dining room 7 nights a week.

However, the family says they cannot afford a care provider. You may have to ask the assisted living facility if it provides a free service to transport clients or ask a neighbor in the assisted living facility to escort Mrs. Scott to the dining room. Finding an affordable solution is one of the challenges to the creativity of the GCM in preparing the care plan.

Care Plan Needs Consensus

Getting Family, Client, and Third Party Buy-In

The GCM always needs to remember that the care plan is about solving the problems and meeting the goals of the client and/or family. Listening to family members, fiduciaries, and legal representatives during the assessment process can help the GCM understand how to craft a care plan that is most likely to be accepted. The greater number of interested individuals who support the plan, the better chance the plan has of being implemented. However, the GCM must seek primary approval from the party who requested the care plan initially and who is paying for the assessment. If the assessment and plan were ordered in a court case by the court, the GCM must provide the answers to the questions the court has asked and should have an attorney review the geriatric assessment before it is submitted to the court. Ask an attorney what to do in this type of situation.

If you have the permission of the client or the client's power of attorney or guardian, and if the client does not make a decision, a way to get support for your care plan from all involved parties may be presenting your care plan at a family meeting or having a conference call with all parties. If not, you may call all parties and present your care plan or fax it to all parties with a follow-up phone call. If you can gain consensus for your care plan by these steps, you have a much better chance of having the family members help the older person accept it, and you have a lesser chance of family members sabotaging the care plan.

Care Plan Needs to Be Impartial Yet Creative

Given the same set of problems, several GCMs may come up with different care plans. It is important that the care plan be suitable to the particular client. Because most clients come to care managers because they or their families have been unable to solve their problems themselves, care plans often involve creative problem solving. A creative care plan is crafted by thinking about the client's identified problems imaginatively and using your experience with and knowledge of community resources to suggest a unique solution. However much creativity it involves, the care plan must begin with standardized assessment tools that have been developed with multiple-choice answers that result in more objective information with which to develop the care plan. Refer to the assessment tools discussed in various chapters for standardized assessment tools. Also, the National Association of Professional Geriatric Care Managers offers, through its GCM Forms Book, standardized assessment tools.

For example, you are asked to consult with a couple. The wife has had Parkinson's disease for a number of years, and the couple lives in a house that they retrofitted for her care with a wheel-in shower, lower counters in the kitchen, no steps, and everything including the laundry on one floor. The husband is now confronted with having an operation that will require 6 to 8 weeks of rehabilitation. They are trying to figure out if they should hire a live-in worker, try to get their current help to commit to 24/7 care for a month, or hire a new agency to fill in the extra hours. You use standardized functional and psychosocial assessment tools to assess their problem. Then, in discussing their options, you suggest the creative solution that both of them move to a facility for 6 weeks because they do not seem very eager to have a live-in.

■ CARE MONITORING: UPDATING YOUR CARE PLAN

Care monitoring is really measuring whether your care plan is working. As an example, consider again Mrs. Virden, who was widowed after 50 years of marriage. The problem you identified in your care plan is Mrs. Virden's social isolation and loneliness. Your solution/intervention is for the GCM to make a weekly monitoring visit and to have a neighbor drive Mrs. Virden to the senior center twice a week. During your first monitoring visit, you find out that the neighbor forgot to take her to the senior center, so you change your care plan to arrange for senior transportation to pick up Mrs. Virden two times a week to take her to the senior center. When you then check with the client to make sure that senior transportation is arriving at the correct time and that she feels comfortable in the van, you are able to state that your plan has succeeded.

Monitor Your Client to Measure Change

GCMs monitor the services they have recommended to find out whether the client's needs have changed, whether the services originally arranged are still appropriate, and whether the client needs new services or needs to stop receiving services. You monitor to find any holes in the care plan, and then rewrite the care plan and follow up to create new interventions.

Monitoring visits are usually done by appointment with the client. However, it may be appropriate to drop in to visit the client or make unannounced visits if your purpose is to oversee the quality of care being provided. For example, you can drop in to observe the care in an assisted living facility outside of regular office hours. When you make a home visit, use a form to record your monitoring visit (see Exhibit 5-3).

The purpose of a monitoring visit is to observe how the client is doing and to see whether the care plan is being implemented. After you have met with the client, you should also speak to any care provider in the home, paid or unpaid. If the client lives in a residential care setting, you could speak to the residential care provider, and if the client lives in a skilled nursing facility (SNF), you could speak to either the director of nursing or the social worker and/or the direct service worker if possible. In addition, in a facility setting, you can review the written record.

In all of these conversations, discuss the previous time period between visits by reviewing historical problems in the care plan. For example, if the older person was wandering but has not wandered for months, ask whether there has been a reoccurrence of wandering. Discuss ongoing psychosocial and functional problems included in the care plan, and probe for any new psychosocial or functional problems, any problems with patient care, any problems with care staff, and any household problems.

During a monitoring visit, check the condition of the environment, cleanliness of the home, and whether there are enough supplies (adult diapers, food, etc.). Check the client's physical condition, mental condition, new medications, and compliance with the current medication regimen. Chart the medications each time you visit. You should then chart on the care monitoring form any specific concerns and actions you plan to take. If you find any changes in the client's situation, update the care plan and make sure the new version is given to the care provider responsible for implementing the plan or to the residence (SNF), board and care, etc.). If you create an updated care plan and no one is aware of the changes, it will, of course, fail to be implemented and your care monitoring will flounder.

New recommendations are integrated into a plan of care as interventions. The goal is to achieve the outcomes that the team has determined are desired despite any changes that might occur in a client's situation. Recommendations must then be communicated to the appropriate care providers and to the client if possible. Periodic reassessment and modification of the care plan are critical to the success of the plan.

Exhibit 5–3   GCM Field Evaluation/Care Management Service

Date: 11/18/04   **Client Name:** Zeke Zeigler
SW Name: Miss Full Charge

(1-excellent   5-poor)

General Home Environment: 1   **2**   3   4   5
Facility was pleasant. Zeke Zeigler was seated in his wheelchair across from the nurses' station next to the lounge. The lounge was busy yet felt organized.

General Home Cleanliness: 1   **2**   3   4   5
The facility was generally clean and free of odor.

Supplies: **1**   2   3   4   5
(food, cleaning supplies, attends, expense $, Ensure, etc.)
Provided by the facility

Client's Physical Condition: 1   **2**   3   4   5
(personal grooming, overall condition, behavior, etc.)

Zeke Zeigler was seated on his chair dressed and ready for his doctor's appt. He was neat and well groomed. Overall he was relaxed.

Client's Mental Condition: 1   2   **3**   4   5
(oriented, moderately confused, very confused)

Zeke Zeigler was alert although he was not oriented to time, place, and person. When Zeke Zeigler entered The Stroke Institute, he read the sign and clearly said "Stroke Institute." While waiting for Dr. Feelgood, Zeke Zeigler read a few words accurately from a magazine, but could not connect words together. During the doctor's visit, he responded clearly when Dr. Feelgood asked his name but started singing when asked about his age, family, or symptoms.

New Psychosocial Problems:
Julia Nimble, social worker at Agility Skilled Nursing Facility, reported that his humming, singing, and general agitation bothered Mr. Zeigler's roommate. However, this behavior did not impact Zeke Zeigler and his relation to the outside world. No other psychosocial problems were apparent. He was pleasant and interacted with the GCM, the nurse, and Dr. Feelgood.

List of Medications:
(include quantity and expiration date)

During this visit, Dr. Feelgood prescribed Seroquel 25mg, 1/2 to 1 tab daily at bedtime to decrease the agitation and allow him to sleep better.

Specific Concerns:
Dr. Feelgood noted that Mr. Zeigler's right hand was contracted and stiff. He suggested botox treatment on his forearm to paralyze the stiffened muscles and decrease the contractures. This will ease the movement of his right hand and also make it easier for a caregiver to dress him. Dr. Feelgood will do the botox treatment at Mr. Zeigler's next appointment.

continues

Exhibit 5–3   GCM Field Evaluation/Care Management Service (continued)

Actions:

GCM rode with Zeke Zeigler in Medical Transport vehicle from Agility Skilled Nursing Facility Care to The Stroke Institute.

GCM sat with Zeke Zeigler during his visit with Dr. Feelgood. Dr. Feelgood took over from Dr. Baseline and spent this visit reviewing symptoms, current therapy, and getting to know Mr. Zeigler.

GCM waited with Zeke Zeigler until Medical Transport came to pick them up. Due to the time of day, we had to wait for over an hour for transport back to Agility Skilled Nursing Facility Care.

Plan:

Return visit was set for Thursday, February 10, 2005 @ 9:45 a.m. During that visit, Dr. Feelgood plans a botox treatment to decrease the contracture of Mr. Zeigler's hand.

Summary of Visit:

Miss Full Charge, GCM accompanied Zeke Zeigler to a doctor's appointment at The Stroke Institute scheduled for 4:30 p.m. Pick-up was scheduled for an hour before the appointment. Zeke Zeigler was seated on his chair dressed and ready for his doctor's appt. He was neat and well groomed. Overall he was relaxed. Zeke Zeigler was alert although he was not oriented to time, place, and person. When Zeke Zeigler entered The Stroke Institute, he read the sign and clearly said "Stroke Institute." While waiting for Dr. Feelgood, Zeke Zeigler read a few words accurately from a magazine, but could not connect words together. During the doctor's visit, he responded clearly when Dr. Feelgood asked his name but started singing when asked about his age, family, or symptoms.

Source: Cresscare, Case Management for Elders, Cathy Cress, Director, 2006.

■ WRITING A GERIATRIC ASSESSMENT AND DESIGNING THE CARE PLAN

The GCM creates the care plan after intake and begins service. At times families, trust officers, attorneys, or other third parties ask the GCM to integrate the care plan into a written report called a *geriatric assessment and recommendations.*

What triggers a written geriatric assessment? A problem. As a GCM, you are a problem solver and you solve an older person's problems through a geriatric assessment. You take the same steps to discover the client's problems and solutions as you use during assessment.

The purpose of a written assessment is to impart to families the information you gathered using the assessment tools to help the family know what the next step in care of the client may be. Occasionally, a written assessment is used by attorneys and judges as an outside professional opinion about how to solve the client's problem: should the person be conserved, should the person move from the home, which adult child would serve best as a guardian?

A written assessment also transmits information from other sources, such as court records, facility records, medical records, and conversations with family members or others that you documented in service notes. Most important, the written assessment communicates all this information in an organized and convincing manner. Here, you are much like an attorney: you are making a case to convince the family, physician, court, and so forth (jury) that the older client has X problems and they can be solved by Y solutions. Last, the purpose of the geriatric assessment is to complete the first significant task the client asked you to do.

Consider Mrs. Hurricane. Her daughter Miss Tornado hires you to write a geriatric assessment because Mrs. Hurricane has had several falls. You begin your written geriatric assessment stating that GCM Care Solvers was hired by Miss Tina Tornado to do a geriatric assessment on her mother Hannah Hurricane because the mother has fallen 5 times at home in the past 2 weeks and refuses to accept care or move to a different level of care.

To begin the written assessment, you take the steps as outlined in this chapter to gather data. You do the assessments. Gathering the information to write the geriatric assessment is done as outlined in Chapter 4, functional assessment, and Chapter 3, psychosocial assessment. Once you have gathered all the information, you must analyze it in a systematic, logical manner. Written assessment questionnaires assist in the categorization of data. Data can be classified according to a number of different parameters, including identified problems, functional deficits, chronic or acute illnesses, and coping mechanisms and deficits. The sorting and classification of data lead to the identification of areas of intervention. Intervention strategies must be individualized in a geriatric assessment. Included in Exhibit 5–4 is an outline of Phyllis Brostoff's assessment and care plan recommendations, which was presented in her report *How to Write a Professional Assessment and Recommendations* at the Geriatric Care Management National Conference in 2004. This can be helpful in categorizing your data into problem types and areas of intervention before you write your geriatric assessment.[3]

Exhibit 5–4   Assessment, Care Plan, and Recommendations Outline

1. Date assessment and care plan and recommendations were prepared: _____

2. Client demographic information:
   a. Name
   b. Address
   c. Phone number
   d. Current living arrangement
   e. DOB
   f. Marital status or primary relationship
   g. Gender
   h. Primary language if not English

3. Information on individual who requested assessment:
   a. Name
   b. Address
   c. Phone number
   d. Relationship to client

4. Informants other than client who provided information, relationship to client, and dates of contact

5. Presenting problem (the problem that precipitated the referral for this assessment)

6. Social network status (include current activities and interests, occupational background, spiritual life, living arrangements, nature and frequency of significant social relationships; describe a typical week in the life of the client such as outings, contacts with others)

7. Physical and mental health/medical status (include current medical diagnoses; medications; name of primary care physician, other specialists, dentist, podiatrist; any problems with sleeping, vision, hearing, elimination, speech,

continues

Exhibit 5–4   Assessment, Care Plan, and Recommendations Outline (continued)

respiration, nutritional status, and diet.) When listing current conditions, observe whether they are stable, worsening, or improving.

8. Activities of daily living status (include assessment of ability to ambulate, bathe, dress, communicate, eat, maintain continence, shave, maintain oral health, toilet, transfer alone or with assistance; if assisted, indicate by whom or with what equipment)

9. Instrumental activities of daily living status (include ability to shop, prepare meals, do housekeeping and laundry, use telephone, manage medication, do own finances alone or with assistance; if assisted, indicate by whom or with what equipment)

10. Legal status (include whether there are signed Health Care and Financial Powers of Attorney and who the agents are in these documents, whether there is guardianship, whether a living will is signed, whether a current will is in place)

11. Financial status (include current income and assets to determine eligibility for state/federal programs or Veterans Administration programs; include how the client is managing daily money matters and whether there is a trust administrator)

12. Insurance coverage (include information on primary and secondary insurance, long-term-care insurance, VA benefits)

13. Summary of concerns and identification of risk factors (specify concerns uncovered in the assessment under the following areas and identify any potential problems you are aware of regarding

possible solutions to these problems, such as client resistance, limited financial resources, or family conflict)

a. Safety concerns (include risks identified in the home setting such as hazards on stairs, in kitchen, in bedroom, in bathroom, in living room)

b. Mental health, behavioral, or cognitive concerns (include outcome of mental status assessments such as depression screens, mini-mental screens, suicide potential, relevant psychiatric history)

c. Driving safety concerns (include whether there is evidence that the client may be driving unsafely)

d. Nutrition concerns (include information on change in weight, unhealthy/unbalanced diet, difficulty preparing food)

e. Fall risks (include information on fear, clutter, medications, balance, strength, specific conditions)

f. Abuse risks (include information on physical, emotional, financial, psychological, neglect, or self-neglect issues)

g. Medications/substance abuse/smoking risks (note any compliance issues, polypharmacy issues, obstacles to attaining medications or taking them appropriately, alcohol or over-the-counter medication abuse)

14. Care plan and recommendations (identify each problem/concern uncovered in the assessment. Explain your rationale for each recommendation, and provide at least two alternatives and the cost associated with each alternative.) Include referrals needed to any medical or other specialists.

Source: "How to Write a Professional Assessment and Recommendations." Phyllis Brostoff at GCM National Conference in 2004.

Writing the Presenting Problem Section

The report always begins with a statement describing the presenting problem. Why did someone ask you to write the assessment? Take the example of Mrs. Hurricane again. Following is a sample Presenting Problem section.

> Tina Tornado contacted GCM Care concerning her mother, Hannah Hurricane, and asked that we complete a geriatric assessment. Ms. Tornado is concerned because her mother has fallen 5 times during the 2-week period from October 15th to October 31. She states Mrs. Hurricane refuses to have help at home and further refuses to move from her home to a higher level of care.

Writing the History Section

The History section follows the Presenting Problem section. It should include a brief history of the client from birth until the time of this current problem. Use the psychosocial assessment form to gather these data. The data should include birth date, where the client grew up, education, job held through most of life, and marriage date. The important part here is to describe this elder as a person who had a life before this major problem or crisis. You do this to give him or her three dimensions. It also gives the attorney and/or family members reading the written assessment a quick history of this person. The history must be brief, succinct, clear, and no more than three paragraphs but contain all relevant information. Following is an example History section.

> Hannah Hurricane was born on September 12, 1918, and grew up in Monterey, California. After Hannah graduated from high school, she attended San Jose State Teachers College. After graduation she worked as an English teacher in the Monterey school system for 10 years. She married Mr. Harold Hurricane in 1942, began to raise her family, and gave up her teach-

> ing career to become a homemaker for more than 50 years.
>
> Mrs. Hurricane has three children: Tina Tornado, James and Steve Hurricane. Steve and James live in Washington, D.C., and Tina lives nearby in Santa Cruz, California. Hannah was widowed when her husband died 13 years ago.
>
> Mrs. Hurricane moved to Park Lane, a residence for seniors in Monterey, after her husband died. Approximately seven years ago, she moved to a condominium in Carmel, where she presently resides. Until recently, she tutored students in English as a Second Language. Mrs. Hurricane also attended social activities and lunches at the Carmel Foundation, a senior center in downtown Carmel. Mrs. Hurricane is a Christian Scientist.

Writing the Functional Assessment Section

Write the chronological history of functional problems that led to the main problem. Describe the health history, including the diagnosis, physician's evaluation, and information from the functional assessment tool. Include present medications and assessment of ADLs and IADLs and home safety. Describe your observations on gait, environment, and so forth as recorded in service notes or a functional assessment form. Following is an example Functional Assessment section.

> Carolyn Hellsapoppen GCM from Care Solvers GCM made a home visit to the client on November 27, 2003, because Mrs. Hurricane had a recent history of five falls. The GCM observed Mrs. Hurricane ambulate. She watched the client arise from the couch and walk to the kitchen with difficulty, assisted by her cane. The Get Up and Go Test was administered by asking Mrs. Hurricane to get up from a kitchen chair, stand still, walk forward 10 feet, turn around, walk back to the chair, and then turn and be seated. The GCM noted Mrs. Hurricane's sitting

balance, transfers from sitting to standing, pace, and stability of walking. Mrs. Hurricane scored a 3 on this test, indicating she needs to be further evaluated by a primary physician.

Mrs. Hurricane's daughter, Tina, reported to Carolyn Hellsapoppen in a phone conversation on November 26, 2003, that her mother had fallen on the dates October 15, 20, 21, 26, and 31. The first two falls happened while she was putting her laundry in the washer, which is located down the stairs on the lower level of the house. The last three falls were reported to have happened in the kitchen, as Mrs. Hurricane rushed to get to a boiling teapot. Ms. Tornado stated that there were no apparent injuries from these falls, but that her mother did lie on the ground for 3 to 4 hours after the first fall. However, in all instances, Mrs. Hurricane was not able to summon help.

Mrs. Hurricane is slightly hard of hearing. The GCM had to repeat some questions before she understood them. She has no hearing aid.

On the home visit of November 27, Mrs. Hurricane told the GCM she was depressed. She identified depression as the cause of her symptoms of a burning sensation in her upper back, neck, and both arms. Mrs. Hurricane stated these feelings come upon her at night and are quite uncomfortable. Mrs. Hurricane also stated to Carolyn Hellsapoppen that she had not seen a physician since these symptoms began.

Mrs. Hurricane was administered a Katz ADL by the GCM, which identified that she needs assistance with bathing because of her balance problems and should be watched on transfers. She is independent in dressing, continence, and feeding. She was administered an IADL test by the GCM.

Mrs. Hurricane is independent in telephone use, managing medication, and financial management. Mrs. Hurricane needs assistance with food preparation, housekeeping, driving at night,

doing laundry, and shopping because of ambulation difficulties and recent falls. A physician's report, received on December 7, 2002, was completed by Mrs. Hurricane's physician, Dr. Olsen. The report stated Mrs. Hurricane has diabetes, high blood pressure, a history of interstitial cystitis, and is noncompliant with doctor's appointments and orders. Mrs. Hurricane was also reported by her doctor to be mentally clear.

Carolyn Hellsapoppen, GCM, reported that Mrs. Hurricane is a non-insulin-dependent diabetic and, according to Mrs. Hurricane, her blood sugar values are "quite high" despite her avoidance of sweets and the use of the prescription drug Glucophage (metformin). She feels this drug has caused a 2- to 3-week bout of diarrhea, which she says is now resolved. She stated to Ms. Hellsapoppen that she has discontinued taking this drug.

As reported to Carolyn Hellsapoppen of GCM Care by Mrs. Hurricane, Mrs. Hurricane had one of her kidneys removed in 1994 and had a urostomy performed in 1990, following several years of interstitial cystitis. Dr. Olsen's physician's report stated this as well. Mrs. Hurricane stated to Ms. Hellsapoppen on her visit of November 27, 2002, that she can usually manage her urostomy well but has had some episodes of skin irritation of the stoma and the surrounding tissue to the point of bleeding. In March 2002, Mrs. Hurricane was admitted to Community Hospital Emergency Room in Santa Cruz. She had an irritation of her urostomy. After treatment, she was released and sent home. There have been no other hospitalizations before this or after this incident, according to Tina Tornado. These periodic irritations of her urostomy prompted Tina Tornado to request a home health aide, who Mrs. Hurricane discharged after two months. Mrs. Hurricane reported to Carolyn Hellsapoppen that she is now using a moisture barrier before applying the urostomy bag and has had good results with it.

As examined by GCM Carolyn Hellsapoppen, RN, on her visit of November 27, 2002, Mrs. Hurricane's lungs were clear; abdomen was soft; ankles were without swelling. Her blood pressure was elevated by 160/100; pulse was 88 and regular; respirations were 20 per minute. She stated that she feels she needs to lose weight. Her daughter Ms. Tornado reported to Amber Helpall, Social Worker for GCM Care, that her mother has lost approximately 20 pounds and weighs approximately 180 pounds. This weight was confirmed on the physician's report. Mrs. Hurricane also stated to Carolyn Hellsapoppen that she is not eating as much as she used to and is losing weight.

As was also reported to Carolyn Hellsapoppen, Mrs. Hurricane's doctor, Mabel Olsen, discharged Mrs. Hurricane as a patient approximately three months ago for missing three medical appointments. According to Mrs. Hurricane and her daughter, Dr. Ted Tittlemouse, endocrinologist, has also discontinued his services as her physician for noncompliance. The doctor recommended she either have 24-hour care or move to a board and care. Carolyn Hellsapoppen of GCM Care recommends that Mrs. Hurricane be evaluated as soon as possible by a new physician because of her elevated blood pressure and the recent falls. The fact that she is a diabetic also puts her at high risk of heart disease, according to Carolyn Hellsapoppen.

On a home safety check the GCM found the following: there is no handheld showerhead installed, no shower chair for safety in the bath. Smoke alarms are not working throughout the house. There are outside obstructions, such as tools and planter boxes, in the pathway that would make it easy to trip and fall. There is no cordless phone, which would prevent the client from rushing to answer phones. Teapot on stove needs to be replaced by an electric teapot so she does not have to hurry to turn it off.

Writing the Psychosocial Assessment Section

Write the chronological history of psychosocial and psychological events that led to the main problem. This could include mental status. If dementia is a big part of the problem, break this out as its own section. The Psychosocial Assessment section should include information about moving from one level of care to another, death of a spouse, substance abuse, economic and legal issues including conservatorships, financial assets, insurance, both informal and formal support systems, activities, spiritual beliefs, recent life changes and life satisfaction, and ethnic background including preferences and needs. Following is a sample Psychosocial Assessment section.

> Mrs. Hurricane has a history of noncompliance with doctors' orders and safety issues. She is a Christian Scientist and, because of her religious beliefs, she prefers to handle her medical problems by prayer first, and medical care second. Mrs. Hurricane and her daughter asked for Carolyn Hellsapoppen's recommendation for physicians in the Monterey area. Carolyn was able to provide them with three names, one being Carl Handsome, MD, an internist in Carmel. Mrs. Hurricane has an appointment with Dr. Handsome on December 13, in one week.
>
> Ms. Hurricane was administered a short portable mental status questionnaire by the GCM, and her score of 1 error indicated she does not seem to need additional evaluation for memory loss. This was confirmed by Dr. Olsen's physician's report. There is no former or present substance abuse.
>
> Upon discussion with Carolyn Hellsapoppen, Mrs. Hurricane stated that she is feeling depressed. The GCM observed she had a flat affect and appeared lethargic, and Mrs. Hurricane stated that she has felt depressed for days. She stated she did not want to go out of the house, hardly wanted to watch her favorite show *Jeopardy* anymore, and does not feel like

going to the Carmel Foundation. GCM Carolyn Hellsapoppen interviewed Miss Service, a social worker at the Carmel Foundation. Miss Service stated Mrs. Hurricane attended until one month ago and repeated calls and follow-up home visits were made to find out what prevented Mrs. Hurricane from attending the foundation. Miss Service said she will work with the family and the GCM to reengage the client in foundation activities. Amber Helpall, social worker, discussed the possibility of Mrs. Hurricane having a pet. Mrs. Hurricane stated she would like one but is unable to have a dog or cat because of restrictions in the condominium complex where she lives.

Ms. Tornado, the adult child who lives closest to her mother, is the primary family care provider. Although Mrs. Hurricane's sons James and Steve live on the East Coast, they have both agreed to offer to their mother whatever support is required, which might include taking her as respite, helping financially, or whatever is suggested by the GCM. Mrs. Hurricane's other social support is her 92-year-old neighbor, Mrs. Charlotte Murphy, who encourages Mrs. Hurricane to go to the Carmel Foundation and visits her most days for tea and conversation. Ms. Hellsapoppen interviewed Mrs. Murphy and Mrs. Murphy stated that Mrs. Hurricane seemed more "down in the dumps lately" and was staying in bed some days instead of watching *Jeopardy*. The two women have watched *Jeopardy* together for several years. Additional social supports were from the Carmel Foundation, where Mrs. Hurricane attended a women's support group, tutored English as a Second Language, and had daily lunches.

Daughter Ms. Tornado has the Durable Power of Attorney for Health Care as well as the Durable Power of Attorney for Finances for her mother. These two documents were established in 1999 to prepare for her mother's future, according to Ms. Tornado. Mrs. Hurri-

cane continues to handle her own finances, but Ms. Tornado "checks everything over" for her mother, according to Ms. Tornado. Mrs. Hurricane has adequate finances (about a million dollars in assets) to pay for care. She has long-term-care insurance through PERS because she was a teacher, plus Medicare and a Medicare supplement.

Mrs. Hurricane asserts that she does her own housekeeping and laundry, and that she needs a cleaning lady only once a week. Mrs. Hurricane's home was very neat and clean, according to the observation of Carolyn Hellsapoppen. However, because of her balance problems, it is recommended that a care provider do the daily light housework for the client. Mrs. Hurricane drives, but she does not drive at night, according to her daughter.

Writing the Medications Section

List all current medications in this section, including dosage. You should get this information from the physician report you send to the client's doctor. You can also find out about all medications by asking the client or client representative if you can look at each bottle of medication in the client's possession. By doing this, you can make a list of current medications and also find medications that are out of date and discover any polypharmacy issues.

Writing the Level of Care Section

In the Level of Care section, you recommend a level of care. You might recommend the same level of care as currently provided with no supports or the same level of care but including additional support systems such as care providers. You might have to recommend the client move to a higher level of care such as moving to an assisted living facility.

Your job as GCM is to be an expert in level of care. After you complete all your assessment tools, you should be able to state exactly what level of care your client needs. Again, evaluating the physical environment in combination with an understanding of the client's ability to perform the ADLs enables a care manager to understand the level of care the client needs. Following is a sample Level of Care section.

> Ms. Tornado is concerned because her mother has fallen five times during the 2-week period of October 15 to October 31. She states Mrs. Hurricane refuses to have help at home and further declines to move from her home to a higher level of care. She would like the GCM's opinion on how to proceed in keeping her mother safe at her present level of care or on a plan to move to a higher level of care.
>
> The GCM recommends that Mrs. Hurricane remain at home where she is in familiar surroundings, has a good neighbor, and is comfortable. If all home safety deficits are followed through and the client is provided assistance with her ADLs of food preparation, housekeeping, driving at night, doing her laundry, and shopping, Mrs. Hurricane can remain in her home with a live-in care provider. However, the GCM recommends that the daughter hire a live-in. Because Mrs. Hurricane is adverse to this level of care, the GCM suggests that she be allowed to counsel Mrs. Hurricane over a period of time to accept this assistance.

Writing the Care Plan Section

The care plan comes next. This care plan should include more details than the care plan you place in the home for care providers and update on an ongoing basis. The care plan in the geriatric assessment must paint a clear picture of the client's needs for a judge, attorney, family member, or third party, and others who are not GCMs. The care plan should be written in clear English, without jargon, and should be concise and readable. Start as stated earlier with the problem you were hired to assess in the first place. Following is a Care Plan example that would be included in a geriatric assessment.

Problem	Intervention
1. Ms. Tornado is concerned because her mother has fallen five times during the 2-week period of October 15 to October 31. She states Mrs. Hurricane refuses to have help at home and further refuses to move from her home to a higher level of care. Ms. Tornado would like GCM Care's opinion about how to proceed with her mother's safety issues.	1. a. Within 1 week, daughter Ms. Tornado to hire live-in care providers for Monday through Friday and Saturday and Sunday who can drive, through a list of home care agencies given to her. b. GCM to visit weekly and as needed to help Mrs. Hurricane to accept care and problem solve with Mrs. Hurricane and care provider. c. Care provider to do standby assist at all times. d. Within 1 week, daughter to arrange for Lifeline alerts through Community Hospital of Mt. Peninsula or other source. e. Daughter to ask physician Dr. Handsome to evaluate reason for falls at next appointment on December 13th.

continues

Problem	Intervention
2. Washer and dryer are located down the stairs and outdoors and are one reason for recent falls.	2 a. Daughter to have care provider do laundry 1 time a week in basement on an ongoing basis.
3. Mrs. Hurricane presently has no primary physician because she has been non-compliant with doctor's appointments in the past.	3. a. Daughter to take Mrs. Hurricane to appointment with Dr. Handsome on December 13th and confirm that he will be Mrs. Hurricane's primary physician.
	b. If Dr. Handsome declines to follow up with Mrs. Hurricane on December 13 appointment, daughter to obtain a primary physician from list given by GCM within 1 week after December 13.
	c. After first appointment on December 13, care provider to keep track of all doctor's appointments and drive Mrs. Hurricane to each doctor's appointment.
4. Alteration in nutrition: recent loss of appetite. Mrs. Hurricane has lost approximately 20 pounds and weighs approximately 180 pounds.	4. a. Daughter to have Dr. Handsome evaluate Mrs. Hurricane's weight loss at December 13 appointment.
	b. Care provider to prepare breakfast and dinner and drive Mrs. Hurricane to the Carmel Foundation for daily lunch on an ongoing basis.
5. Alteration in urinary elimination: client has a urostomy.	5. a. Daughter to ask Dr. Handsome to evaluate Mrs. Hurricane's urostomy and urinary problems at December 13 appointment.
6. Alteration in bowel elimination: medication side effects of diarrhea.	6. a. Daughter to ask physician to evaluate urinary medication side effects at December 13 appointment.
7. Mrs. Hurricane. has elevated blood pressure.	7. a. Daughter to ask Dr. Handsome to evaluate elevated blood pressure and monitor blood pressure at December 13 appointment.
	b. Care provider to prepare low-salt meals on an ongoing basis.
8. Pain: Mrs. Hurricane complains of burning sensation and pain in back and neck.	8. a. Daughter to ask Dr. Handsome to evaluate present pain and burning sensation at December 13 appointment.
9. Mrs. Hurricane is a non-insulin-dependent diabetic and her blood sugar values are self-reported as "quite high" despite her avoidance of sweets and the use of the prescription drug Glucophage (metformin), which she has discontinued using.	9. a. Daughter to ask Dr. Handsome to evaluate diabetes and present diabetic medications for side effects at December 13 appointment.
	b. Care provider to prepare diabetic meals on an ongoing basis.

Problem	Intervention
	c. Care provider to monitor sweet intake and chart on an ongoing basis.
	d. Daughter to call Carmel Foundation and order diabetic meals week before client returns to Carmel Foundation.
	e. Daughter to investigate a diabetic support group for Mrs. Hurricane at Dominican Rehab Services held one Tuesday a month.
10. Mrs. Hurricane is hard of hearing and has no hearing aid.	10. a. GCM to take client to an audiologist to have hearing evaluated and to get possible prescription for hearing aid within 1 month.
11. Depression: Mrs. Hurricane expressed being depressed to the GCM, and she is no longer engaged in social activity that enhances her quality of life.	11. a. Daughter to arrange for mother to see mental health provider Martin Skirt at Community Hospital within 2 weeks to evaluate level of depression and assess for possible medications.
	b. Daughter to instruct care provider to drive Mrs. Hurricane to Carmel Foundation daily for lunch and socialization as soon as care provider is hired.
	c. GCM to contact social worker Miss Service at Carmel Foundation to find new activities that would benefit client or a continuation of old activities such as women's support group 1 week before client begins attending.
	d. GCM to work with Carmel Foundation social worker to make sure Mrs. Hurricane is engaged in activities and to work with any barriers the client may have in attending activities on an ongoing basis.
	e. Within 1 month, GCM to call Monterey School District to find out whether client could continue to tutor English as a Second Language if care provider accompanied her to site.
	f. Care provider to take Mrs. Hurricane to plays at Forrest Theater, to SPCA to visit animals, and to other activities suggested by GCM to engage Mrs. Hurricane in activities that improve her quality of life and increase her social engagement.
	g. Care provider to drive Mrs. Hurricane to have lunch with daughter one day a month, hopefully on day the client attends the diabetic support group in Santa Cruz.

continues

Problem	Intervention
12. Home safety issues that may lead to more falls include these: shower lacks safety bars, shower lacks handheld showerhead, smoke alarms are not working, outside obstructions are in pathway of client. Client does not have cordless phone and may rush to answer phone. Client fell rushing to take teapot off stove.	12. a. Daughter to arrange for shower bars to be installed in bathroom outside of shower on both sides, within 1 week. b. Daughter to arrange to have handheld showerhead installed within 1 week. c. Daughter to get a shower chair for mother at medical supply store or Carmel Foundation within 1 week. d. Daughter to arrange for repair person to hook up smoke alarms within 1 week. e. Daughter to have handyman remove outside obstructions in pathways, such as tools and planter boxes, within 1 week. f. Daughter to order cordless phone so mother does not have to rush to answer phone, within 2 weeks. g. Daughter to buy electric teapot that automatically turns off, within 2 weeks.
13. Mrs. Hurricane states that she cannot drive at night.	13. a. Daughter to take mother to have a thorough eye exam at an ophthalmologist within 1 month. b. Care provider to drive Mrs. Hurricane to all night events on an ongoing basis.
14. Mrs. Hurricane is opposed to medical treatment and thus is noncompliant because of her Christian Science beliefs.	14. a. GCM to contact the local Christian Science foundation in Monterey and make arrangements for a church member who specializes in working with elders to help problem solve so Mrs. Hurricane's health, safety, and spiritual issues can all be met. b. Care provider to drive Mrs. Hurricane to Christian Science services once a week.
15. Daughter is stressed by caregiver burden.	15. a. Daughter to consider attending on first and third Fridays caregiver support group through Del Mar Caregiver Resources in Santa Cruz, where she lives.
16. Mrs. Hurricane's care plan needs to be monitored on an ongoing basis.	16 a. To monitor care plan, care provider, activities, health issues, spiritual issues, and compliance issues GCM will visit Mrs. Hurricane every week for the first 2 months and then every other week after that if Mrs. Hurricane is stable. b. GCM to reevaluate weekly whether daughter is able to do all tasks and to take over tasks daughter wishes to delegate.

Narrative Explanation of Care Plan

After the actual care plan, include a narrative explaining the care plan. For example, if the care plan states that Mrs. Hurricane is depressed and needs to see a mental health provider to be evaluated for depression and possible medications, you can insert the additional information that Mrs. Hurricane has only one friend in her informal support system and that a care provider should be hired. You can explain some of the things the care provider can do to allay the client's depression, such as taking Mrs. Hurricane on visits to the Monterey County SPCA because Mrs. Hurricane likes animals but cannot have one and taking Mrs. Hurricane to plays at the local theaters.

■ EVALUATING THE GERIATRIC ASSESSMENT

Proofread the first draft of the geriatric assessment to make sure you have all the correct information, that the information is well written, grammatically correct, and spelled correctly. The following subsections describe some tools to help you accomplish this.

What Makes You a Good Detective?

When you complete the first draft of your geriatric assessment, go back and check that all elements are in place. In other words, did you gather all the clues? Did you talk to every person who could give you a point of view about the crisis? In Mrs. Hurricane's case, the daughter, the two other adult children, the friend, the Carmel Foundation social worker, and Mrs. Hurricane's former primary physician were involved.

Check that every line of your assessment tool was completely and accurately filled out. This is where you keep track of your clues. Too many GCMs are messy, leaving lines in assessment forms unfilled or skipping over lines or writing in haste. Don't miss any clues. As stated earlier, look at your assessment tools to make sure you slowly and meticulously sift through clues, leaving no stone unturned in your efforts to ensure that all evidence has been taken into account before reaching conclusions and announcing them. Following that, ask yourself these questions: Did you distill the sifted information into your care plan? Does your care plan have complete and well-written problems? Does it have complete and well-written solutions? Is your care plan measurable? Does your care plan tell the reader who will accomplish the solutions?

What Makes a Good Written Assessment?

In a workshop titled *How to Write a Professional Assessment and Recommendations*, Phyllis Brostoff discussed the 4Cs of writing a geriatric assessment that are invaluable in checking your document.[3] The first is *clarity*—facts are presented clearly. In Mrs. Hurricane's geriatric assessment, you would not say, "Mrs. Hurricane looked depressed." You would state, "When visiting Mrs. Hurricane on November 1, 2002, Mrs. Hurricane stated to the GCM that she was feeling depressed."

The second C is *cohesiveness*. This means organization. For example, don't put information about the client's depression in the home management section of your geriatric assessment. Follow the guidelines in Exhibit 5–5. Do not commingle sections. Write a tight outline, follow it, and make your written assessment cohesive.

The third C is *completeness*. You have conducted multiple assessments, but have you filled in every line like a good detective? Have you answered every question fully? With Mrs. Hurricane, did you answer the question of why she was having falls? The answers were many: having no care providers, having to walk down a flight of steps to the laundry, having no portable phone, having a teapot that could not turn itself off, not attending the Carmel Foundation where she had supervision, and so forth.

Exhibit 5-5   Elements of a Geriatric Assessment

Problem

Brief client history from birth to crisis that prompted GCM to intervene

Written summation of functional assessment

Written summation of cognitive assessment

List of all medications

Written summation of psychosocial assessment

Written summation of home environment assessment

Written summary of any other pertinent assessment

Care plan

Written explanation of the care plan

Summary of recommendations

The fourth C is *coherence*. Your geriatric assessment must lead to logical conclusions. In the beginning of Mrs. Hurricane's geriatric assessment, her daughter Ms. Tornado wanted you to find out why her mother had multiple falls and what level of care her mother belonged in. You need to offer a solution to these beginning problems in your conclusion section—why is Mrs. Hurricane falling and where should she live?

Next, determine whether the items included in the geriatric assessment are actionable. When editing the first draft of your geriatric assessment, use Phyllis Brostoff's criteria to help you create an actionable care plan.[3] The solutions in your geriatric assessment must be actionable, which means they should be affordable, acceptable, and doable.

- Are solutions affordable? In your geriatric assessment, you discovered that Mrs. Hurricane has about $1 million in assets and Ms. Tornado, who is durable power of attorney for finances, is open to spending the money on care and services for her mother. So it seems you have an affordable care plan.

- Are solutions acceptable? Will Ms. Tornado pay for a 7-day live-in? Ask her. Will the daughter carry through with all the interventions you are recommending to her? Did you discuss these recommendations with her? Will Mrs. Hurricane be noncompliant with another doctor? Will she accept a care provider? You can check whether some of these interventions are acceptable just by asking the client and/or family members. Whether interventions like the ones created for Mrs. Hurricane are acceptable will depend on whether the GCM can work with the client during care monitoring visits and the quality of the care provider. Some of these interventions take time to become acceptable to the client.

- Is your plan doable? Can Ms. Tornado get Mrs. Hurricane to the mental health assessment at Community Hospital? Will Ms. Tornado follow through, or is her relationship with her mother so strained that Mrs. Hurricane might not go with her? Would it be better to have the GCM take Mrs. Hurricane?

Did You Sell Your Services Well?

Your written geriatric assessment is your geriatric care management product. If you were selling a car, you would never put a vehicle on the car lot with smashed windows, torn seats, and an empty tank. If you sold a car to someone, you would not deliver the car late. So in your geriatric care management work, do not be sloppy. Check to see that you have gathered enough information to evaluate and solve the problems you were hired to solve without making errors. Don't present questionable or unfounded information in your written assessments. If you cannot check the facts, don't include them in the document, or make clear the source of the information and how reliable that source is. Do not include poor spelling, bad grammar, and awkward sentence structure. Have someone who knows how to write and edit review your document, even if you are a good writer. Organize your information by following the outline presented in this chapter. Base your conclusions on facts, not assumptions.

Also, make sure that there is coherence between problems you have identified and interventions you are recommending. For example, if you are dealing with the problem that Mrs. Hurricane is depressed, don't simply recommend she go to a women's support group. Although that might help, a more complete recommendation would be for Mrs. Hurricane to be assessed by a mental health professional. Include the name of the professional, his or her phone number and address, and a recommended time frame for the appointment as part of your recommendation.

Do not be subjective. Always be objective. "I thought she appeared depressed" should be reworded as "On the GCM's visit of 6/6/06, GCM observed Mrs. Hurricane had a flat affect, appeared lethargic, and stated that she has felt depressed for days. She stated she did not want to go out of the house and hardly wanted to watch her favorite show *Jeopardy* anymore." Also, do not be vague—present measurable statements: "She should be evaluated for symptoms of depression by Martin Skirt, LCSW, within 2 weeks," not "She should see a mental health professional."

■ CONCLUSION

Once the assessment is completed, mailed out to the party who requested it with copies sent to the other relevant individuals, and discussed with all concerned parties, the job of the GCM may be finished or just begun, depending upon whether the GCM is asked to carry out the care plan. In this chapter's example, Ms. Tornado may say she will move forward with all the GCM's suggestions, or she may say she will wait on some. At times, the client or family may resist the changes recommended in the plan and decide that their connection with the GCM is finished. If and when a crisis arises in the life of the client, the GCM may be called upon again to become involved, adjust the plan to fit the needs of the current situation, and implement and manage the care plan. If this occurs, because the GCM has already acquired so much information about the client, the GCM is usually able to provide relatively quick assistance. In either case, the GCM has provided the client and family with a comprehensive blueprint of how to proceed and hopefully has assisted them in seeing the value of using professionals for consultation and assistance.

■ NOTES

1. National Institutes of Health. Consensus Conference on Geriatric Assessment Methods for Clinical Decision-Making. October 19, 1987. Available at: http://www.nlm.nih.gov. Accessed April 4, 1999.

2. American Geriatrics Society. Comprehensive Geriatric Assessment Position Statement. October 1996. Available at: http://www.americangeriatrics.org. Accessed March 15, 1999.

3. Brostoff P. *How to Write a Professional Assessment and Recommendations*. Presented at: Geriatric Care Management Conference. October 2004; Austin, TX.

completing old business to welcome the new year. Thus, at a particular point in time, the Japanese American may be more "Japanese" than at others. Other ways to assess the degree of acculturation are discussed in the following sections.

Length of Time Since Immigration and Circumstances of Relocation

The length of time the elder/family has been living in the United States and the circumstances of immigration are important in assessing acculturation status. How long has the elder been in the United States (one year or decades)? Why did he or she come? For example, Vietnamese immigrants arrived in essentially two "waves" to escape communist oppression and economic hardship. Did the elder arrive with the first group of relatively well-educated, well-to-do Catholic immigrants who worked with the U.S. Forces in the mid-1970s? Or did the person arrive with the second wave of essentially mixed, less-educated rural/urban refugees (e.g., boat people)? Was the elder imprisoned in a reeducation camp or did he or she spend time in a refugee camp in Malaysia, Thailand, or Indonesia? Have the family members been reunited or are they separated? Are the elders "followers of children"?[9]

Personal Preferences

Other indicators of acculturation include personal preferences for language usage, food, media, service providers, and socialization. The GCM can ask which language is preferred and used primarily in the client's home. Food preference is important particularly when long-term-care residential options are being considered. Does the elder prefer ethnic food on a daily basis (e.g., rice with every meal) or a variety of food choices? Ethnic media is also an indicator of acculturation. Does the client prefer an ethnic newspaper or television/radio station? Does the elder prefer someone from

the same ethnic group? It should not be assumed that the elder prefers a service provider from the same ethnicity—but for those who are less acculturated or monolingual non-English-speaking, this is frequently the case. Finally, does the ethnic elder prefer to socialize exclusively with others from the same ethnic group or does it matter? The most effective way to obtain this information is to ask the client. Although family members may be helpful in ascertaining this information, even close family members frequently make assumptions about an elder's personal preferences that are not entirely accurate.[10]

Ideally, every effort should be made to locate providers who can communicate with the elder in the person's language of choice. However, if this is not possible, trained interpreters should not be used as interpreters. Because of the sensitive nature of many medical/social service encounters, young children or family members should not be used as interpreters. Additionally, a "cultural guide," a knowledgeable person from the elder's particular ethnic community who is familiar with the culture and beliefs of the traditional society, could also be consulted.

■ COHORT HISTORY

A *cohort* is a group of people born around the same time, generally within a 5-year time span. A cohort analysis considers the historical experiences, both positive and negative, that have influenced the lives of elders today. The GCM should consider the ethnic elder's background when doing an assessment to gain insights about the client's values, beliefs, behaviors, relationships, and preferences.[9] Specific examples follow; however, each individual is unique and may not have experienced or perceived these events in the same way.

Many Mexican American elders have experienced the long-term effects of discriminatory immigration policies that have exploited Mexican laborers for decades. For example, the

Bracero program was started to ease the U.S. labor shortage during World War II by welcoming short-term contract laborers and promising them citizenship as well as other benefits. However, depending on the U.S. economy, this program fluctuated over time and the informal immigration policies resulted in *Braceros* sometimes confused with "illegals," culminating in raids and mass deportations. Because of fear, confusion, and broken promises, many *Braceros* did not apply for citizenship even if they were eligible.[9] Despite these inequities, Mexican American elders have contributed to U.S. society economically, socially, and culturally.

The majority of today's U.S.-born African American elders faced institutionalized racial discrimination when they were young in the form of the Ku Klux Klan, Jim Crow laws, segregated schools, anti-miscegenation laws, and the Tuskegee Alabama Syphilis Experiment. As a result, black elders may distrust the system that supported such injustices. Despite the discrimination, African American elders have the legacy of the civil rights movement; the one million plus men and women who served in segregated units during World War II and the Korean and Vietnam Wars; Harlem Jazz and gospel music as well as the work of such leaders as the Rev. Dr. Martin Luther King.[9]

Similarly, other immigrants have also experienced discrimination and hardships. Older Japanese Americans remember World War II when 120,000 individuals of Japanese descent, most of them U.S. citizens, were incarcerated by the U.S. government in wartime relocation centers. Filipino World War II veterans were recruited to serve in the US Army and Navy in exchange for U.S. citizenship; however, this promise was revoked in 1945. It was not until the 1990s that the Veterans Equity Bill was passed, which granted the aging veterans immediate citizenship but only upon resettlement on the U.S. mainland.

Many Jewish elders are survivors of the Holocaust. American Indian elders faced decades of abuse, including relocation of the young to reservations and boarding schools, the termination of 100 tribes, and subsequent forced urbanization.[9] In the 1970s and 1980s, Muslim refugees from Afghanistan fled the war with Russia and are now aging in the United States.[11] These are just a few examples of significant events that ethnic elders carry in their memories.

Despite the injustices, all of these elders have contributed enormously to the U.S. society, economy, culture, and way of life.

Cohort history also considers migration patterns and resettlement within the United States. Decades ago, African American elders moved from the Deep South to work in the industrial plants of the North where there was greater economic security. The largest populations of Hmong elders in the United States reside in California and Minnesota where the earliest refugees were assigned. The greater San Francisco Bay Area in California is home to the largest populations of Portuguese from the Azores (Portugal); Afghanis from Afghanistan; Sikhs and other South Asians from India; South Vietnamese; Chinese from Taiwan; and Filipinos from the Philippines. The location of resettlement communities was largely because of ethnic enclaves where lay referral networks and service providers helped immigrant families adapt to the foreign ways.

It is impossible for a GCM to know all the historical events that influenced all the different groups living in the United States today. However, knowing where to look for information and what resources are available is a necessary and important skill. (See the section titled "Resources" later in this chapter.)

■ FAMILY VALUE SYSTEMS IN ETHNIC COMMUNITIES

Ethnic/Cultural Group Norms

Ethnic elders/families may have value orientations that differ from mainstream society. In the United States, the focus is placed on individualism—Americans are socialized to be independent, autonomous, aggressive, opportunistic, and in control of various aspects of their lives from birth to death. Assertiveness in communication is encouraged along with the mandate to question authority and demand individual rights. However, many cultures promote values and behaviors diametrically opposed to these highly regarded American norms.

In other societies, the focus may not be on the individual but on the immediate or extended family, the tribe, or the entire village.[12] The benefits and burdens, the good and bad, are experienced by, and reflect upon, the family unit rather than individual family members—children are warned not to bring shame upon the family. Some cultures stress nonconfrontational behaviors, whereas others teach deference to authority. An understanding of these differences helps to enhance communication between clients and providers.

Communication Styles

The GCM must learn to establish trust and rapport with the ethnic elder. Early on, respect must be shown in an appropriate manner and the elder made to feel as comfortable as possible. This can be done by addressing the elder as Mr. or Mrs., taking time to chat before starting to discuss business, and listening carefully when the elder is speaking. Methods of communication may also vary by ethnic/cultural group. For example, many older Asians perceive that asking questions of a health professional is insulting to the provider and implies that the information has not been explained clearly or adequately. Other elders were taught deference to authority and unquestioning compliance because of the provider's expertise. Asking a question may also make the elder feel "stupid" or embarrassed. Hence, the Asian elder may shake his or her head in the affirmative; however, the nod means "yes, I hear you" and not

"I understand" or "I agree." In some cultures, direct eye contact may be perceived as threatening. In others, standing or sitting too close may be uncomfortable and inappropriate.[13]

End-of-Life Decisions

There may be cultural differences in end-of-life decision making as a result of underlying cultural values regarding disclosure of a terminal illness and life-sustaining medical treatment. With the widespread availability of advanced medical technology in the United States, people are encouraged to do everything possible to seek a cure for a life-threatening medical condition. However, there are others for whom quality of life is more important than length of life. Providers must realize that quality of life differs for each individual.

There are some societies such as Japan where a terminal illness may not be disclosed to a patient and it is culturally inappropriate to discuss impending or imminent death.[14] For instance, among some Chinese, it is considered bad luck to discuss death because such talk may cause death to occur. Sometimes the ethnic elder is not expected to make the health care decision and the responsibility may be based on a family hierarchy. For instance, in many Filipino families there may be a designated decision maker, who is not the patient (e.g., the oldest son or a daughter/son who is a health professional), to express the wishes of the elder/family. Other end-of-life decisions are based on religious tenets. In many Catholic immigrant communities, there may be strong resistance to an advance directive because this document would indicate "loss of hope" or be interpreted as suicide, which is against church doctrine. These beliefs may affect the use of services such as hospice.

Many providers are not aware that alternative clauses for advance directives are available from the various religious traditions that convey religious intent and attitudes toward end-of-life issues (e.g., Christian Science, Jewish, Roman Catholic documents). Additionally, if a provider cannot discuss end-of-life preferences directly, other types of documentation (e.g., personal values charts) may be collected over time.

■ ETHNICITY, AGING, AND HEALTH

Health Disparities

Significant racial and ethnic differences in the health status of older adults have been documented in the United States. A recent panel convened by the National Academies on race, ethnicity, and health in later life attempted to explain some of the differences.[15] In the past, most research focused on black–white differences, which revealed that even though life expectancy is increasing and overall health status is improving among older adults, blacks continually experience lower life expectancy than whites.[15] In general, blacks and American Indians/Alaska Natives are less healthy than older whites are, and Hispanics and Asians tend to be healthier.[15] There are many groups for which there is little to no information available, particularly the recent foreign-born immigrants from Southeast Asian, Eastern European, and Latin American countries.

The underlying determinants of these differences have remained elusive because of the many complex factors that influence health. Furthermore, relatively little research has focused on older adults.[15] Health status in ethnic communities is influenced by macrosocial factors (e.g., socioeconomic status, institutions, politics, residence, family); behavioral risk factors (e.g., smoking, exercise, alcohol use); cumulative prejudice and discrimination; stress (both personal and environmental); health care access and quality (e.g., cost, availability); lack of culturally competent services; adaptive health behaviors (e.g., coping, social supports); health care behaviors (e.g., utilization, help seeking, self-care); and genetics. Furthermore, these factors must be considered across the life course because early behaviors influence health in later years.

Health Risks and Health Status

Providing detailed information regarding the health status and risks among ethnic elders is not possible in this limited space—however, a brief discussion of major health risks is necessary. This material is based on the four federally designated racial/ethnic categories; therefore, caution must be taken to avoid generalization to specific subpopulations. To begin, Hummer et al. summarized overall differences in mortality:[16(p14)]

> Blacks generally have worse health than other groups. American Indians and Alaska Natives, especially those on reservations, are also less healthy than other groups except blacks. Whites are usually taken as the standard against which other groups are compared, but they are not necessarily in the best health. Hispanics appear to be healthier than whites on a number of measures, though not all. Asians are generally in better health than any other group.

It is noteworthy that among the oldest-old, those 85 years and older, there appears to be a mortality crossover in some populations—black elders live longer than whites do and there is some evidence that American Indian/Alaska Native mortality falls below that of Hispanics and Asian/Pacific Islanders.[15]

In general, the six leading causes of death among ethnic elders is similar to whites—heart disease, neoplasms (cancers), cerebrovascular disease, lower respiratory conditions, influenza and pneumonia, and diabetes.[15] When compared to data on the health of whites, self-report of the most common diseases and health conditions by ethnic elders reveals that older blacks have more hypertension, diabetes, strokes, kidney disease, and dementia/Alzheimer's disease.[17]

Among Hispanic elders, non-insulin-dependent diabetes mellitus is a significant problem particularly among Mexicans and Puerto Ricans, as are hypertension and cardiovascular disease, cognitive impairment, and affective disorders.[18,19] The major health problems of elderly American Indian/Alaska Natives include Type II diabetes mellitus, high blood pressure, tuberculosis, heart disease, cancer, and liver/kidney disease. Additionally, when compared to the general U.S. population, American Indian/Alaska Natives have high death rates from alcoholism, tuberculosis, and accidents.[20]

Overall, Asian/Pacific Islanders have a lower prevalence than whites do for heart disease, cancer, and cardiovascular disease, but it depends on the subgroup.[4] Asian Indians, Chinese, Filipinos, and Japanese tend to have better health status than whites do,[21] whereas Native Hawaiians and Samoans tend to have worse health.[22] However, distinct differences exist within groups—for instance, breast cancer incidence is twice as high among Japanese as among Vietnamese women, whereas cervical cancer is seven times as high among Vietnamese as among Japanese women.[23]

Health Beliefs

Some cultures perceive illness and healing from a different perspective than mainstream elders do. Given the diverse number of cultures in the United States, numerous explanations exist for various medical conditions. The patient/client's perception of the source/cause of an illness carries broad implications for the acceptance of prescribed therapies and adherence to treatments as well as the utilization of medical/social services.

Western vs. Traditional Systems of Health Beliefs

The Stanford Geriatric Education Center (SGEC) has categorized culturally based health belief systems from documented informa-

tion.[24] Health belief system origins and some of the major characteristics are shown here:

- Biomedical model (Western, Allopathic)—practiced in the United States, based on medical research studies
- American Indian—mind–body–spirit integration, spiritual healing, use of native plants, respect for nature/environment
- African/African American—integration of American Indian, Christian, other European traditions, occult/spiritual illness, religious healing
- Asian—combination of Chinese medicine, Japanese Kampo, Korean Hanbang, and Southeast Asian medicine; balance of yin/yang, vital energy (*chi*); Taoist and Buddhist influence; Indian Ayurvedic medicine shaped by Hinduism and mind–body–spirit integration; Hmong beliefs involve healers, spirits, loss of soul
- Latin American—biomedical model blended with Native American, European, African beliefs
- Other European American—folk and religious healing practices, herbs, osteopathy, homeopathy

Caution must be taken because medical pluralism is common in self-care. The SGEC has identified three overlapping sectors in health care: the professional sector (organized Western or other healing traditions), the popular sector (self-treatment, family care), and the folk sector (other practitioners and healers).[24] In ethnic families, these sectors frequently overlap and the patient may or may not inform the provider.

Meaning of Health and Illness

In ethnic communities, the source of an illness or medical condition may be attributed to biomedical causes and/or reflect an alternative belief system. For example, in some cultures, illness is believed to be caused by evil spirits or demons rather than disease pathology. The best way to obtain information is to ask the individual. Kleinman recommends the following questions[25]:

1. What do you think caused your problem?
2. Why do you think it started when it did?
3. How does your sickness work on your body?
4. How severe is your sickness?
5. How long do you think it will last?
6. What are the problems your illness has caused you?
7. Do you know others who have had this problem? What did they do to treat it?
8. Do you think there is any way to prevent this problem in the future?

The answers to these questions serve as a basis for adherence to treatment interventions. The health professional should be aware that some medical terms to identify a medical condition may not exist in another language. This is particularly true of mental health problems because of the associated stigma. For example, a study of Vietnamese family caregivers of elders with Alzheimer's disease revealed there was no word in Vietnamese for dementia and the symptoms were considered a normal part of aging.[26] Similar findings were noted among Hispanic family caregivers.[27]

Ethnic Family Caregiving

Caregiving among ethnic families has not been well studied. However, ethnic family caregivers describe a cultural mandate toward eldercare at home, regardless of the circumstances, as a result of values such as filial piety (duty or obligation for parental care). Thus, placing an elder in a nursing home may be perceived as abandonment, an act that brings shame upon the family unit.

The degree of stress/burden experienced by a family caregiver depends on a number of factors. These mitigating factors include the family relationships such as the strength of the bond between the caregiver and care recipient and the express needs of the elder such as type of care, intensity, duration, and prognosis. Caregiver needs are also important such as willingness to provide care, available time, other family/work commitments, financial means, skill level, social and other support, personality, and acculturation. In general, although ethnic families desire to care for their elders at home, the demands of modern society may discourage eldercare.[10]

Depending on the ethnic group, there may even be a reluctance to use available services. Support groups may be perceived as discussing private family matters in public. Respite care may be linked to shirking responsibility. Other caregivers may feel guilty for seeking assistance.

Elder Abuse

There is a paucity of information on elder abuse (EA) in ethnic communities. Overall, incidence of mistreatment is underreported, particularly if the perpetrators are family members.[28] Other reporting problems are systemic, such as the absence of a consistent definition for EA across states.

In the mainstream U.S. population, the primary forms of EA are physical, psychological, emotional, financial, verbal, neglect, and self-neglect with physical abuse being the most common. Elder mistreatment is caused by a web of factors such as lack of information about EA, caregiver stress/burden, dysfunctional family relationships (retaliation, unresolved conflicts, lack of close bonds), exploitation caused by economics, mental illness (substance abuse), and vulnerability.[29] There is a belief that EA does not exist in ethnic communities because of the respect for elders taught early in life. This is not true because elder mistreatment can occur in any family, but the type of abuse may vary.

Generally speaking, ethnic elders live with family members because of cultural values such as filial piety, love, and respect; economic necessity; and poor health. The expectations for family care make it difficult for an elder to believe that a relative would take advantage of his or her dependence and vulnerability.[28] Ethnic elders are reluctant to report mistreatment and tend to consider the intent, circumstances, and nature of the harm and ultimately condone abusive behaviors to avoid bringing shame upon the family. Elders may also have different perceptions of abuse.[28] For example, in a study using hypothetical vignettes, a Korean adult child could spend a parent's money without permission, which is considered financial abuse in the United States. However, the parent may condone the act because (1) the child must have needed the money badly or for a very good reason, and (2) the adult child will inherit the money anyway.[30] There is also evidence that psychological and emotional abuse is more common in some ethnic families. Tomita found that persistent extreme silence was used by one Japanese daughter-in-law, which literally stripped her mother-in-law of personhood within the family.[31]

There is a need for outreach and education about EA among ethnic families and providers and improvements in the service delivery system.[28] Because of the complexity involved in such EA cases, creative and culturally appropriate interventions must be developed and used. Furthermore, cultural and family values and relationships must be considered and incorporated into EA interventions such as ways to overcome the stigma of having private family matters addressed by outsiders.

Spirituality

Spirituality is discussed at length in Chapter 14. Similar to mainstream populations, ethnic elders come from a wide array of religious traditions and belief systems. In assessing an ethnic elder, a GCM must use a holistic approach that considers the mind, body, and spirit; this necessitates some assessment of spiritual practices and beliefs.[32]

Spirituality is most important to quality of life because it defines a meaningful life and gives an individual's existence value and purpose.[32] Many ethnic families rely on spirituality when faced with adversity, and it can serve as a coping mechanism and provide support, hope, comfort, and guidance. Some health care providers believe that spiritual support assists in the healing process.

The role of spirituality appears to be similar across cultures. As mentioned previously, the best way to assess spirituality is to ask the client. What is important in life? What about the future? How is quality of life defined? This interaction can enhance the quality of an ethnic elder's existence.

Health Literacy

Another area of growing concern in ethnic communities is *health literacy*—the skills to access, read, process, understand, communicate, and act upon basic health information to make informed health and long-term-care decisions.[33] An increasing body of research exists on this topic; however, very little attention has been paid to older immigrant populations. The GCM must have some indication of the health literacy skills of the ethnic client, particularly if recommendations to health care providers and other services are to be made.

The goals of health literacy extend beyond simply having educational materials translated into other languages. Monolingual, non-English-speaking clients may be unable to make medical appointments, use public transportation, understand insurance benefits and billings, comprehend directions, read instructions for a treatment regimen, and/or to report back on progress.[34] Some ethnic elders are functionally illiterate in their native countries, unable to read or write in any language—some languages have no written form. Particularly troublesome are cases involving informed consent because the medical terminology and concepts are daunting to older adults.

Current efforts to improve health literacy in foreign-born populations include increasing practical health literacy topics in English as a Second Language (ESL) courses, providing tutors to assist in teaching health communication, and developing materials using different media (e.g., videos, audiotapes) to accommodate varied learning styles. Immigrant elders also require assistance navigating the complex U.S. health care system. One frustration is the insufficient number of trained, linguistically and culturally competent medical interpreters even though federal law requires an interpreter be available in all settings that accept federal funds. Although telephone language banks are increasingly available, they may lack regional familiarity and personal attention required in medical encounters.[35] This is particularly important when body language and other indirect forms of communication are necessary for accurate diagnosis and treatment. The GCM can advocate for professional interpreters on behalf of ethnic clients and their families.

■ BARRIERS TO SERVICES AND PROGRAMS

Ethnic elders frequently encounter barriers to services and programs that tend to be structural or conceptual.[4] Structural barriers are built into the bureaucracy and include affordability and the high costs of health/social services; the absence or availability of services in ethnic communities; access issues such as inconvenient hours; low-quality services; the lack of information and outreach; and service providers that disregard diversity. Conceptual barriers are the personally unacceptable and inappropriate aspects of the service delivery system. Conceptual barriers include sociocultural factors (e.g., personal preferences); discrimination or prejudice experienced in the past; lack of knowledge about available options such as screenings to prevent illness; attitudes toward the use of various services; and the culture of

the health/social services systems per se. These barriers prevent ethnic elders from having access to needed quality services.

■ RECOMMENDATIONS

The following recommendations for the GCM can enhance the quality and appropriateness of geriatric care management services.

- Ask questions about the personal preferences and specific needs of ethnic elders; listen closely to their responses.
- Be aware of your own values, biases, and gaps in knowledge about ethnic aging.
- Learn as much as possible about the backgrounds of the ethnic clients.
- Be sensitive and accepting of differences in values, beliefs, and behaviors.
- Use trained language interpreters and cultural guides if necessary.
- Modify assessment instruments to incorporate personal experiences, beliefs, and needs of ethnic families.
- Refer clients to culturally competent service providers.
- Advocate for education, outreach, information/referral in ethnic communities.

CASE STUDY

Objectives

1. The first objective of this case study is to illustrate the sensitivity to cultural differences that the GCM must have when working with an ethnic client. The GCM must be sensitive to traditional cultural practices such as the Japanese way of showing gratitude to those who provide assistance or services.

2. The second objective is to show that the GCM working with an ethnically diverse client may maximize the use of community resources (both mainstream and ethnic-specific) to

accommodate the client's needs and preferences.

In October 2004, a discharge planner from the ABC Hospital called the professional GCM at the Japanese American Senior Agency (JASA), a culturally sensitive social service agency for older adults, to ask for assistance in finding a caregiver for Mr. Ken Takaki. The hospital received a call from a Dr. Bob Edward, Mr. Takaki's friend, reporting that the caregivers from the local home care agencies were not meeting Mr. Takaki's needs. Mr. Takaki did not feel comfortable with the caregivers (ethnic/racial issues), and he was not used to eating the food that the caregivers prepared for him (food preference issues). Mr. Takaki prepared only Japanese food and was not fond of American food.

Mr. Takaki was an 84-year-old *Nisei*, a second-generation Japanese American. His *Issei* (first-generation) parents immigrated to Hawaii, where Mr. Takaki was born. He was bilingual and spoke Japanese with his parents and English among his friends. After his father's death when he was 15, Mr. Takaki left Honolulu and moved to California with his mother in search of a better-paying job. World War II broke out in 1942 and all people of Japanese descent living on the West Coast were incarcerated in War Relocation Authority camps. Mr. Takaki and his mother were no exception and were evacuated to Topaz, Utah.

In 1946, after returning to San Francisco from the camp, his mother became very frail and needed constant care at home. Mr. Takaki took a job as a janitor cleaning a dental office near his home at night for Dr. Edward, which enabled Mr. Takaki to care for his mother during the day. Mr. Takaki never married and lived with his mother until she passed away peacefully at the age of 74. He worked for Dr. Edward until the doctor retired in 2000. Although Mr. Takaki had a heart attack in 1987 at the age of 65, he continued working. He had very little social life, and his only enjoyment was an annual week-long trip to Reno. In September 2003, he found blood in his urine and in December 2003, he had a prostatectomy. Mr. Takaki stayed at a local board and care facility, RN Home, for six months and was discharged on July 1, 2004.

The JASA GCM referred Mr. Takaki and Dr. Edward to several Japanese caregivers, who were bilingual in Japanese and English and could cook Japanese food. Dr. Edward contacted the first caregiver, Ms. Chieko Saito, and they both interviewed her at Mr. Takaki's residence. Both liked her and hired her, four hours a day, twice a week starting right away. She was to do the housekeeping and laundry, shopping, food preparation, medication reminders, assist with walking, and so forth.

Mr. Takaki was very pleased with Ms. Saito's services. However, after a couple of weeks, Ms. Saito called JASA and reported that Mr. Takaki bought food for her every time they went grocery shopping, spending twice the amount of money he should. She did not feel comfortable taking groceries from him. If she refused the food, he did not buy his own groceries. Ms. Saito was aware that Mr. Takaki was on a fixed income; however, he used his ATM card. Mr. Takaki's attitude reflected the traditional Japanese custom of showing gratitude to those who provide services even though Ms. Saito was paid to provide care.

After discussion with Dr. Edward, who had Mr. Takaki's power of attorney for finances and health care, a care plan was developed that used both mainstream and Japanese community services. Meals-on-Wheels and JASA's home-delivered Asian meals fulfilled Mr. Takaki's dietary needs, thereby eliminating Ms. Saito's cooking responsibilities. She did not have to take him grocery shopping, which eliminated his excess spending. Ms. Saito no longer felt guilty and Mr. Takaki's independence remained intact. Mr. Takaki continued to be ambulatory and exercised by walking four long blocks four times alone. He was engaged in the community, read the Japanese newspaper, watched Japanese TV programs, and rented Japanese videos.

In January 2006, JASA received a call from Dr. Edward that Mr. Takaki was rushed to ABC Hospital because he became disoriented while at a nearby restaurant. His cognition appeared to be declining and he required 24-hour care. Dr. Edward asked JASA if there were any Japanese care homes for Mr. Takaki. A few facilities were Japanese-owned; however, there were no vacancies at that time. Dr. Edward and the JASA GCM visited a board and care facility, Grace's Care Home, and arranged for Mr. Takaki's care. While there, the home tried to accommodate his personal preferences—he continued to receive the Japanese newspaper, watched Japanese TV, and the Filipino caregiver cooked Asian, but not Japanese, food at least three times a week.

For about a month, there was no problem and Mr. Takaki seemed happy with his new home. The Filipino caregiver took him out three times a week for a walk. However, Mr. Takaki became bored with the suburban environment where his care home was located. He was used to walking around his house daily, which was in the center of the city. He also missed his favorite Japanese foods and videos. To further accommodate Mr. Takaki's needs, a new care plan was established whereby the JASA GCM located some nearby Japanese/Asian grocery stores, listed his favorite Japanese foods in both Japanese and English, and asked the caregiver to buy and prepare some of the food for him. The JASA GCM arranged with a Japanese video store to mail a list of available Japanese videos to Mr. Takaki, so he could order the ones of interest. The JASA GCM also contacted the local county library to mail a list of its Japanese books. Mr. Takaki could call the library for a monthly bookmobile delivery to his care home. Mr. Takaki was occupied watching Japanese videos, reading Japanese books, and enjoying a taste of Japanese food.

The next step was to motivate Mr. Takaki to do some activities outside the care home to maintain his ambulatory abilities and avoid further decline.

Conclusion

1. The JASA GCM working with this ethnic client was sensitive to traditional cultural practices. Traditionally, Japanese people express their gratitude to service providers and others. In Mr. Takaki's case, buying groceries for Ms. Saito was probably the only way he could express his appreciation even though he paid for her services. To avoid Mr. Takaki's overspending, the JASA GCM changed Ms. Saito's responsibilities for meal planning/cooking by substituting community programs (mainstream and ethnic home-delivered meals).

2. The GCM working with an ethnic client must use community resources (both mainstream and ethnic). To meet the needs of a homebound elder is always a challenge. However, if the elder is from a different ethnic/cul-

tural group, it can be a daunting task depending on the barriers faced by the client and the providers. Although Mr. Takaki did not have any language barrier, he still preferred Japanese foods and activities, which the GCM considered in the assessment. To satisfy and fulfill Mr. Takaki's needs, the GCM hired a Japanese-speaking caregiver; requested both mainstream and ethnic home-delivered meals; arranged for a subscription to an ethnic newspaper; used a Japanese video mail service; arranged for a bookmobile delivery from the local library; and gave instructions to the Filipino caregiver about purchasing and preparing the client's favorite Japanese foods.

CARE MONITORING

Objectives

1. The first objective of this case is to illustrate that, ideally, a GCM working with an ethnic client should speak the client's language and have an understanding of the client's cultural background and preferences.
2. The second objective is to show that the GCM should be aware of available agencies and resources that serve various ethnic communities.

Ms. Debbie Martin, discharge planner at Richmond Hospital, called the JASA about Mr. Jiro Ikeda. Mr. Ikeda was hospitalized after a neighbor found him disoriented in his truck in front of his home. He was diagnosed with dehydration caused by heat exhaustion and fatigue. Mr. Ikeda was a 74-year-old Japanese *Shin-Issei* (newcomer) who came to the United States as a typhoon

refugee after the Immigration and Naturalization Services Act of 1965, which increased Asian immigrant quotas. He graduated from a Japanese high school. Although he had been living in the United States for more than 40 years, he could not understand, speak, or write in English because of his limited social network of Japanese-speaking associates. He worked as a gardener all his life, never married, lived alone in a small rented house, and had no social life. Mr. Ikeda had no relatives in the United States.

According to Ms. Martin, Mr. Ikeda was very cooperative at the hospital, followed doctors' directions, and was well-liked. His only support system appeared to be his employee, Mr. Jorge Martinez, who worked for Mr. Ikeda for seven years. While Mr. Ikeda was in the hospital, Mr. Martinez took care of Mr. Ikeda's business and house, along with a friend, Ms. Elena Sanchez. Mr. Martinez was from Mexico and Ms. Sanchez came from Honduras. Mr. Martinez could not read or write in either Spanish or English and Ms. Sanchez had limited English language capability, and most of the time, they communicated in Spanish. Mr. Martinez and Ms. Sanchez had purchased a three-bedroom house and were willing to take Mr. Ikeda in as soon as the house was available. They were not planning to charge Mr. Ikeda any rent because he had given Mr. Martinez all his customers.

The JASA GCM, who was bilingual in Japanese and English, met with Ms. Martin, Mr. Ikeda, Mr. Martinez, and Ms. Sanchez at the hospital. Mr. Ikeda had had a thorough psychosocial assessment, and the GCM also did a functional assessment. Ms. Martin explained Mr. Ikeda's physical and psychological status in English and limited Spanish. Mr. Ikeda's physical condition was good and he was ambulatory. His cognition was fair, although he sometimes became confused and had mild dementia. He also needed assistance with some instrumental activities of daily living (IADLs). They concluded that Mr. Ikeda was ready to be discharged as long as he had 24-hour care. After thorough discussion, agreement was made on the following care options:

1. The GCM would do a home assessment and, if it was acceptable and safe to return home, the GCM would recommend a Japanese-speaking caregiver from JASA's caregiver directory two times a week, four hours a day until Mr. Ikeda's condition improved. The other three days, Mr. Martinez would have Mr. Ikeda accompany him on his job, so that Mr. Ikeda could give advice. On weekends, both Mr. Martinez and Ms. Sanchez would watch over Mr. Ikeda. Payment would be discussed at a later time.
2. If his home was not safe enough for Mr. Ikeda to live by himself, the GCM would search for a board and care facility to aid in Mr. Ikeda's recovery.

Mr. Ikeda did not remember how much money he had in the bank. The JASA GCM contacted Ms. Maria Lopez, at Kyoto Bank, to get Mr. Ikeda's account information. Ms. Lopez, who spoke Spanish, also agreed to be a translator for Mr. Martinez and Ms. Sanchez to help Mr. Ikeda.

The GCM made a care monitoring and assessment visit. The condition of the house was totally uninhabitable and the house was located between several busy streets, which posed a health hazard. Windows were broken and walls

were damaged. None of the utilities were functioning. Therefore, the first plan was not an option.

The GCM informed Mr. Ikeda that he could not go back to his old home and that he needed to move out of the house. The GCM located a facility, Sierra Home, which accepted tenants for respite care on a monthly basis at a fixed rate ($2,000). Mr. Ikeda agreed to move into the care home when he was discharged from the hospital.

As soon as Mr. Ikeda moved, the GCM received several calls from the owner, Mr. Ray Chang, complaining that Mr. Ikeda did not sleep at night and moved furniture around. He was also incontinent and needed to wear pads. This information was all new to the GCM because the discharge planner had not mentioned these problems.

The GCM made a care monitoring visit to Mr. Ikeda the next day. Mr. Ikeda explained it would take a month to get used to the new place. He did not know why he could not get to the bathroom on time. He liked the food and had no problems. Mr. Chang said he would take Mr. Ikeda to his doctor and have him prescribe medication to help him sleep through the night.

A few days later, the GCM received another call from Mr. Chang reporting that Mr. Ikeda was taken to the doctor, but that he was still wandering and incontinent. Mr. Chang said that Mr. Ikeda wore a diaper, only to tear it off during the night and urinate on the floor. The GCM visited Mr. Ikeda again only to find out that because of his Japanese cultural background, he was not honest in his initial response. In Japan, information that might hurt someone else's feelings should be withheld, particularly if the person is trying to help (*enryo*). However, Mr. Ikeda's behavior revealed his true feelings. He actually did not want to stay in the home because he was uncomfortable with the Asian caregiver.

Mr. Ikeda stated that he wanted to move out of Sierra Home and move in with Mr. Martinez. To make sure that Mr. Martinez and Ms. Sanchez were responsible individuals, the GCM contacted Ms. Lopez from Kyoto Bank to act as a translator. Ms. Lopez, Mr. Martinez, Ms. Sanchez, and the GCM had a meeting. Mr. Martinez left Mr. Ikeda's checkbook with Ms. Lopez. Mr. Martinez explained their intent to care for Mr. Ikeda in their new house, but he did not want to assume the responsibility for Mr. Ikeda's financial matters. The following care plan was developed.

1. Mr. Ikeda would move in with Mr. Martinez. Ms. Sanchez was to care for Mr. Ikeda on Mondays, Tuesdays, and Thursdays, and Mr. Martinez would watch over him on Wednesdays and Fridays. Both would share the responsibilities on weekends.
2. Maria was to keep Mr. Ikeda's checkbook and the JASA GCM was to help with check writing until other options could be investigated.

A couple of days after Mr. Ikeda moved, the GCM made a care monitoring visit. Mr. Ikeda looked happier and was cleaner. The house was spacious, clean, and orderly. However, Mr. Martinez reported that Mr. Ikeda did not sleep well and was incontinent at night. The GCM made an appointment with Mr. Ikeda's primary care physician and accompanied him to the doctor.

Subsequently, the GCM proposed that JASA become Mr. Ikeda's representative payee and also became Mr. Ikeda's agent for his durable power of attorney for finances and health care.

■ RESOURCES

The following are resources for further information about ethnicity, aging, and health. However, this is not a comprehensive listing of all that is available.

1. Stanford Geriatric Education Center
   c/o VAPAHCS
   3801 Miranda Avenue, Building 4
   (182B-SGEC)
   Palo Alto, CA 94304
   Phone (650) 494-3986; fax (650) 494-3617
   http://sgec.stanford.edu

   Materials available:
   a. Preventive screenings recommended for all elders
   b. Immunization and prophylaxis recommended for all elders
   c. Counseling recommended for all elders
   d. Examples of translated standardized instruments
   e. Monographs and curriculum materials on aging, ethnicity, and health in specific disciplines (nutrition, social work, spirituality, and many other fields)

2. Cross Cultural Health Program (cross-cultural health care and training programs for medical interpreters)
   http://www.xculture.org/index.cfm

3. Culture Clues (tip sheets designed for clinicians)
   http://depts..washington.edu/pfes/cultureclues.html

4. Diversity Rx (promotes language and cultural competence to improve quality of health care)
   http://www.diversityrx.org

5. Ethnomed
   http://ethnomed.org/

6. Health Literacy Resource Center (health literacy information and training)
   http://www.cahealthliteracy.org/healthliteracyresourcecenter.html

7. Office of Minority Health Resource Center
   http://www.omhrc.gov
   1-800-444-6472

8. World Education (English as a Second Language resources for health professionals and others)
   http://www.worlded.org

■ INTRODUCTION TO ASSESSMENT AND PLAN OF CARE FORMS

The following Initial Assessment and Plan of Care Forms (Exhibits 6-1 and 6-2) are based on several existing geriatric care management tools currently used by both mainstream and ethnic-specific social service agencies and geriatric care management providers. These instruments were created for use with ethnic elders, including recent immigrants. The forms are comprehensive, but not all inclusive, because it is impossible to include all the different ethnic/cultural groups in one template. The purpose of these samples is to stimulate awareness of the diversity found in the elderly population and increase sensitivity to differences that exist.

The following Web sites can help the GCM to reflect upon his or her own cultural competence:

http://www.aafp.org/fpm/20001000/58cult.html
http://www.ncccurricula.info/assessment/index.html

Exhibit 6-1   **Initial Assessment Form**

Date: _____

Client Name: First: _____   Middle: _____   Last: _____

How to Address Client: _____

How Client's Family Members Address Client: _____

DOB: _____   Sex: ❑ Male   ❑ Female

Ethnicity/Race: _____

Street Address: _____

City: _____   State: _____   Zip: _____

Phone Numbers: Home: (   ) _____   Cell: (   ) _____

Live Alone: ❑ Yes   ❑ No   Marital Status: _____

Client needs assistance in: ADL   ❑ Eating   IADL   ❑ Preparing meals
                                    ❑ Dressing   ❑ Shopping
                                    ❑ Bathing   ❑ Managing medications
                                    ❑ Toileting   ❑ Managing money
                                    ❑ Getting in/out of bed   ❑ Using telephone
                                    ❑ Walking   ❑ Doing heavy housework
                                                               ❑ Doing light housework
                                                               ❑ Transportation ability

Primary Language: _____   Secondary Language: _____

Language Proficiency:

English:	❑ Good	❑ Fair	❑ Not good
Primary Language:	❑ Good	❑ Fair	❑ Not good
Secondary Language:	❑ Good	❑ Fair	❑ Not good

Exhibit 6–1   Initial Assessment Form (continued)

Educational Level: Home Country: _____ Years   In the U.S.: _____ Years

Interpreter Need: ❑ Yes   ❑ No

Interpreter Availability: ❑ Yes   If yes, who would it be? _____
                             ❑ No

Place (Country) of Birth: ❑ U.S.A.   ❑ Other   If other, which country? _____
                             Year when client moved to the U.S.: _____
                             Age when client immigrated to the U.S.:   _____ years old
                             Reasons of immigration: _____

Cultural Needs: _____

Food Preferences (including Ethnic Food): _____

Dietary Needs: _____

Religious Preferences: _____

Emergency Contact Name: _____   Relationship: _____
Address: _____   Phone: (   ) _____
City: _____   State: _____   Zip: _____

Emergency Contact Name: _____   Relationship: _____
Address: _____   Phone: (   ) _____
City: _____   State: _____   Zip: _____

Caregiver Name: _____   Relationship: _____
Address: _____   Phone: (   ) _____
City: _____   State: _____   Zip: _____

Financial Resources: ❑ Social security   ❑ Supplementary security income (SSI)
                        ❑ Pension   ❑ Help from family members
                        ❑ Other

Insurance: ❑ Medicare   Policy #: _____
                        ❑ Private Health Insurance   Policy #: _____
                        ❑ Private Dental Insurance   Policy #: _____
                        ❑ Long-term Care Insurance   Policy #: _____
                        ❑ Other   Policy #: _____

Hobbies: Currently enjoy doing: _____
                        Used to enjoy doing: _____
                        Family activities: _____

Reasons for the initial contact:
_____
_____
_____
_____
_____

Exhibit 6-2   Plan of Care Form

Date: _____

Name of Client: _____

Name of Care Manager: _____

Name of Agency: _____

Address: _____

Phone Number: ( ) _____   Cell Number: ( ) _____

Fax Number: ( ) _____   E-mail: _____

Ethnicity/Race of Care Manager: _____

Linguistic competency besides English: _____
(Name of Language)
❏ Speak ❏ Read ❏ Write

Name of Social Worker: _____

Name of Agency: _____

Address: _____

Phone Number: ( ) _____   Cell Number: ( ) _____

Fax Number: ( ) _____   E-mail: _____

Ethnicity/Race of Social Worker: _____

Linguistic competency besides English: _____
(Name of Language)
❏ Speak ❏ Read ❏ Write

Client - Personal Information

Client Name: First: _____ Middle: _____ Last: _____

How does the client prefer to be addressed? _____

How does the client's family address him/her? _____

DOB: _____   Sex: ❏ Male ❏ Female

Ethnicity/Race: _____

Street Address: _____

City: _____   State: _____   Zip: _____

Phone Numbers: Home: ( ) _____   Cell: ( ) _____

Former Occupation: U.S.A. _____   Other than U.S.A. _____

Live Alone: ❏ Yes ❏ No   Marital Status: _____

Other Living Arrangement: _____
_____
_____
_____

Exhibit 6–2   Plan of Care Form (continued)

Has the client had any change in residence in the past year?   ❏ Yes   ❏ No

If yes, how and why? _____

Does the client wish to remain at home?   ❏ Yes   ❏ No

Has the client had any life event or traumatic experience
in the past year (hospitalization, move, etc.)?   ❏ Yes   ❏ No

If yes, what, when and why? _____

Names, Addresses, and Phone Numbers of Children:

Name: _____   Relationship: _____
Address: _____   Phone: ( ) _____
City: _____ State: _____   Zip: _____

Name: _____   Relationship: _____
Address: _____   Phone: ( ) _____
City: _____ State: _____   Zip: _____

Name: _____   Relationship: _____
Address: _____   Phone: ( ) _____
City: _____ State: _____   Zip: _____

Current Care Arrangements among Family Members: _____
_____
_____
_____

Preferable Language: _____
Interpreter needed: ❏ Yes   ❏ No
Names of Interpreters: _____
Cultural Needs: _____
Food Preferences (including Ethnic Food): _____
Dietary Needs: _____
Religious Preferences: _____

Emergency Contact Name: _____   Relationship: _____
Address: _____   Phone: ( ) _____
City: _____ State: _____   Zip: _____

Emergency Contact Name: _____   Relationship: _____
Address: _____   Phone: ( ) _____
City: _____ State: _____   Zip: _____

Caregiver Name: _____   Relationship: _____
Address: _____   Phone: ( ) _____
City: _____ State: _____   Zip: _____

continues

Exhibit 6–2   Plan of Care Form (continued)

Medical Information

Primary Physician: _____   Phone: ( ) _____

Hospital: _____   Phone: ( ) _____

Interpreter Available: ❏ Yes ❏ No

Dentist: _____   Phone: ( ) _____

Interpreter Available: ❏ Yes ❏ No

Pharmacy: _____   Phone: ( ) _____

Interpreter Available: ❏ Yes ❏ No

Name of Health Insurance: _____
Address: _____
Phone Number: ( ) _____   Fax Number: ( ) _____
Policy #: _____

Name of Dental Insurance: _____
Address: _____
Phone Number: ( ) _____   Fax Number: ( ) _____
Policy #: _____

Name of Long-term Care Insurance: _____
Address: _____
Phone Number: ( ) _____   Fax Number: ( ) _____
Policy #: _____

Physical Health Symptoms: _____
_____
_____

Mental/Cognitive Symptoms: _____
_____
_____

Scheduled Medication

Name of Medication	Dosage	Time of Day	Instruction

Exhibit 6–2   Plan of Care Form (continued)

Does the client have a Durable Power of Attorney for Health Care? ❑ Yes ❑ No

    Name of the person/agent: _____ Relationship: _____

    Address: _____

    Phone Number: ( ) _____ Fax Number: ( ) _____

If no, who will make the client's health care decisions?

    Name of the person: _____ Relationship: _____

    Address: _____

    Phone Number: ( ) _____

    Name of the person: _____ Relationship: _____

    Address: _____

    Phone Number: ( ) _____

Does the client have a Do-Not-Resuscitate Order (DNR)? ❑ Yes ❑ No

If no, who will make decisions on behalf of the client?

    Name of the person: _____ Relationship: _____

    Address: _____

    Phone Number: ( ) _____

    Name of the person: _____ Relationship: _____

    Address: _____

    Phone Number: ( ) _____

Personal Care

	Needs Assist	Devices
Ambulation		
Bathing		
Dressing		
Feeding		
Foot Care		
Grooming		
Medication		
Oral Care		
Skin Care		
Toileting		
Transfers		
Vision Care		
Other Care		

continues

Exhibit 6–2   Plan of Care Form (continued)

Meal Preparation

Food Preferences (including ethnic food): _____

_____

Dietary Needs: _____

_____

Breakfast: _____
        Time: _____
        Eating Arrangements: _____
Lunch: _____
        Time: _____
        Eating Arrangements: _____
Dinner: _____
        Time: _____
        Eating Arrangements: _____
Snacks: _____
        Time: _____
        Eating Arrangements: _____
Meals-on-Wheels (MOW) requested?   ❑ Yes   ❑ No

        MOW: ❑ Yes   ❑ No   Which days? _____

        Ethnic MOW: ❑ Yes   ❑ No   Which days? _____

Is the client able to receive MOW without assistance?   ❑ Yes   ❑ No

Time of MOW delivery: MOW: _____   Ethnic MOW: _____

Additional Meal Instructions:_____

_____

Housework

	Need Assist	Frequency/Instructions
Dishwashing		
Dusting		
Kitchen cleaning		
Bathroom cleaning		
Floor cleaning		
Laundry		
Vacuuming		
Other Housework		
Other Housework		

Exhibit 6–2   Plan of Care Form (continued)

Schedule of Activities

Daily Activities:

    Morning: _____

    Afternoon: _____

Hobbies: _____

_____

Outside Group Activities: _____

_____

Religious Activities: _____

_____

Exercises: _____

_____

Additional Arrangements (such as ethnic video, mobile book programs, etc.):

_____

_____

_____

Finances

Is the client able to manage his/her finances without assistance?   ❏ Yes   ❏ No

Does the client have agents (representative payee, conservator, power of attorney for finances, etc.)

    Finances?   ❏ Yes   ❏ No

    Name of the person/agent: _____   Relationship: _____

    Address: _____

    Phone Number: (   ) _____   Fax Number: (   ) _____

If no, who makes financial decisions for the client?

    Name of the person: _____   Relationship: _____

    Address: _____

    Phone Number: (   ) _____

    Name of the person: _____   Relationship: _____

    Address: _____

    Phone Number: (   ) _____

■ CONCLUSION

The objective of this chapter is to increase awareness of the complexity of issues and barriers that confront ethnic elders and their families today. Immigrant elders and their families are unique additions to the tapestry of life in the United States, and this cultural pluralism has contributed much to our society. For the GCM to render appropriate assistance to this diverse population requires knowledge about the backgrounds, beliefs, and preferences of ethnic clients and highly developed skills to guide them in the right direction.

■ NOTES

1. US Census Bureau. *Census 2000 Summary File 1 (SF1) 100-Percent Data.* Washington, DC: US Census Bureau; 2000.

2. US Census Bureau. *We the People: Aging in the United States. Census 2000 Special Reports.* Washington, DC: US Census Bureau; 2004.

3. Levinson D, Ember M. *American Immigrant Cultures: Builders of a Nation.* New York: Simon and Schuster Macmillan; 1997.

4. Kagawa-Singer M, Hikoyeda N, Tanjasiri SP. Aging, chronic conditions, and physical disabilities in Asian Pacific Islander Americans. In: Markides KS, Miranda MR, eds. *Minorities, Aging, and Health.* Thousand Oaks, CA: Sage Publications; 1997:149–180.

5. Mutran E, Sudha S. Ethnic and racial groups, similar or different, and how do we measure? *Res Aging.* 2000;22(6):589–598.

6. Spector RE. *Cultural Diversity in Health and Illness.* 5th ed. Upper Saddle River, NJ: Prentice Hall Health; 2000.

7. Barresi CM, Stull DE. *Ethnic Elderly and Long-Term Care.* New York: Springer Publishing; 1993.

8. Kitano HHL. *Generations and Identity: The Japanese American.* Needham Heights, MA: Ginn Press; 1993.

9. Yeo G, Hikoyeda N, McBride M, Chin S-Y, Edmonds M, Hendrix L. *Cohort Analysis as a Tool in Ethnogeriatrics: Historical Profiles of Elders from Eight Ethnic Populations in the United States.* Palo Alto, CA: Stanford Geriatric Education Center; 1998.

10. Hikoyeda N, Wallace SP. Do ethnic-specific long term care facilities improve resident quality of life? In: Choi NG, ed. *Social Work Practice with the Asian American Elderly.* New York: Haworth Press; 2001:63–82.

11. Morioka-Douglas N, Sacks T, Yeo G. Issues in caring for Afghan American elders: insights from literature and a focus group. *J Cross-Cultural Gerontol.* 2004;19:27–40.

12. Fugita SS, O'Brien DJ. *Japanese American Ethnicity: The Persistence of Community.* Seattle, WA: University of Washington Press; 1991.

13. McBride MR, Morioka-Douglas N, Yeo G. *Aging and Health: Asian and Pacific Islander American Elders.* Palo Alto, CA: Stanford Geriatric Education Center; 1996.

14. Braun KL, Pietsch JH, Blanchette PL. *Cultural Issues in End-of-Life Decision Making.* Thousand Oaks, CA: Sage Publications; 2000.

15. Bulatao RA, Anderson NA. Racial and ethnic disparities in health and mortality among the US elderly population. In: Anderson NA, Bulatao RA, Cohen B, eds. *Critical Perspectives on Racial and Ethnic Differences in Health in Later Life.* Washington, DC: National Academies Press; 2004.

16. Hummer R, Benjamin MR, Rogers RG. Racial and ethnic disparities in health and mortality among the US elderly population. In: Anderson NA, Bulatao RA, Cohen B, eds. *Critical Perspectives on Racial and Ethnic Differences in Health in Later Life.* Washington, DC: National Academies Press; 2004.

17. Hayward MD, Crimmins EM, Miles TP, Yang Y. The significance of socioeconomic status in explaining the racial gap in chronic health conditions. *Am Sociol Rev.* 2000;65:910–930.

18. Pleis JR, Coles R. Summary health statistics for US adults: National Health Interview Survey, 1998. *Vital Health Stat.* 2002;10:209.

19. Manly JJ, Mayeux R. Ethnic differences in dementia and Alzheimer's disease. In: Anderson NA, Bulatao RA, Cohen B, eds. *Critical Perspectives on Racial and Ethnic Differences in Health in Later Life.* Washington, DC: National Academies Press; 2004.

20. McCabe M, Cuellar J. *Aging and Health: American Indian/Alaska Native Elders.* 2nd ed. Palo Alto, CA: Stanford Geriatric Education Center; 1994.

21. Kuo WH, Porter K. Health status of Asian Americans: United States, 1992–04. *Advance Data from Vital Health Statistics*, No. 298. Hyattsville, MD: National Center for Health Statistics; 1998.

22. Hoyert DL, Kung H. Asian or Pacific Islander mortality, selected states, 1992. *Mon Vital Stat Rep.* 1997;45(suppl 1): 1-64.

23. Miller B, Kolonel L, Bernstein L, Young Jr JL, Swanson G, West D, et al. *Racial/Ethnic Patterns of Cancer in the United States, 1988–1992.* Bethesda, MD: National Cancer Institute; 1996. NIH Pub. No. 96-4101.

24. Levkoff S, Chee YK, Reynoloso-Vallejo H, Mendez J. Culturally appropriate geriatric care: fund of knowledge. In: Yeo G, ed. *Core Curriculum in Ethnogeriatrics.* 2nd ed. Palo Alto, CA: Stanford Geriatric Education Center; 2000.

25. Kleinman A. *Patients and Healers in the Context of Culture.* Berkeley, CA: University of California Press; 1980.

26. Yeo G, Tran JNU, Hikoyeda N, Hinton L. Conceptions of dementia among Vietnamese American caregivers. In: Choi NG, ed. *Social Work Practice with the Asian American Elderly.* New York: Haworth Press; 2001:131–154.

27. Villa ML, Cuellar J, Gamel N, Yeo G. *Aging and Health: Hispanic American Elders.* 2nd ed. Palo Alto, CA: Stanford Geriatric Education Center; 1993.

28. Tatara T. *Understanding Elder Abuse in Minority Populations.* Philadelphia: Brunner/Mazel; 1999.

29. Rittman M, Kuzmeskus LB, Flum MA. A synthesis of current knowledge on minority elder abuse. In: Tatara T, ed. *Understanding Elder Abuse in Minority Populations.* Philadelphia: Brunner/Mazel; 1999:221–238.

30. Moon A. Elder abuse and neglect among the Korean elderly in the United States. In: Tatara T, ed. *Understanding Elder Abuse in Minority Populations.* Philadelphia: Brunner/Mazel; 1999: 109–118.

31. Tomita SK. Exploration of elder mistreatment among the Japanese. In: Tatara T, ed. *Understanding Elder Abuse in Minority Populations.* Philadelphia: Brunner/Mazel; 1999:119–142.

32. Barton J, Grudzen M, Zielske R. *Vital Connections in Long-Term Care: Spiritual Resources for Staff and Residents.* Baltimore, MD: Health Professions Press; 2003.

33. Ratzan SC, Parker RM. Introduction. In: Selden CR, Zorn M, Ratzan SC, Parker RM, eds. *Natural Library of Medicine Current Bibliographies in Medicine: Health Literacy.* Bethesda, MD: National Institutes of Health; 2000. NLM Pub. No. CBM 2000-1.

34. Williams MV, Parker RM, Baker DW, et al. Inadequate functional health literacy among patients at two public hospitals. *JAMA.* 1995;274(21):1677–1682.

35. Gordon D, Yoshida H, Hikoyeda N, David D. *Patient Listening: Health Communication Needs of Older Immigrants.* Philadelphia: Temple University Center for Intergenerational Learning; 2006.

■ SUGGESTED READINGS

Adler RN, Kamel HK, eds. *Doorway Thoughts: Cross-Cultural Health Care for Older Adults.* Sudbury, MA: Jones and Bartlett Publishers; 2004.

Cress C. *Handbook of Geriatric Care Management.* Gaithersburg, MD: Aspen Publishers; 2001.

Gallo JJ. The content of geriatric care. In: Fulmer T, Gallo JJ, Paveza GJ, eds. *Handbook of Geriatric Assessment.* 3rd ed. Gaithersburg, MD: Aspen Publishers; 2000:1–12.

Goode TD. *Promoting Cultural and Linguistic Competency Self-Assessment Checklist for Personnel Providing Primary Health Care.* Adapted from: *Promoting Cultural Competence and Cultural Diversity for Personnel Providing Services and Supports to Children with Special Health Care Needs and Their Families.* Washington, DC: Georgetown University Center for Child and Human Development; 2004.

Kane RJ, Kane RA, eds. *Assessing Older Persons: Measures, Meaning, and Practical Applications.* New York: Oxford University Press; 2000.

Mouton CP, Esparza YB. Ethnicity and geriatric assessment. In: Fulmer T, Gallo JJ, Paveza GJ et al, eds. *Handbook of Geriatric Assessment.* 3rd ed. Gaithersburg, MD: Aspen Publishers; 2000.

PART 3

The Business of Geriatric Care Management: Beginning, Expanding or Adding, and Managing a Geriatric Care Management Business

CHAPTER 7

How to Start or Add a Geriatric Care Management Business

Cathy Jo Cress

A new geriatric care management business must spring from the intersection of three streams: your passion, your competence, and market opportunity. To start a geriatric care management business, the adage to "know thyself" becomes critical. Are you passionate about geriatric care management? You will need passion to sustain you when the situation gets tough—which it does in all beginning businesses. You must have the core competence *both* to be a geriatric care manager (GCM) and to run a business. Good GCMs with no business acumen frequently fail in business. You must also have the market opportunity. If no older people live in your community, you may not be in the right place to start a geriatric care management business. If 10 other GCMs are practicing in your town, that may limit your own market opportunity. Finally, you need to assess why you want to start this type of business in the first place. Are you motivated by the financial gains? by community recognition? by a need to make a difference? Use Exhibit 7–1 to assess your motivations, abilities, and personality to help you decide whether starting a geriatric care management business is a wise choice for you.

■ ENTREPRENEURIAL RISKS

There are several types of geriatric care management businesses. In 1999, the most common type was the owner-run business. However, new models have appeared, for example, the corporate models of Senior Bridge, LivHOME, and ResCare, which integrate home care and geriatric care management practices. There are also GCM models pairing GCMs in business with physicians, attorneys, and accountants; and GCMs who specialize in such areas as relocation of older adults or death and dying.

This chapter focuses on starting a geriatric care management business and also discusses how to add a geriatric care management practice onto an existing business or not-for-profit agency.

■ STARTING A BUSINESS IN GERIATRIC CARE MANAGEMENT

According to a survey done by the National Association of Professional Geriatric Care Managers in 1997, 80% of all geriatric care management businesses were owner run, and 20% were run by nonowners.[1] Entrepreneurial people who do not mind some risk usually start owner-run businesses. Starting a geriatric care management business is not for the faint

Exhibit 7–1   Know Thyself

Going into business for yourself requires certain personal characteristics. Not everyone is suited to be a business owner. Take some time to think about your motivations, personality, and abilities.

As a first step, ask yourself why you want to own your own business.

1. Freedom from the 9–5 work routine?
2. Being your own boss?
3. Do what you want when you want to do it?
4. Improve your standard of living?
5. Boredom with your present job?
6. Having a product or service for which you feel there is a demand?

Although no answer is wrong, some are better than others. Be aware, however, there are tradeoffs. For example, as a business owner, you can escape the daily 9–5 routine, but you may replace it with a 6 am–10 pm routine.

Do you have the personal characteristics typical to an entrepreneur? Try to be objective in the following self-analysis. Remember, it's your future that is at stake!

1. Are you a leader?
2. Do you like to make your own decisions?
3. Do others turn to you for help in making decisions?
4. Do you enjoy competition?
5. Do you have will power and self discipline?
6. Do you plan ahead?
7. Do you like people?
8. Do you get along well with others?

Think about the physical, emotional, and financial strains you will encounter when you start your new business.

1. Are you aware that running your own business may require working 12–16 hours a day, six days a week, and maybe even Sundays and holidays?
2. Do you have the physical stamina to handle the workload and schedule?
3. Do you have the emotional strength to withstand the strain?
4. Are you prepared, if needed, to temporarily lower your standard of living until your business is firmly established?
5. Is your family prepared to go along with the strains they, too, must bear?
6. Are you prepared to lose your savings?

Certain skills and experience are critical to the success of a small business. Since it is unlikely that you possess all the skills and experience needed, you will need to hire personnel or contract for services to supply those you lack. There are some basic and special skills you will need for your particular business. Identify your strengths and weaknesses with the following questions.

1. Do you know what basic skills you will need to have a successful business?
2. Do you possess those skills?
3. When hiring personnel, will you be able to determine if the applicants' skills meet the requirements for the positions you are filling?
4. Have you ever worked in a managerial or supervisory capacity?
5. Have you ever worked in a business similar to the one you want to start?
6. Have you had any business training?
7. If you discover you don't have the basic skills needed for your business, will you be willing to delay your plans until you've acquired the necessary skills?

of heart. Many new businesses are started every day, only to be boarded shut within a few years.

People considering beginning a geriatric care management business should first find out whether they are comfortable with the level of risk inherent in starting a new business by honestly answering the questions in the self-assessment (Exhibit 7–2). Entrepreneurs share many personality traits, including high energy, aggressiveness, a love of ambiguity, a zest for problem solving, and monumental self-discipline.

After completing the general self-assessment, you should consider whether you are suited to own a business, even if you are an experienced and skilled GCM. In a presentation to the 1998 National GCM Conference in Chicago, Elizabeth Bodie Gross and Linda Fordini Johnson outlined the skills and personality traits GCMs should have as follows[2]:

- Have they worked as care managers? Have they worked with older adults or had education or training in geriatrics or gerontology? These experiences help prospective GCMs know what to expect and whether they like the work.
- Do they have a business background? Do they know accounting, have they ever had to meet a payroll, and can they tolerate not being paid the first few

years? Can they do another job while also being a GCM? Many budding GCMs hold other jobs for years until their geriatric care management practice can make enough money to support them.

- Do they have the energy to run a 24-hour-a-day, 7-day-a-week business? Can their family tolerate calls night and day? Can their family accept this invasion of privacy and family life? Will their children suffer from receiving less attention?

In the beginning, running a geriatric care management business can be lonely. Often, the entrepreneur is the entire business, doing all the jobs, including billing, seeing clients, marketing, being on call 24 hours a day, and perhaps even running to the bank to borrow more money to cover operating expenses. Often, the entrepreneur sees much less of his or her family because the GCM is consumed by running the fledgling operation. Often, GCMs face initial criticism or rejection of their services if they do not have already established sources of client referrals. (Chapter 10 discusses marketing in more detail.) Finally, to be successful, the entrepreneur needs to seek out the advice of experienced professionals, listen to it, and be willing to adapt and change as needed.

Exhibit 7–2   Are You Entrepreneur Material?

- Are you a leader?
- Are you a self-starter?
- Do you make decisions easily?
- Do you like competition?
- Do you get along well with different types of people?
- Are you good at planning and organizing?
- Do you have the physical and emotional strength to run a business?
- Do you have the drive to maintain your motivation in times of trouble and slowdowns?
- Can your family survive on a more limited income the first few years of your business?
- Do you have self-discipline?

So, what are the rewards of running a geriatric care management business? According to Kraus, the dividends for many GCM entrepreneurs are as follows[3]:

- Finding an outlet for their creativity
- Working on a flexible schedule
- Earning the respect of their community by offering a service that gives great support to older people and their families
- Doing a variety of tasks every day
- Interacting with many other professionals in a variety of disciplines, through assessment, marketing, and interacting with clients
- Meeting other like-minded people through joining the National Association of Professional Geriatric Care Managers and the Case Management Society of America (CMSA) and exchanging new and creative ideas about geriatric care management and running a geriatric care management business
- Working in an up-and-coming discipline

Another way for people to find out whether they really want to start a geriatric care management business is to talk to working GCMs. Prospective GCMs can try one or more of the following options to learn from the experience of working GCMs:

- Attend a GCM or CMSA conference to meet GCMs and talk with them about their practice.
- Go to the GCM or CMSA Web site to find names of nearby GCMs, and then make an appointment to meet with a GCM in person to discuss his or her business experience (see Appendix A for contact information).
- Buy tapes, compact disks (CDs), and manuals that discuss starting a geriatric care management business.
- Buy products that help you start a professional geriatric care management business such as the GCM Toolbox, offered

through GCM Products on the Web site (http://www.caremanagers.org). You don't have to reinvent the wheel, but instead use materials that have already been tested in the field and found to be useful.

Prospective GCMs can and should try to learn from the experiences of others who have been down the path before.

■ TYPES OF GERIATRIC CARE MANAGEMENT BUSINESSES

This section discusses three different types of organization a geriatric care management business may choose: solo practices, partnerships, and corporations. For more information, refer to the workbook *The Business of Becoming a Professional Geriatric Care Manager* offered in the GCM Tool Box on the Web site listed above.

Solo Practices

Most GCMs begin their business as a solo practice. They choose a legal entity known as a sole proprietorship, which means that the business is owned and controlled by a single party. In a sole proprietorship, the proprietor is always responsible for any legal or financial liabilities that occur during the course of business. In a 1997 survey of GCMs, Knutson and Langer found that 45% of all GCMs were organized as sole proprietorships.[1]

A sole proprietorship is probably the easiest and most common type of business to start. It is appropriate for an individual or one person. There are few legal restrictions (compared with those that come with partnerships and corporations) and few legal papers to complete, with the exception of a business license or a fictitious business license in some states. Any profit is taxed at the individual's personal tax rate. There are no separate income tax forms to complete; the individual can put the business revenues and losses on Schedule C of his or her personal 1040.

Sole proprietors have relative freedom from government taxes and regulations. There are many other advantages to starting a geriatric care management business as a solo practitioner. It is easier to maintain control and be flexible because the GCM makes all the decisions and is able to respond quickly to client requests and business needs. Another advantage is financial, in that 100% of the profits go to the owner rather than profits being split between multiple owners. In addition, solo practitioners can dissolve the business more easily if they decide being a GCM is not for them, which might be a distinct advantage if the owner decides to close the business.

There are also many disadvantages to being a solo practitioner. Multiple tasks are involved in running a geriatric care management business, including marketing, bookkeeping, managing human resources, counseling, and being on call. A sole proprietor must either do all of these jobs or outsource some of them, which can be expensive. Many times, sole proprietorship leaves a GCM exhausted, with no salary to boot.

Another negative is that sole proprietors have to be on call 24 hours a day, 7 days a week because this is the nature of being a GCM; the only alternative is to outsource some time to an employee or another GCM. If the GCM becomes ill or cannot practice for any reason, there is no one else to bear the burden of the cases or to run the business. Having an agreement with another GCM who you can fall back on is a possibility, but client service will be less consistent.

Sole proprietorship can also pose tough financial issues. In this business form, the owner has unlimited or 100% liability, so creditors can come after the owner's personal assets. The owner has 100% of the risk, so his or her personal assets are at risk. It is much more difficult to borrow money for this type of ownership, and few lenders are willing to

make ongoing business loans to a sole proprietorship. Sole proprietors may have a hard time getting long-term financial capital, which can affect their ability to grow. However, because a sole proprietor is also the only one making the decision to spend money, it may be less necessary to seek loans or credit.

Finally, sole proprietors have no one to lean on in times of crisis. Having a colleague to bear the burden of care and decision making means that a GCM gets feedback, support, and respite from the pressure that is an inevitable part of being a GCM and being a business owner.[4] Future GCMs should consult with an attorney and an accountant before deciding on whether to choose this form of business organization. An attorney can help with many issues, including a right of survivorship agency agreement in case of the GCM's death or disability. An accountant can explain tax requirements for recording business expenses and profits, Social Security, and employee wage withholdings.[5]

Partnerships

Some GCMs prefer to have a partner. There are two legal types of partnerships. First, there are general partnerships, where the business has two or more owners. All individuals are liable if the business defaults, no matter what percentage of the business each individual owns. Each partner must report income or loss in the business. Second, there are limited partnerships, where one partner simply invests in the business but does not make business decisions. In this case, the investing partner is liable for only the amount of the investment. Before deciding on setting up a partnership, you should see an attorney and an accountant to decide whether a partnership is the best option and which type of partnership to choose.

Partnerships have their advantages. Partners share financial, administrative, on-call, and emotional burdens. If you have to take time off, you should be able to rely on your partner to cover your cases and respond to new referrals. Compared with corporations, partnerships are relatively easy to set up and are flexible in that a limited number of people make decisions. Lending sources tend to prefer partnerships to sole proprietorships, although partnerships are still less appealing to lenders than corporations.

There are also disadvantages. Unlike corporation owners, partners have unlimited liability. Like sole proprietors, partners may still have an unstable business life, with fluctuating incomes and exhausting schedules. If something happens to one partner, the partnership may be dissolved. If a partner decides to leave, it may be hard on the other partner because buying out a partner can be legally and financially difficult.

Wendy Marks and Carol Westheimer gave a workshop at the 1995 GCM conference entitled "Partnerships: The Good, the Bad, and the Ugly. Why Do They Succeed or Fail? Or Everything You Wanted to Know About Marriage Without Sex But Were Afraid to Ask." According to Marks and Westheimer, partnerships are as delicate as marriage, and people need to think carefully before becoming partners. As Marks points out in her 1996 article about partnerships in the *GCM Journal*, people should first assess whether they are suited to be in a partnership.[6] Some individuals, according to Marks, have problems sharing tasks with other people, whether they are equals, subordinates, or superiors. People with this very domineering personality type are probably not suited for partnerships. Partners are meant to bear a mutual burden and make mutual decisions. Some people have a hard time sharing leadership duties and think of everything in terms of "mine" or "yours," which can cause the same types of problems in a business partnership as in a marriage.

Marks also suggests understanding the relevant skills of both people considering a partnership. This list may include bookkeeping, care management, geriatric assessment, marketing, payroll, hardware and software support, administration, and human resources management. A skill map can identify which partner has which skills. Marks points out that areas that are not covered by either partner as well as areas that are covered by both partners are of concern in establishing a partnership.

Another step is to assess how long a commitment each partner can make to the fledgling enterprise. If one partner plans to retire in 5 years and wants to stay in the partnership only for that long, and the other wants to make a 20-year commitment, the mutual venture may need to be reassessed. Does one partner want to have another child in a few years? Does one partner expect to relocate anytime soon? People should assess the present commitment to the partnership, and then anticipate what the partnership will look like 2, 5, and 10 years down the line. There may be a period where one partner would be running the business alone, and this may not seem agreeable to the other partner.

Next, the partners should list the tasks that their business will require to make it operate well. These tasks can include marketing, being on call on a 24-hour basis, paying bills, doing accounts receivable and accounts payable, and handling human resources. Both partners should decide what level of commitment they have to each task. One partner will have to do each task, or the partners will have to outsource the task. For example, if neither partner understands bookkeeping, the partners will have to hire a bookkeeper.

According to Marks, the ideal partnership has two people who are equally committed. If there is a different level of commitment, then partners may want to explore splitting the profits accordingly (a person who does 40% of the work gets 40% of the profits). This needs to be thought out and explored with an attorney.

What all this leads to is exploring whether the potential partners have a similar vision for the future of the business. In addition to writing a business plan, the partners each may also want to write down a 5- or 10-year plan for his or her involvement in the business, and then compare their visions. If the forecasts are similar, great. If they are different, the partners can negotiate and try to agree. Are both partners willing to share the evening and weekend responsibilities in this around-the-clock business? Resentment can build if someone is unfairly shouldering more of the burden.

The best GCM partners make decisions objectively and are comfortable with change. They learn from their mistakes and are not afraid to fail. If one partner cannot stomach failure, that person may blame the other partner rather than see the errors as a way to learn what does and does not work in the business. Together, good GCM partners are prepared for and able to survive a crisis because crises are inevitable parts of new (and ongoing) businesses. An adjunct to this is the "worst nightmare" scenario: partners should consider what they would do if the business failed, because, realistically, this is not an unlikely occurrence. What contingency plans might be set up? Would the partners survive without blaming each other?

Being partners in a business also means spending many hours together working very hard. People considering a partnership need to make sure that they can comfortably spend that much time with another person. Many partners have tested the waters by going off and "playing" with each other (e.g., by taking a trip together). This helps them gauge their compatibility. Partners should also make sure they have compatible values, according to Marks.[6] If one partner believes that earning a profit is immoral and the other partner embraces capitalism, there will be problems. If one partner believes in spending all avail-able funds and the other is fiscally conservative, there will be problems. Partners may complete some kind of values assessment and compare the results. Potential partners may also, as Marks suggests, interview friends, family members, and colleagues to see how their potential partner's values mesh with their own. An accountant can help partners assess their beliefs about finances (e.g., should you have credit cards, what the limits should be, what constitutes abuse of those cards), and then compare the responses for compatibility. If the responses are not compatible, the partners may try to negotiate, may rethink the partnership, or may decide not to proceed with the partnership.

As Marks points out, partners should also discuss their commitments to their families, because geriatric care management is such a time-intensive business. Are the family members on both sides willing to accept the partners' absences? This needs to be assessed before the partnership begins. Can each partner devote the same amount of time to the business? If not, should one partner get more money? If the imbalance cannot be resolved, the partnership should be reconsidered. Exhibit 7–3 contains a quiz that sums up many of the points discussed here. Potential partners should take the quiz before formalizing the partnership.

In 1996, Marks sent out a survey about partnerships to GCM members. She found that most GCM partnerships consisted of two people. Most partnerships did not have adequate insurance; usually, they had life insurance but not disability insurance. Only half of the partnerships had formal contracts. However, most partners who felt their business was successful had formal agreements and terms of partnership. Most respondents felt good about being a partner.[6] As these survey results suggest, formal partnership agreements may help partnerships succeed, and insurance is important.

Exhibit 7-3
Partnership Quiz

❑ Do you both have the entrepreneurial qualities to survive the first 5 years of a business?

❑ Is either one of you unable to share tasks with anyone else?

❑ Can you both commit to this company for the next 7 years?

❑ Do you both have all of the following traits?

   ❑ Honesty
   ❑ Risk-taking ability
   ❑ Ability to withstand failure
   ❑ Ability to withstand rejection
   ❑ Capacity to share
   ❑ Ability to argue strongly and courteously lose
   ❑ Ability to forgive
   ❑ Ability to survive a crisis

❑ Do you both look at each other as someone with whom you could spend long periods of time?

❑ Can you both say "no" to a plan but "yes" to a person?

❑ Do you both have a similar vision of the future?

❑ Do you both have the finances to cover expenses until you turn a profit?

❑ Can you both survive failure?

Corporations

The third and most complex form of business organization is the corporation. If you decide to form a corporation, you need to hire an attorney.

Setting up a corporation offers several advantages. Corporations are considered legal entities that exist apart from the shareholders. If a founder or stockholder dies, it does not affect the business's legal status. Liability is limited to the assets of the corporation; therefore, the personal assets of the shareholders are not affected if the corpora-

tion becomes insolvent. This is the advantage of establishing a corporation when starting a business. Ownership is easily transferred, so if the founder wants to relocate or retire, he or she simply has to sell his or her stock in the company.

Another advantage is that banks and lenders are more open to lending to a corporation that has a good track record or a new corporation that has sufficient equity and promise. However, as a precaution lenders will still most likely ask for collateral and/or personal signatures from the stockholders. The corporate form of ownership can also offer certain advantages with regard to fringe benefits such as health insurance, stock plans, or pensions.

But choosing the corporation business form also has its drawbacks. First, it is more expensive to start a corporation than it is to start a sole proprietorship or a partnership because of the legal costs. And, unlike sole proprietorships and partnerships, corporations may be exposed to regulation by state, local, and federal governments and require more assistance from attorneys and accountants.

In a C corporation, another limitation is double taxation. C corporate profits are taxed once to the corporation and again as income when the profits are distributed to the stockholders. So, the stockholder pays taxes on his or her salary and any share he or she might have of the distributed profits. Corporations are also required to have bylaws, may be required to hold stockholders meetings, and must keep records.

Another form of corporation is an S corporation. In an S corporation, both income and losses are passed directly to the individual shareholders, rather than the corporation; therefore, they are taxed at only the shareholder's rate. Because new businesses generally lose money in the first year, this can be a distinct advantage to the shareholder. Any loss can be applied against any other personal income, thus reducing the amount of income tax levied. However, it is necessary to consult an attorney to find out whether you can qualify for an S corporation status.[7]

Attorneys help with many essential corporate functions, including the following:

- Filing articles of incorporation in the state where the business is located
- Issuing stock
- Organizing the election of directors and officers as required under the laws of the state
- Drawing up bylaws
- Helping devise procedures for conducting stockholder meetings, keeping records of these meetings, and creating stock and by/sell agreements

It is also essential to have an accountant to set up the corporation's books, ensure that all taxes are paid fully and on time, and provide other advice on the proper keeping of the corporation's books.

■ CREATING A BUSINESS PLAN

After choosing which form a business will take (sole proprietorship, partnership, or corporation), future GCM business owners need to write a business plan (see Exhibit 7–4). Writing a business plan clearly organizes all of the ideas about the GCM business in a focused description of the products the geriatric care management business will sell, who will buy these products, who the competition is expected to be, and how your products are similar to and different from that of the competition.

Why do this? First, a business plan makes ideas concrete and ordered, turning subjective dreams into objective goals. It also lists the obstacles that a business might face. It explains, step by step, how a person's entrepreneurial dream will become a reality.

In addition, a written business plan is required if you need to borrow money to start the business. Bank loan officers and other funding sources expect to see a fully developed, written business plan. Merrily Orsini, in her workshop titled "Doing Good Makes Cents: Advanced Business Practices," presented at the 10th annual national GCM conference in 1994, emphasizes the importance of having a business plan at every stage of a geriatric care management business, but particularly in the beginning.[8] A business plan makes you think through the whole business you envision, not just individual parts. It helps you evaluate whether you should be in business. It gives you a way to evaluate your daily business operations. And, finally, it gives you a tool you must have if you expect to find investors or seek a loan or line of credit with a bank.

Why Plan

The future comes no matter what. Planning helps you to anticipate the future and make well-informed decisions. Planning is the first step in business management. Without it you may have no business. You should write this plan yourself if you expect to be successful in owning your own geriatric care management business based on your ideas and efforts. Of course, you may well want to have someone else review your business plan, but the bottom line is that businesses that do not have a written business plan have a much higher failure rate than businesses that have a written plan. Increase your chance of success in your

Exhibit 7–4
Outline of a Business Plan

I.	Business
II.	Products and services
III.	Industry
IV.	Location
V.	Market
VI.	Competition
VII.	Marketing
VIII.	Operations
IX.	Personnel
X.	Finances

geriatric care management business— write a business plan.

Prior to developing a business plan, you need to consider many personal abilities and skill sets. You should consider referring to the workbook *The Business of Becoming a Professional Geriatric Care Manager*, available in the GCM Tool Box on the GCM Web site, and answering the questions in the section titled "Prior to Developing Your Business Plan."

Your GCM Business Plan

When developing a business plan, several sections are key to making your plan successful. The first key section is value proposition.

1. Value Proposition

The first section of a geriatric care management business plan should state your value proposition. It begins by describing the business in general terms. Include a description of the background of the principals. Résumés of the principals can be included as an attachment to the plan. This section also explains how you plan to use your business plan and why the plan is being written (e.g., to attract investors, to show how the operation will work, to show that the business is financially feasible, to clarify your business operation, to create a guide for managing your business, etc.).

Start with your mission statement, which should state the core of your business in a few sentences. The mission statement should reflect the goals and values of your organization. It should be short, focused, perhaps only 20 words, written in the present tense, in positive terms and without qualifiers.

2. Industry

Next, describe the geriatric care management industry because it is a relatively new industry that must be described to bankers and other investors who may not be aware of it or the niche market it fills. Helpful information to describe the geriatric care management industry is available on the Web site (http://www.caremanager.org), including what a GCM is, how many GCMs are in the country, how long the profession has been around, the financial performance of the industry, the role of government regulation, and so forth. You might add a history of the geriatric care management industry (see Chapter 1, "Overview and History of Geriatric Care Management") and describe the growth patterns of the GCM industry and of the GCM organization.

3. Current Situation Analysis

If you are already operating an existing and related business, for example, a home care company, you should describe that business, including key indicators such as revenue, profitability, number of customers, and so forth. Include a brief history of the existing business, why it has been successful, key points of the business's growth, profitability patterns, and how the existing business has changed over time. You should also explain how the addition of a geriatric care component will enhance or fit in with your existing business operations.

4. Market Assessment

Next describe the customers you intend to serve. Start with a definition of your ideal client. Example: Woman, 85 years old with chronic care needs who has an income or liquid assets of $500,000 or more.

Again, you want to list the customers who will reward you the most financially. How many of these ideal clients are in the area you wish to serve? You need do an analysis of the age and income levels. Generally, geriatric care management customers are over age 85 or are disabled younger people with incomes in the range of the top 10% in your community. Your customers are also the local overstressed adult children of clients, long-distance caregivers with family members who need help and live in your community, and third parties who may hire you as a GCM such as trust officers, attorneys, conservators, or guardians.

You need to do market research to define the size of the market in the area where your business will be located (e.g., how many people over age 85 live in San Luis Obispo, California, how many third-party target markets such as trust departments are in the town?). This type of demographic information may be available from U.S. Census Bureau reports, local Area Agencies on Aging, local chambers of commerce, local hospitals, and even members of the local media who have done their own surveys. You can use the Internet to retrieve U.S. Census data in your area, and in addition you can Google the State Department of Aging, find your local Department of Aging, and then find all senior services that may have data on older people in your area.

The Market Assessment section also contains all your target markets besides older people and their families. These would be defined as client representative or third parties. They include targets who you expect to refer older people and their families to you, including physicians, elder-law attorneys, trust officers, senior services information and referral agencies, hospital-based care managers, and so forth. You can use the Internet or the yellow pages to track the number of third parties. For example, if you want to know the number of elder-law attorneys in your community, Google "National Academy of Elder Law Attorneys" and enter the zip code of the location and border areas where you intend to start your business, and you will find a list of elder-law attorneys.

The Market Assessment section should also include your own research into the needs of the area. Who else is providing similar or related services in your target market? Why do you think the local target market needs this business? Will older people in the area be able to afford your services?

Finally, calculate the total market opportunity in your geographic area in terms of the expected total market and how much you believe your business can earn from that total possible market.

5. Problems Faced by Your Target Market

GCMs are problem solvers. What problems do you intend to solve in your market area? You need to describe the specific problems you are expecting to solve. For example, a problem you may expect to be a major focus of your care management practice is the needs of long-distance caregivers who live in your geographic area but whose elderly family members live elsewhere. These long-distance caregivers may require help in managing their own burnout and finding resources where their elderly family members live. Another example could be the needs of chronically ill adults over age 85 who need supportive services arranged for them, and then monitoring of these referrals to ensure the best continuum of care. A third possibility is meeting the needs of trust officers who do not want to be available 24/7 and who want to contract with a trained care manager to visit their customers on a regular basis to monitor customer needs and report back to the trust officer. A final example would be the needs of elder-law attorneys who need a thorough geriatric assessment to present to court in conservatorship or guardianship cases.

6. Your Unique Solution to These Problems

This section of your business plan describes in more detail the geriatric care management products or services you expect to provide. Why should people buy these services from you? What makes your business unique and special? How do you intend to charge for your services? What do you expect your fees to be and how will they be organized; for example, will you charge by the hour or by the product? Even though the geriatric care management business sells services, you can think of services as products: for instance, geriatric assessment might be one product, and placement assistance another product.

Here is an example of a geriatric care management product and how you would describe it in this section of your business plan: Care Management Plus example: "Care Management Plus is a weekly monitoring service for chronically ill elders. It includes a monitoring visit to the older person, a monthly report, phone support as needed by the family or client representative, and e-mail communication with family members, third parties, and client representatives (attorney, trust officer, conservator, etc.). Additional visits to solve a crisis or as requested by the family or family representative are also included in this package."

Why should people buy it? Client representatives should buy this product to assure themselves, the courts, or other third parties or family members that all the older client's needs are met, any crisis is resolved, and all interested parties are communicated with daily, weekly, and monthly.

What makes this product unique and special? Families in our town have no other services like Care Management Plus. Conservators, elder-law attorneys, third parties, and families have no other means to monitor ongoing care or the client's current status, or to solve emergencies as they arise.

How much does it cost to provide Care Management Plus? We pay a GCM $25.00 an hour to cover a caseload of between 5 and 10 clients who each require on average 4 hours a week of the care manager's time.

What does Care Management Plus cost for the customer? We expect to sell the care manager's time for $100.00 per hour, which covers payment of all required taxes, training and supervision, charting, and so forth.

7. Competition

When describing your market and the total market opportunity in the area, you need to estimate the money you expect your business to earn. Next, you need to describe what share of that expected opportunity you believe your business can expect to attract. To do this you need to assess your competition.

Are there other geriatric care management businesses in the area? Do home health agencies in the area offer care or case management? Are there physician practices offering geriatric care management? You can do research into these issues in a variety of ways, including by using the local phone book or the Web sites of CMSA or the National Association of Professional Geriatric Care Managers.

Once you have identified the competition, you need to describe any traits you believe your new business shares with the current competition. What differentiates your new business from the competition? Do you expect the new business to woo customers or referral sources away from the competition? Would you expect to offer lower prices, better or different services? You might consider doing a survey of your expected competition. A competition survey is used to find out what your competitors are doing that is different, better or worse, and then use that information to your benefit. For a sample competition survey see Chapter 10.

To compare your geriatric care management business to others in your area and to describe your competition you can make a comparison chart ranking your new business against the competition. You can do a competitive analysis with the help of any of the Small Business Development Centers throughout the country. See Appendix A, Contact Information, to find your local or regional Small Business Administration (SBA) Center. When updating your business plan, you may also redo this competition survey yearly.

8. Sales Plan

GCMs rarely see themselves as salespersons. However, this is a fatal error. You may have a product, but to make money from that product, you have to sell it. In the beginning you yourself may have to sell your geriatric care management product. To begin to put together a sales plan you need to identify who makes the decision to buy your geriatric care management products. With older adults over age 85, the buying decision is generally made by the adult children or the third party (trust officer, etc.). Many times young older adults (65–85 years of age) make their own buying decisions.

You then need to identify what criteria the person making the buying decision uses to evaluate your geriatric care management product. For example, you have to figure out whether the decision to purchase your Care Management Plus product is made by the adult child based on price, features, or availability. How will you give your customer, the adult child, enough information to say yes? Does this buying decision require personal contact in intake by a GCM, a Care Management Plus sell sheet you dropped off at the parent's physician's office, word of mouth, paid advertising, or public relations such as a story about your services submitted and published by the local paper? Describe your sales plan. (Please refer to Chapter 10's section "Setting Yourself apart from Competition" for more information.)

9. Operations

Where will your business be located? This section of the plan discusses the place where the company will do business. Some beginning geriatric care management businesses start in the GCM's home office. Some GCMs prefer to rent an outside space. You need to make that decision. If finances are a critical factor, you might choose a home office. You have to consider whether location is a factor in getting customers. If you are going to have a business address, is the office going to be in a certain part of town because that's where the customers are? Perhaps the business will be near a hospital or a large assisted living facility that offers services for older people. Geriatric care management businesses are not like clothing stores or other merchandise-based businesses, which need to be located in areas with considerable foot traffic (e.g., malls, busy streets). But locating next to a long-term-care discharge unit might increase business.

Describe where you will be located and what the square footage will be. Include blueprints that show accurate diagrams of the floor plan, including where staff, furniture, and customer access are located. Add photos of the location. Then describe the occupancy cost of the location by month and by year, listing rent, property tax, maintenance and repairs, insurance, utilities, telephone service, and other expenses that may apply to your location.

Next, describe how your geriatric care management product is created and delivered. Your product is created by your expertise as a GCM. Refer to your résumé or those of your GCM staff included in the value proposition for information on expertise and experience. Refer to your sell sheets, presentation folders, brochures, intake folders, case files, and all hard-copy descriptions of your products to describe how these products will be delivered. Describe which staff member will take these marketing tools out to your target market representatives (physicians, elder-law attorneys, discharge planners, etc.).

Who actually delivers the product, your geriatric care management services? Your staff of GCMs or perhaps just yourself in the beginning? Create a flowchart that shows all steps of delivery from the time a customer calls to inquire about your geriatric care management products and services, through intake, and onto delivery of your products and services (e.g., employee Miss Help monitors 85-year-old Mr. Bottomly weekly as part of the Care Management Plus product package).

You might refer to quality control of your product—do you have customer satisfaction letters or surveys that are sent out on a regular basis or after a customer closes the case? If not, develop one.

Describe when the office will be open and when GCMs will be on call. Describe a typical day in your GCM office. Include a blueprint for the upcoming days, weeks, and months of geriatric care management operations, defining how and when the entrepreneurs will carry out the tasks necessary to run the business and serve the clients. Give a clear picture of how many people are needed to run the business. The section should also describe the following:

- All equipment and supplies to be used in running the business (e.g., a computer system, a printer, a telephone, a pager, a cell phone, a BlackBerry device)
- The business's recordkeeping system and how much it will cost to operate (i.e., how client information will be tracked and whether it will be stored in case files, computerized records, on the Web or in another storage system)
- The business's accounting and billing system (is it manual? computerized? outsourced?) and how much it will cost to operate
- How stock is divided in the business agreements and the business succession in case of the loss of key personnel
- Which professionals the business will need to use (e.g., an attorney, an accountant, a cleaning person)

10. The Management Team

In this section, describe who the key players are in your geriatric care management business, both existing and new. The professional experience of the owner and key employees must be described. Each person's daily role in the business is explained. The business's organizational structure (e.g., sole proprietorship, partnership, or corporation) is also noted.

Then describe the key players in your business. Is it just you or you and a business partner? Describe who is on this team and how they are uniquely qualified to make this business happen. Include a résumé of all people on the management team that shows the background that makes them qualified to run this business. For example, you may have 15 years of experience working with seniors and your partner is a Certified Public Accountant with 15 years of small business experience.

11. Building a Financial Model

In building a financial model, start with the first year and project out 2 to 5 years. Estimate your annual revenue, and then calculate your gross margin potential (selling price of your geriatric care management products; for example, Care Management Plus will be sold to the customer for $100 an hour, and cost of goods sold will be $25.00 an hour to staff plus employment taxes plus overhead expenses). Calculate your margin. You must make a profit and sometimes that means raising fees. Include how much money is needed to fund the venture and a history of the owner's finances. Also, mention people who will offer audits of the business's success or failure, such as an accountant.

Sometimes it is helpful to get expert advice on these financial matters. The SBA has small business development centers all over the United States to help small businesses get started. Local chambers of commerce can provide information about where local small business development centers are located. The Service Corps of Retired Executives (SCORE) can also provide assistance. There are also consultants who specialize in helping geriatric care management businesses get started. The GCM and CMSA Web sites may be able to direct you to these consultants.

Appendix A contains contact information for all these organizations.

12. Funding Requirements

What cash will be available to launch the business? Does that include your own money? How much will be needed over the next 18 months? Are there already identified sources of funding? These are the first questions a lender will ask. If you are looking for investors, how much of the company are you willing to sell and at what price? Again, consult your local SBA center or SCORE counselors for help here. Don't begin your business without this critical financial advice.

13. Financing a Geriatric Care Management Business

According to the SBA, 80% of new entrepreneurs start their businesses without any commercial loan or debt financing.[9] Banks are usually hesitant to make loans under $50,000 because the loan is not cost-effective for the bank.

Because small businesses often need less than $50,000 and frequently have difficulty finding banks to lend them money, they look for other financing. Serious lenders and investors want to finance new businesses with a track record and an excellent business plan. New business owners with some background in geriatric care management, social work, or nursing will probably have an easier time satisfying lenders and investors.

The SBA lists the following sources of financing that new care management practices often use:

- Personal savings
- Personal credit (including credit cards and personal lines of credit)
- Loans from friends and family members
- Loans from informal investors
- Home equity loans (especially in areas where home values have risen considerably)

- Financing from credit unions (which tend to be more open to lending to alternative or new borrowers)
- Financing through city and county economic or community development programs
- Bank loans or lines of credit
- Investors' angels or venture capital
- Donors, such as a nonprofit organization

The SBA itself is another source to consider. It has loan programs of its own and lists of local economic development offices that may have loan programs for start-ups that respond to local economic development needs. Some of these programs offer loans and provide information and technical assistance on starting a business.[8]

14. Getting Funded

Now that you have written your business plan, you need to use it to get funded. Before you submit it to any bank, angel, or informal investor, you need to take several more steps. Prepare all the marketing material for your business opportunity. Write a letter of introduction, write an executive summary (limited to two pages in length), and create a presentation about your geriatric care management business opportunity (use Microsoft Office PowerPoint or another electronic slideshow application).

Then, identify prospective funders, make initial contact through personal referral if possible, and make an initial deal presentation using your business plan and all your marketing materials. If the investor is interested, secure a term sheet or loan agreement, which will form the initial framework for the transaction, and which is usually prepared by the legal team and includes purchasing terms if agreed upon and outlines how many shares you are selling and at what price, if this is your plan. You will then go through the long and sometimes painful process of due diligence and negotiate a final agreement. The last step hopefully is when you accept the check to begin your geriatric care management business. Do not go through these last steps without an attorney and accountant on board and make certain to use the help of your local SBA, SCORE, or other advisory source.

■ PROFESSIONAL CONSULTANTS

Professional consultants are a very important asset in setting up a geriatric care management business. Many of these consultants may not require a capital outlay but provide consultation based on the business's future earnings. Even if consultants do charge from the beginning, businesses are usually smart to invest in expert advice because consultants help businesses avoid costly mistakes and make better choices (e.g., an attorney can help a new business avoid lawsuits, an accountant can help the business owner develop figures to help get funding from the bank, a geriatric care management business consultant can help a business owner come up with excellent geriatric care management services/products to make the business really grow). This section discusses the role of different professional consultants in helping establish a new geriatric care management business.

Attorneys

A new geriatric care management business needs an attorney, and not just any attorney. The attorney should have considerable experience in working with small businesses. The attorney can help set up the legal business entity, help the business decide how to register or get licensed, help the business meet Internal Revenue Service (IRS) requirements (e.g., whether the business needs an employer identification number), offer advice on whether the business should employ staff or independent contractors, and help the business obtain a fictitious business name. Attorneys can help you along the way to getting funded by making sure your business opportunity meets all legal requirements and reviewing any deal you are offered. Ongoing, an attorney is essential to managing and reviewing legal problems that may come up and monitoring the growth of your company.

Accountants

The business needs an accountant, possibly one that is a CPA. The accountant helps with setting up the business plan by assisting with the financial arrangements. Owners need help determining the funding requirements of the new business, including how much cash is needed to open the business, the terms under which the business will obtain the money, and the type of money desired (loans, personal savings, etc.). Business owners also need to decide with accountants what type of accounting system to use.[9] An accountant can also offer advice on what types of business records to keep, including a cash receipts journal, a cash disbursement journal, a sales journal, a purchase journal, a payroll journal, and a general ledger. There are many accounting software packages out there, and many cost under $300. Unless the geriatric care management business owner is an accountant, has a degree in business, or has owned businesses before, getting help from a professional accountant is important.

Consultants in the Geriatric Care Management Field

Most new geriatric care management businesses can benefit from assistance from a specialist in the industry. A professional consultant can help a business owner gain a thorough understanding of geriatric care management, which can help the business owner develop services. The consultant can help with the business plan and be on call in case a crisis occurs. Contact the National Association of Professional Geriatric Care Managers or CMSA for referrals to these consultants.

Bankers

Bank representatives can help new geriatric care management businesses as well. Even though banks do not operate the way they used to, with one-to-one relationships between bank representatives and customers, some banks (especially small-town banks and credit unions) do have representatives that handle small business loans and can work with the business on an ongoing basis. Ted Turner, now famous for developing CNN, has many secrets to his success, including incredible energy, an ability to fail and pick himself back up, and unbelievable vision. But he also had an uncanny ability to work with bankers and borrow money. Owners who find a bank to loan them money should also try to develop a long-term relationship with a representative at that bank, for assistance with both future lines of credit and direct deposit for employees and payroll. Credit unions are sometimes a good choice and more open to a new industry such as geriatric care management.

Insurance Brokers

Insurance brokers also provide new geriatric care management businesses with an important service. See the section titled "Business Insurance" later in this chapter for more information on the contribution of these professionals.

Free Advice

Other sources of advice and assistance are free. One is the IRS. It offers new business owners many free materials and workshops, including information about recordkeeping, tax reporting, and hiring employees and independent contractors. (Business owners should, of course, also work with their attorneys and accountants in determining their tax reporting requirements.)

Another source is the local chamber of commerce, an excellent resource for information on what help is available to new businesses in a particular area. Chambers of commerce can point the way to local small business development centers. In addition to helping businesses get started, chambers of commerce can help businesses grow. Many case management services across the country, like other small business owners, have joined the chamber of commerce to develop relationships to further their business. Some chambers have newsletters that announce new businesses, and chambers usually have mixers where businesspeople can meet each other, talk, offer support to each other, and exchange business cards. Owners might ask local chambers if it would be possible to celebrate the opening of their businesses at one of these mixers.

Professional Associations

Professional associations are another helpful resource. The National Association of Professional Geriatric Care Managers and CMSA, as stated previously, have a wealth of resources to help geriatric care management businesses get going. New business owners must seriously consider joining one or both industry-specific organizations and purchasing their start-up materials. These associations also put new business owners in contact with (1) more experienced professionals who can either act as mentors or simply offer advice about setting up a business and avoiding pitfalls, and (2) other new business owners with whom you can form an informal support group, and (3) products to help you start and run your geriatric care management business.

These associations also have regional and local chapters that offer start-up information and information about ongoing areas of interest in the field (e.g., Alzheimer's). Owners should also consider attending the regional and national conferences of the National Association of Professional Geriatric Care Managers and CMSA. These events usually include presessions covering issues that owners of fledgling geriatric care management businesses need to understand. Tapes and CDs of presessions and regular sessions are also available, as are tapes or CDs that cover start-up business issues.

The national association of GCMs offers a Care Manager's Resource section on its Web site that can help you research other professional associations that might be helpful to your practice. It has an entire GCM Toolbox with a kit of information to help you start and grow your new geriatric care management business that covers many of the issues in this chapter through tapes, manuals, and copies of presentations. Exhibit 7–5 summarizes this section and lists the individuals as well as groups and agencies that can help a new geriatric care management business get off the ground.

■ DEVELOPING PROCEDURES AND FORMS

Any geriatric care management business needs procedures to run smoothly, efficiently, and legally. New business owners need to have many procedures in place, from how to do a geriatric assessment to how to open, manage, and close cases; store records; open and close the office; and set up and maintain a filing system. The business owner must write out how each procedure will be done. For instance, if

Exhibit 7–5   Groups to Help a Geriatric Care Management Business Get Started

Individuals
Accountants
Attorneys
Bankers
Chambers of commerce
Consultants specializing in geriatric care management

Groups and agencies
Insurance brokers
IRS
Professional associations
SCORE

the owner is unable to run the business for some time, someone else will need to take over, and unless procedures are written out, inconsistency and other trouble will result. (See Chapter 13 on preparing for emergencies.)

The National Association of Professional Geriatric Care Managers publishes procedure manuals (GCM Policies and Procedures) that can help new business owners get started. These general procedures need to be tailored to each business, and a consultant can provide assistance if necessary—the expense of using a consultant may be worth it in the end. A local chamber of commerce can provide names of consultants who can help. A comprehensive GCM Forms Book is available on the GCM Web site. You can take these forms and tailor them to your own agency and also adapt some forms suggested in this book for assessment tools.

■ BUSINESS INSURANCE

Business insurance is taken out to protect people from professional, business, and personal liabilities or risks created by a private practice. Both start-ups and mature geriatric care management practices need business insurance. It protects assets, prevents loss of income, provides expenses in case of illness, provides coverage for errors and omissions, and meets requirements for third-party reimbursement. As in legal and accounting matters, it is best to hire the services of an insurance broker to provide advice about what type of insurance coverage a business needs and help businesses with claims. Because geriatric care management is a very new field, business owners should make sure to talk to an insurance broker who understands the needs of businesses in the field.

Beginning geriatric care management businesses need the following types of insurance:

- **Professional malpractice insurance.** This insurance protects a business and its employees for any (subject to the policy conditions) act, error, or omission that arises out of the performance of professional services to others. Policies may also be extended to cover independent contractors.

- **Business liability insurance.** This insurance covers bodily injury, property damage, product liability, and job completion in the general operation of a business. Personal endeavors are excluded. A business can also decide to insure the building in which it operates as well as improvements or personal property for either replacement value or actual cost. Other options include coverage for loss of business earnings, accounts receivable, and valuable papers and records.
- **Workers' compensation insurance.** This insurance offers disability coverage for work-related illness or disability for employees. All business employees must be covered under a workers' compensation policy.
- **Business overhead insurance.** This insurance is designed to cover loss of income caused by the disability of a principal in a business. It is based on the monthly expenses of the business, not its earnings.
- **Social Security Disability Insurance and other disability insurance.** Social Security Disability Insurance is paid through payroll taxes and provides a minimal income after a period of 6 months of disability if the disability is expected to last 1 year or more. In various states, short-term disability insurance is available. Long-term disability provides monthly benefits after the 26-week short-term disability benefits are used up.[5]

■ SETTING UP AN OFFICE

A geriatric care management business needs an office. Many GCMs start practicing out of their homes. In this era of telecommuting, running a home office may be even more feasible if space is available. Using a home office eliminates the expense of renting office space but may be too distracting. Crying babies, complaining children, and laundry that just has to be done can get in the way of being a GCM.

Whatever the choice of office location, it is helpful to make a timeline listing all tasks that need to be completed before the business can open: renting office space or refurbishing a home office; getting insurance; recruiting and hiring staff; ordering a system to handle telephone calls, voicemail, and paging; arranging for a security system and cleaning people; arranging for an answering service or setting up an on-call system; buying office equipment; making arrangements with suppliers of items such as office supplies; arranging for credit cards; ordering brochures; and so forth. The new business owner should estimate how long each task will take, put each task on a timeline, and give him- or herself a deadline of opening day. Exhibit 7-6 shows a sample timeline.

If there is no space for a home office or working at home seems too distracting, entrepreneurs need to contact a realtor and look for a small space to rent. They might want to consider renting 400 to 600 square feet with a small reception area, so clients are not walking right in on conversations with other clients. The realtor and an attorney can offer advice about how long a lease to take and what terms the lease should have.

Offices should be as professional as possible. Having administrative assistants and other staff members helps. An administrative assistant answering the phone is much more professional than using an answering machine. An administrative assistant can also help process paperwork in a professional and timely manner. Good staff can actually help a business make more money. When an owner does everything alone (e.g., answering the phone, seeing clients, doing the billing, responding to emergencies), a business may not make as much

Exhibit 7–6   Sample Timeline of Startup Tasks

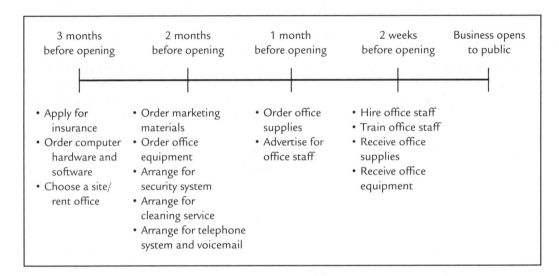

money as it would if tasks were handled by others. The business makes money off billed GCM time, and if a GCM spends a lot of time away from clients, less time is being billed.

Also, doing everything alone can send a GCM into a cycle in which too many care managers find themselves: people with human services backgrounds are so accustomed to emergencies that they become "adrenaline junkies." However, when a business involves dealing with clients' emergencies, the business itself should not have daily emergencies of its own. An owner who does everything alone may eventually find him- or herself in this cycle.

■ HIRING GOOD STAFF MEMBERS

Hiring staff members is an art. Well done, this art can help a business considerably. Poorly done, this art can lead to trouble, making the owner a care manager to staff as well as to clients.

Before advertising for employees, an owner should write job descriptions. A sample job description appears in Exhibit 7–7. The description should list the qualifications applicants should have and the responsibilities and tasks

of the position. A human resources consultant can offer assistance in writing job descriptions. Sample GCM job descriptions are also available through the national association's Web site, in the GCM *Policies and Procedures Manual.*

Advertising for staff should occur at least 3 to 4 months before opening your office. An ad should run for at least a full week. It takes another week or two to interview staff. It then may take 2 weeks or a month until someone is on board as a new employee because he or she may have to give notice somewhere else. You then need to train your staff, which can take up to a month. Again, using the services of a human resources consultant can help you tailor your advertising timeline to your agency's needs. GCMs who belong to the National Association of Professional Geriatric Care Managers can now advertise for staff on some regional Web sites. There also may be gerontology or employment Web sites in your area on which you can advertise for staff.

A business owner might want to put together a professional policy manual, which might include policies and procedures regarding paydays, vacation, and time off as well as all policies required by the Department of Labor

Exhibit 7-7   Sample Job Description

ADMINISTRATIVE ASSISTANT

QUALIFICATIONS:

Minimum	**Desired**
Excellent Communication Skills	AA in Business
Administrative Skills	Case Management Experience
Organizational Skills	Home Health Care Experience
Typing/Filing Skills	Desktop Publishing Skills
Computer Experience/Knowledge	
Dependable	
Self Starter	

SUMMARY STATEMENT:

The Administrative Assistant is responsible for general operations of office procedures.

Answers telephones

Opens mail

Prepares and distributes all monthly charting

Prepares and maintains Client Data Books

Prepares and maintains all Client Charting Books

Prepares and maintains all Case Site Charting Books

Prepares and maintains blank charting files

Prepares and maintains completed charting files

Opens and closes all new intake files

Opens and closes all CMP, PP, CA, and GA cases

Takes minutes at staff meetings

Inputs, copies, and mails all monthly reports

Retrieves messages from answering service twice daily

Takes on-call every third weekend

Creates emergency list

Maintains filing system

Creates and edits Care Staff Newsletter and quarterly marketing Newsletter

---

(e.g., sexual harassment, nondiscrimination). Sample policy manuals are available in bookstores and through the SBA.

Employers should take care that they are meeting the legal standards for employment. An attorney can help the owner draw up legal contracts to sign with employees. The employer–employee relationship should begin on solid ground, which means making everything clear in a contract.

■ BILLING

Billing customers is key to keeping a geriatric care management business afloat. A billing system needs to be set up and functioning well before a business opens. A good accountant can help a business set up an appropriate billing system.

Catherine C. Thompson did a survey of the national association's members in 1994, and the results were published in an article in the *GCM Journal* in 1996.[10] She found that GCMs handle billing in many different ways. The frequency of billing seemed to depend upon how much business the GCM did. Thompson suggested that low-volume businesses could probably manage with quarterly billing, but that high-volume businesses would do better with more frequent billing. Billing statements used by GCMs ranged from bills handwritten on standard forms purchased at office supply stores or business stationery to bills done on the computer. Timeslips, Quicken, and QuickBooks seemed to be the most popular software used to assist with billing, but many GCMs used customized billing programs. Most GCMs billed for their phone calls, often at the same rate as they charged for care management ($20 to $150 per hour). Many GCMs billed more for phone calls with the GCM than for phone calls with a clerical person. Some GCMs did not bill for messages left but billed for long-distance consultation or cell phone calls. Some had no differentiation between types of phone calls and billed for all. One-fourth billed for all staff conference time, half did not bill for any conference time, and a quarter billed for some conference time. The GCMs who did bill for staff conferences charged them at their current rate for geriatric care management. The great majority of those surveyed billed for travel time. Some billed at their regular rate, and some billed at half of that rate. Mileage was billed in addition to the travel time by some of the responders. Others responded that they billed for mileage and not for time. The mileage rate varied from $0.22 to $0.50 per mile.

GCMs reported several problems in the survey. Some complained about the need to train staff on handling billing (i.e., installing and using billing software) or learning to do this themselves. Others complained that clients wanted detailed bills and that adding detail to bills was tedious and time-consuming. Some reported that clients did not pay or were slow to pay. GCMs surveyed wondered whether they should charge interest on unpaid bills.

Thompson points out that careful contracting is key to successful billing; a good attorney should draw up client contracts for a new business. Contracts should address issues such as telephone time, mileage, billing for staff conferences, and different billing rates for different staff members. Another issue to address is whether to get a retainer before rendering services. In addition to a sound contract, Thompson emphasizes how important it is to have clearly stated fees. Everyone should understand how much each service costs and about how many hours it will take to render that service. A business should have in place not just a client contract but a service description before opening its doors. Thompson recommends looking for templates in the GCM forms manual.

Thompson does not address cash flow in detail but does note that most business professionals are advised to bill as soon as possible and pay bills as late as possible without incurring late fees. Whatever an owner decides to bill for (phone calls, staff conferences, travel time, etc.), he or she needs to remember that this is a business, not just a community service, and the business is supporting the owner and any staff members. Unbilled time is uncollected revenue, which creates more stress for the owner and staff members. Many GCMs come into the field from human services, where they have never billed; they may feel guilty about billing.

Designing time cards to capture billable time is important. If no one involved in the business can handle the billing, it should be outsourced. Getting a good bookkeeper or billing/payroll service to do billing may be helpful. Without proper billing, the business and its personnel will not have the money necessary to function.

◼ INTEGRATING A GERIATRIC CARE MANAGEMENT BUSINESS INTO ANOTHER PRACTICE, BUSINESS, OR AGENCY

Throughout the United States, geriatric care management practices are slowly merging with for-profit agencies and private practices, including law practices, trust departments, physician offices, accountant offices, and the practices of a myriad of other professionals who deal with the needs of older people. GCMs offer these practices one central and very important skill: the ability to do geriatric assessment. GCMs assess the older client in his or her home and bring back to the trust officer, attorney, accountant, physician, or other professional helpful information about the client's health and psychosocial status as it is in the home setting. Other professionals may see the client in the home but do not assess the client's functioning based on the home environment.

Integrating with Physicians

Because older patients represent such a large segment of most physicians' practices, GCMs are naturally helpful to physicians. As the skills of the GCM are increasingly recognized as an important part of solving chronic health problems, physicians' practices may become more open to having GCMs on staff. In 1992, the John Hartford Foundation funded a 5-year initiative to come up with better approaches to caring for the frail elderly.[11] Part of the study looked at how case management became integrated into physicians' practices. In general, the study found that integrating a GCM into a physician's practice worked well. The GCM was able to work closely with the family and patients because the GCM had access to the patient that neither the staff members nor the physician had. The physician's busy office staff found it a relief to "hand off" the older patients when problems involved accessing the continuum of care in the community or dealing with complex family problems. Physicians in the study found the GCMs' home visits very helpful; GCMs could alert the staff to potential patient problems early on, before they became a crisis, so physicians treated patients in half the time, an outcome that impressed the physicians.

The study found that integrating the GCMs into the physicians' practices initially required GCMs to overcome the resistance of the office staff by making a good first impression. Whether the physician accepted the case manager depended on learning and appreciating the value of case management before the GCM was really integrated into the patient's care. GCMs had to build trusting relationships with both the office staff and the physicians before they were fully accepted into the practices.

Integrating with Attorneys

Attorneys have slowly begun to integrate GCMs into their practices. Elder-law attorneys in particular stand to benefit from involving a GCM in their practice. Both elder-law attorneys and GCMs serve aging clients, have long-term relationships with their clients, and address conservatorships, medical planning, elder abuse, powers of attorney, and geriatric planning. Attorneys understand law as it applies to older people, and GCMs understand psychosocial and health issues as they apply to aging, making these professionals a very good match.

GCM time is not billed at as high a rate as attorney time. GCMs often see clients before attorneys do, reducing the amount of time that clients need to spend with high-cost attorneys. Very few attorneys employ GCMs at this point, but many may look into employing GCMs because of the benefits of such an arrangement, including one-stop shopping for the client.

Benefits to the elder-law attorney are many. If the attorney handles conservatorships, the GCM can assess competency. This can be very helpful when the attorney may suspect that a person petitioning for conservatorship has a questionable agenda in getting the older person conserved or whether the person should be conserved or make legal decisions; financial abuse is often involved in these cases. GCMs also have valuable knowledge of the continuum of care in the community when cases need to be referred to psychiatrists or medical social workers. GCMs can not only assess the level of confusion but help create care plans to deal with the confusion (either the primary GCM or another GCM can then take on the older person's care).[12] GCMs employed by attorneys have also been helpful in making placement suggestions in cases where the attorney serves as guardian, attorney in fact, or health care agent.

Advance planning for times when the client is unable to make medical or personal care decisions is another area where having a GCM on staff in an attorney's firm can be helpful. GCMs can help clients formulate the questions to which they need answers. Older clients may be confused about the various options available to them. The GCM can have a discussion about the medical planning needs of the client before the client sees the attorney, thereby helping the older client be better prepared to work with the attorney. The specific needs of the client will determine how the GCM will be of assistance in this area. For example, if the client is fully capable of making decisions and is seeking assistance for the future, the discussion will be about hypothetical situations. If the client is already in poor medical health and needs assistance, the GCM can facilitate communication between the client (and/or family) and the attorney about these often difficult and private matters through precounseling. This reduces the time the attorney needs to spend with the client and raises the quality of medical planning. In a similar way, GCMs can help clients sort through personal feelings about will making and power-of-attorney appointment.

Caregiver education is another general area where the GCM can really benefit an elder-law practice. A GCM on staff can help to educate families, older people, and third parties about Medicare. Medicare benefits are little understood and, unfortunately, the majority of older people and their families still believe that Medicare will cover long-term care. Having a GCM educate clients about what Medicare will and will not cover is very helpful to a law firm because the GCM's time, again, can be billed out less expensively. Clients and their family members quickly come to understand Medicare's limitations and benefits and can do better long-term-care planning, saving themselves money and making smart choices. GCMs can also educate clients and their families about managed care. As more and more older people are going into managed care plans, this education can be very helpful.

Some law firms have used GCMs as part of the general legal team helping an older client. GCMs can do telephone checks on older clients, make home visits, go with older clients to physician appointments, consult with physicians and other health care consultants about clients, consult with staff and caregivers in a client's facility, or serve as a liaison between the client and family and friends. All these standard geriatric care management tasks enhance the legal firm's services.

Integrating with Accountants

Accountants and GCMs have begun to work together in both formal and informal relationships. Accountants and GCMs both deal with older people, have clients who are in the upper income brackets, have long relationships with clients, have a strong ethical code, and can work with other professionals to meet their clients' goals. Unless accountants specialize in elder-care services, they do not always have extensive knowledge about entitlements such as Medicare and Social Security and can benefit from a GCM's understanding of these entitlements. Accountants understand taxes, long-range financial planning, and resolution of financial problems, while GCMs understand psychosocial issues and the continuum of care, especially managed care systems. All in all, the professions are complementary.

Because long-term care is so costly and considerable financial planning must be done to make it affordable, accountants are a wonderful resource to older people facing long-term-care planning and decision making. Because long-term-care planning hinges on the client's ability to pay for his or her care or have it covered by insurance or third-party payment, accountants and GCMs can complement each other by helping the older client come up with options for long-term care based on the client's finances and the care options available in his or her community. This pairing will benefit the accounting firm and the accounting firm's clients, who will be able to do one-stop shopping.

The accountant and the GCM need to be able to work together, have open lines of communication, and have mutual trust and confidentiality, according to Rona Bartlestone and George Lewis, who have presented workshops on this type of collaboration.[13] The American Institute of Certified Public Accountants (AICPA) has encouraged accountants to move into the elder-care field. AICPA has established an ongoing task force to communicate with AICPA members about elder care. It offers five 8-hour courses on elder care (available in self-study or group-study formats) for accountants and is working on creating more. In addition, AICPA has published a guide called *Eldercare: A Practitioner's Resource Guide*. Another guide, *Guide to ElderCare Engagements*, is published by Practitioners Publishing Company. The AICPA also has an elder-care marketing kit for accountants. AICPA suggests that accountants create relationships with GCMs as well as other specialists such as elder-law attorneys. The accountants can then refer clients to the GCMs and the clients can hire the GCMs independently.

Like physicians and attorneys, few accountants have GCMs on staff. However, accountants are interested in expanding the relationship between the professions and have reached out to the National Association of Professional Geriatric Care Managers to speak at its conferences and begin collaborating.

GCMs and Managed Care Organizations

Many people believe that managed care plans seek to maximize profits and minimize quality. Improving everyone's perception of the quality of managed care is a challenge that managed care organizations face. In the market-based environment, consumer choice, consumer satisfaction, and client health outcomes will affect the success of managed care organizations. Geriatric care management may help improve older people's perceptions of managed care.

The fee-for-service system that managed care has been replacing did not always, according to Rosalie Kane, give older people fair access.[1] That system was not ideal, although many people today talk about it as if it was. Older people need to fairly compare managed care with the fee-for-service system.

Managed care has tried to contain spiraling costs and ensure greater fiscal responsibility. It has also tried to provide a less fragmented health care system. Reducing fragmentation, which both managed care and case management can do, was critical to curbing the health care cost crisis.[2] In the fee-for-service system, the costly acute care environment (i.e., the hospital) was used more often than it needed to be. Both managed care organizations and GCMs have tried to replace this acute care model with the continuum of care model. The continuum of care model does not simply treat illness but encourages wellness. So, managed care, like GCMs, moved away from filling beds to treating clients in an appropriate environment, such as in the community.[3] Therefore, managed care and geriatric care management have much in common. Staff GCMs could greatly enhance managed care's present tarnished image, helping the plans increase consumer satisfaction and improve consumer outcomes. Unfortunately, GCMs have only just begun to work with managed care.

GCMs and Trust Departments

Mellon, a well-respected financial services firm, discovered the advantages of having an expert on aging working with them and their clients. GCM Catherine C. Thompson worked in the Mellon Bank trust department for 21 years. Catherine served as the Social Service Consultant and Professional Geriatric Care Manager for Private Wealth Management of Mellon Financial Services. Ms. Thompson was responsible for each incapacitated person with a guardian account in conjunction with the trust officer for each account. She also worked with any trust clients referred by the trust officer. In addition, her expertise was solicited by the trust officers to handle unusual circumstances where the skills of a care manager are essential.

The use of a care manager by the bank is considered a good business decision. It embodies the bank's commitment to quality service to the community. It also saves time and money for the bank to have a person skilled and knowledgeable in the psychosocial area handle health- and care-related situations, leaving the trust officer to deal with the financial areas. Mellon found that caring for the personal needs of trust customers as well as financial needs is very much appreciated by trust customers and their families. Providing that extra personal attention helps to keep the clients happy and increases business. The GCM is able to provide a care plan to the trust officer who is dealing with a client with incapacity or other issues. The care manager assists in providing an accurate diagnosis of a client's problems and recommends a course of care for the current and future needs of the client. Even experienced trust officers do not have the training and experience necessary to deal with the medical, psychological, and social issues when planning for the clients.

The costs of long-term care and the effect that longevity will have on clients have big impacts on clients' financial situations. Many people are now living into their 90s. The trust officer and the care manager together can consider the impact of the possibility of increased longevity on individual clients with particular types of health care issues and particular financial situations. The care manager can manage chronic illness and even save money for clients by protecting their health and well-being. Working within a trust department or as an outside consultant, the care manager and the financial officer can form an alliance that benefits the trust officer, the client, and the care manager

GCMs and Corporate Models

In the past decade, two national corporate geriatric care management models, Senior Bridge and LivHOME, have emerged. These models have grown throughout the United States by acquiring smaller GCM businesses and integrating them into the larger corporate model. They are both geriatric care managed home care models, employing care providers. The future may bring more corporate players into the geriatric care management industry.

GCMs Specializing in One Area

Geriatric care managers have also evolved into specialized geriatric care management practices in the past 5 years. GCM Peter Belson runs a nonprofit care management agency that provides care management to adult and adolescent (older than age 12) populations who have developmental, psychiatric, or traumatic brain injury–related disabilities (or combinations thereof). They offer geriatric care management for elders who have lifelong, severe, persistent mental illness, who have not been well served by other GCMs.

Many GCMs have begun primarily to serve dementia clients in their practice. Many GCMs focus their practice on elder move coordination. (See Chapter 16.) Some new GCM practices specialize in death and dying issues. This diversification of the geriatric care management field will probably continue in the next decade with even more specialties emerging.

■ CONCLUSION

Starting a geriatric care management business is no easy task. Many decisions must be made, many tasks must be completed, and many systems must be put in motion before the business's opening day. Once the business opens, the hard work continues.

In the future, many GCMs may find themselves no longer running their own businesses but integrated into the businesses of physicians, attorneys, accountants, managed care organizations, corporations, and other entities that can benefit from GCMs' great input.

■ NOTES

1. Knutson K, Langer S. Geriatric care managers: a survey in long-term/chronic care. *GCM J.* 1998;8:9.

2. Gross EB, Johnson LF. The development of a case management business: the changing paradigms. Presented at: The National Association of Professional Geriatric Care Managers Conference; October 22–24, 1998; Chicago, IL.

3. Kraus A. Before you leap: a start-up guide for the beginner. Part I: Do you have the soul of an entrepreneur? *GCM J.* 1993;3:2–10.

4. Brostoff P, Stewart H. Basic components of private geriatric care management, Part II. Presented at: The National Association of Professional Geriatric Care Managers; October 14–17, 1992; Tucson, AZ.

5. Dolen L, Rubin E, Charnow J, Cress M. The business of becoming a private geriatric care manager. Presented at: The National Association of Professional Geriatric Care Managers; October 17–19, 1992; Tucson, AZ.

6. Marks W. Partnerships: the good, the bad, and the ugly. Why do they succeed or fail? *GCM J.* 1996;6:6–9.

7. Burstiner I. *The Small Business Handbook: A Comprehensive Guide To Starting and Running Your Own Business.* New York: Prentice Hall; 1989.

8. Orsini M. Doing good makes cents: advanced business practices. Presented at: The National Association of Professional Geriatric Care Managers Conference; October 19–22, 1994; Paradise Island, Bahamas.

9. US Small Business Administration, San Francisco District. *Women's Small Business Start-Up Information Package.* Denver, CO: SBA Publications.

10. Thompson CC. Billing and invoicing options for geriatric care managers. *GCM J.* 1996;6:15–19.

11. Netting FE, Williams FG. Geriatric case managers: integration into physician practices. *Care Manag J.* 1999 Winter;1(1):3–9.

12. Miller AH, Karasov MA. Elder law and elder care. Presented at: The National Association of Professional Geriatric Care Managers Conference; October 21–24, 1999; San Diego, CA.

13. Bartlestone R, Lewis G. CPAs in partnership with care managers. Presented at: The National Association of Professional Geriatric Care Managers Conference; October 21–24, 1999; San Diego, CA.

Chapter 8

After the Start-up: Issues for Mature Care Management Organizations

Phyllis Mensh Brostoff

■ INTRODUCTION

As Chapter 7, "How to Start or Add a Geriatric Care Management Business," made clear, the new geriatric care management business has very particular concerns. It must define itself, decide who it serves, and establish its place in the community. After this flurry of start-up activities, methods of operation have been established and relationships have been initiated. Eventually, the business comes to a point at which initial premises are reexamined, systems are refined, and directions are reconsidered. If the owner decides to go beyond a one- or two-person business model, new organizational systems must be developed. If the owner decides to expand significantly, he or she begins a period of adding staff and working him- or herself out of jobs they previously had done. To decide how to proceed, the mature geriatric care management business needs to do periodic reassessments and adjustments.

■ DEFINING A NICHE

The organization's niche is defined by the services it provides and the population it serves. When contemplating growth, the maturing geriatric care management organization may be ready to consider expanding or changing the population it serves and the services it offers. Just as a functional assessment of a new client guides a geriatric care manager (GCM) in planning initial services, and periodic reassessment keeps GCMs responsive to changing client needs, a reassessment of the type of clients served and the services provided can offer guidance in developing a plan for growth and development for the organization.

Organizations finding themselves at this crossroads should answer the following questions about the clients they have served:

- What are the geographical location and pattern of the population being served (e.g., within a given city, which neighborhoods have the highest density of older people or older people in certain income brackets)? A breakdown by zip code can be a useful tool.
- What is the average income of the clients you have served?
- Are the clients primarily living at home (alone? with spouses or family members?) or in institutions?
- How functionally dependent are the clients?
- Is there a focus on long-term care, short-term care, or a mix—what is the average length of service of the clients you have served?
- Are services primarily short-term consultations or long-term, ongoing care management?

- Is care coordinated to help the client remain at home, or is the primary focus on helping clients transfer to assisted living or skilled care facilities?
- Are services provided in assisted living or skilled nursing facilities?
- Are fiduciary services such as bill paying, guardianships, or conservatorships provided?
- What services has the organization actually provided to the clients it has served since it began?
- What services have proved to be economically viable and which ones are money losers?

Having answered these and any other relevant questions, the geriatric care management organization can assess its patterns of service to clients, the demographics of the clients it has served, and determine whether services should be added, dropped, or shared with other providers.

■ MODELS OF GERIATRIC CARE MANAGEMENT

Geriatric care management has evolved largely as a private professional practice shaped by the unique skills and orientation of the GCM conducting the practice and the identified needs of the clients served. The GCM practicing alone may continue indefinitely or as long as the individual's strength and health allow. Some GCMs practice with other professionals such as elder-law attorneys, certified public accountants, or physicians (as described in Chapter 7).

In the late 1970s, when geriatric care management was beginning to be recognized as a distinct practice specialization through the federally funded community option Medicare/Medicaid waiver programs, care management was defined as a broker model. The care manager employed by a governmental unit or nonprofit organization was

expected to assess the client, define the service mix the client needed, order those services for the client from vendors with whom the organization had contracts, and then monitor the quality of care provided by those vendors.

In the early 1980s, when private pay care management began to develop, it was the expectation of the entrepreneurs who opened up these private practices that they would be paid directly by their clients. In fact, when the National Association of Professional Geriatric Care Managers was founded in 1986, it was called the National Association of *Private* Geriatric Care Managers, reflecting the expectation that all of the members would be providing care management as a business, on a fee-for-service basis. However, as these businesses matured, it became clear that a major service the private care manager found herself providing to clients was finding competent, reliable caregivers to work for them. Care managers typically screened and recommended these caregivers, charging their regular hourly rates for this service. However, hiring private caregivers required families to pay the required taxes, obtain needed liability insurance, and other payroll-related expenses. Care managers found that it was sometimes difficult to supervise the caregiver she had screened and recommended to the family because she was not the employer and could not discipline or fire the caregiver. In addition, families and third parties (trust companies, attorneys) did not want to bother with the payroll-related tasks. Care managers began to hire their own caregivers, and the care managed home care agency model was born.

Brokerage, or Free-Standing Care Manager, Model

In the brokerage, or free-standing care manager, model, the care manager service is the only service provided. All of the assistance needed by and arranged for clients, including caregivers, are provided by other businesses or organizations. The GCM assesses the client's level of functioning and living situation, explores options, develops a plan of care, and, if the case goes beyond the assessment and recommendation phase to ongoing care management, the GCM arranges for whatever service the client needs, which might include caregivers, shopping, transportation, emergency response, and so forth. The GCM monitors and coordinates the care that is provided by all of these independent sources. The care manager, by constantly monitoring the services clients are receiving, is in a position to be knowledgeable about the quality of care of the services she is monitoring. In large part, it is the expertise gained by this interaction with the service community that the GCM is selling.

Care managers who provide only care management services sometimes find that they specialize in short-term consultations. Other care management practices find that clients come to them to research and recommend alternative living arrangements when they no longer can remain in their own homes. Another specialization of a mature care management practice is working with the probate court and trust and estate attorneys in disputed guardianship cases, where the expertise of a care manager can assist in untangling complex family disputes and "dueling" powers of attorney. Finally, mature care management–only practices generally have long-term monitoring roles with clients whose care they may oversee for many years. A mature care management–only practice may also find that it is asked to do presentations to local civic organizations, or teach a class in gerontology or services to the aged at a local university. These opportunities may provide some additional income to the sole practitioner or an excellent means to market the care manager's expertise, even if there is little or no compensation for the program.

Integrated Models

There are a number of integrated models of mature care management practices paired with one or more related services. The most common one is the care managed home care practice, which employs caregivers directly, as described earlier. However, there are also mature care management practices that combine care management with selling insurance-related services, usually long-term care insurance. Another combination of services is care management and employee assistance and/or eldercare in the workplace programs. These services may be provided primarily via the telephone, or they may be combined with in-person assessments and family consultations, or "brown bag" programs in workplaces to provide education and support to employees. Combining care management and becoming a corporate guardian and/or conservator has also proved to be a successful model for the expansion of mature care management practices. These practices vary greatly across the country because guardianship and conservator systems are governed by each state and/or municipality, rather than a uniform system throughout the country. In addition to these examples of care management practices integrated with other significant services, some care managers provide emergency response services through one of the national systems such as LifeLine or ResponseLink.

However, no matter what other service the care management practice also operates, the GCM still begins with a client assessment, identifying options, and developing a plan of care. Care managers who practice in the most ethically sound manner provide clients with information about other options if the client needs one of the other services the care management organization provides, unless it is clear that the client came to the organization for one of these other services, and receives the care management as an enrichment, rather than the service the client sought from the agency originally.

Choosing a Model

After a geriatric care management business is well established, the owner is often confronted with a dilemma—if she has been successful, she may find herself with more business than she can handle on her own. Or she may find clients asking her to provide one of the other services mentioned earlier. The business owner must then decide if she wants the business to grow, which might be just through hiring another professional GCM. This is a relatively easy decision to make because it does not require building an organization. However, even this decision requires the care manager owner to develop some additional business expertise, including developing a contract for the care manager employee, setting expectations regarding productivity, agreeing on reporting systems, providing equipment, and supervising the employee. For some care managers, this is clearly not what they want to do. One-person care management businesses can thrive, and these practitioners have found creative ways to allow themselves vacations and time off, usually by pairing with another sole practitioner with whom they have developed a collegial relationship.

However, for care managers who want to build an organization, any of the service combinations identified earlier can be chosen, based on the care manager's own interests, background, and expertise. Because the care managed home care model is the most frequent model for growth chosen by GCMs, this model will be the one that is most extensively discussed in this chapter. However, no matter which model is chosen, much of the following information is relevant.

■ MAINTAINING A CONSISTENT ORGANIZATIONAL IMAGE

As an organization grows beyond a single person, maintaining a consistent philosophy and approach to service is essential. The chief executive officer (CEO) must convey to all new employees—whether they are caregivers, administrative/clerical staff, or professional GCMs—the guiding philosophy and values of the organization. Defining and maintaining the image of the organization is an ongoing task for the CEO of any growing organization.

The image of the organization is based on everything the public sees and hears about the organization, including the following:

1. The physical appearance of the people who work for the organization
2. The appearance and location of the offices occupied by the organization
3. The observable behaviors of all the employees of the organization
4. The reputation of the organization
5. The collateral material (e.g., logo, letterhead, brochure, print advertising) produced by the organization
6. The training and experience level of the staff

Reputation depends partly on the professional training and orientation of the organization's leading GCMs. GCMs may have been trained as social workers, nurses, gerontologists, psychologists, health administrators, or educators. Whatever their professional background, all GCMs should project their competence as seasoned professionals capable of conducting autonomous, independent practices in which the welfare of the client is the highest priority. This image can be projected by having well-organized protocols, an attitude of caring and helpfulness, and respect for the client's need for autonomy and self-determination.

In mature geriatric care management organizations that employs several GCMs, each GCM will have unique skills and strengths, and each will have weaknesses. Regular, consistent, supportive supervision is critical to ensuring high-quality service. At a minimum, GCMs should have the following characteristics and attitudes:

- Be professionals who are perceived as being friendly, caring, and cooperative people experienced in serving the client population
- Be licensed and/or credentialed by their professional group or the standard-setting bureau of their state
- Approach client needs and problems in an organized, thorough manner
- Be flexible and creative in exploring client options and developing unique care plans
- Assist clients and families in making decisions without imposing their own opinions or being judgmental
- Understand their value as professionals and charge for their time accordingly
- Not take on tasks that can be completed by paraprofessionals or nonprofessionals
- Be an integral part of the community by participating in community organizations
- Receive regular, consistent, supportive supervision

In care managed home care agencies, the caregivers must understand that the work of the organization is carried out through them and behave accordingly. They are the eyes and ears, heart and hands of the organization. As the mature geriatric care management organization grows, and, in care managed home care businesses, the number of caregivers increases, regular and ongoing training must be planned. Orientation to the geriatric care management organization's procedures, protocols, safety precautions, and care guidelines should be required for all new employees.

Every member of an organization contributes to the image of that organization, and it is the responsibility of each person to project an image congruent with the mission of the organization. Although appropriate professional behavior is the most important factor, it is also important for employees themselves, their cars, and the organization's offices to look clean and neat. When all employees look

and behave in a professional manner, the organization's reputation will be enhanced.

■ MARKETING

To thrive and grow, mature care management organizations must refine their marketing approach by examining their marketing philosophy periodically and updating their marketing plan. If the organization has an annual strategic planning meeting, marketing is an appropriate topic for discussion. If the organization is a smaller or part-time practice, choosing a new marketing strategy may simply mean deciding to develop a new brochure and update marketing materials. In larger organizations, additional marketing materials may be needed, targeting specific segments of the community.

Marketing Philosophy

Three best practices in geriatric care management provide the basis for marketing care management—providing education, building goodwill, and developing positive relationships. The first best practice is education. Marketing can educate older people, their families, and professionals who serve older people about the spectrum of services geriatric care management provides. The second best practice is the building of goodwill. The community's goodwill toward the organization is one of the greatest assets an organization can have. Though it may seem to have little to do with the financial standing of the organization, goodwill is in fact a vitally important element of an organization's equity. The third best practice is the primacy of relationships. A marketing philosophy focused on relationship building is most consistent with the care management values that drive the organization. It is also most congruent with the way in which services are delivered: through a relationship between the GCM and the client. The clinical and marketing functions of a geriatric care management organization ideally have the same focus: relationship building. Marketing conducted from the perspective of relationship building can demonstrate to potential clients the quality of relationships available to them. Prospective clients choose providers of elder care who they trust, with whom they feel safe, and who they view as competent professionals. It is through a relationship that prospective clients develop this trust. These three threads—education, building goodwill, and building relationships—form the fabric of a positive and effective marketing philosophy.

Marketing Plan

This section discusses marketing plans for mature geriatric care management organizations—organizations that have already had marketing plans in their start-up phase. Seven elements of a marketing plan that a mature organization might look at are discussed:

1. Definition of services and target profiles
2. Market research
3. Community development
4. Advertising
5. Public relations
6. Inquiries and the intake process
7. Tracking and learning

The beginning geriatric care management organization will have become involved in at least some of these seven elements. But most start-up organizations lack the financial and human resources to invest in the development of a full-blown marketing plan. As the organization grows, new challenges and opportunities appear. Additional resources may become available. An annual review of the marketing plan and assessment of the organization's functional capacity are critical to an organization's success.

Definition of Services and Target Profiles

A marketing plan for a mature geriatric care management organization begins with a redefinition of services and a profile of the target markets. For whom do we do what? The organization must clearly redefine the features and scope of its services. Only then is it able to differentiate its services from other services provided in the community. Does the organization provide geriatric care management only? Does it provide caregiving services? Does it contract out for caregivers or employ its own? Are services subsidized or are they paid for privately?

What is the profile of the target market? There are generally three target audiences: the older clients themselves, their families and relatives, and professionals in the community who refer older people to needed services. The question then becomes, which target market does the organization wish to reach?

Older people themselves may resist services and be among the last to admit they need assistance. The older person may or may not be making the decisions about purchasing care management services. The decision maker may be a family member, a trust officer, or a conservator. Marketing efforts must be directed to educate older people about geriatric care management as an alternative to institutional care. What is the profile of the specific kind of older person the agency wishes to serve? What is the person's age range, income level, and level of education? What are the person's levels of cognitive and physical functioning?

The adult children or relatives of the older person are frequently the ones initially to reach out for services. Although geriatric care management as a professional service has been in the marketplace for more than 20 years, many families do not know it exists, much less what it can provide. Education for this segment of the target audience is a vital function of marketing. Information about the availability of care management services, what specific services a given organization provides, and how these services are differentiated from other services offered to older people in the community needs to be clearly explained to this group. The care management organization must understand the demographics of this target audience. Are its members well-educated, upper-income professionals with busy careers and young families of their own? Do they live out of town or out of state?

The third target market is other professionals who serve older people and their families. These professionals are valuable potential referral sources and frequently participate as members of the support team for the older person. This group includes trust and estate and elder-law attorneys, financial planners, geriatric physicians, psychiatrists, trust officers, private fiduciaries, hospital discharge planners, members of the clergy, and other community organizations that provide services for older people. What is the profile of this population in the community where the geriatric care management organization is and the communities it serves? A geriatric care management company serving an upper-class suburb will target a different kind of professional than a nonprofit agency providing care management services to low-income older people.

Market Research

The second step in updating a marketing plan is to develop a market research strategy. This research strategy will enable the geriatric care management organization to redefine the needs of those residing in its market area. A sense of the character and lifestyle of the older people in the community will guide the practitioner so that services may be tailored to appeal to the individual community's older residents and their families.

Demographic information can often be obtained from the Area Agency on Aging. Census data can be obtained on the Internet. Chambers of commerce and other local planning bodies may also have valuable information.

When looking at demographic data, geriatric care management organizations should ask a number of questions. How many older people reside in the organization's service area? In what zip codes are they concentrated? How many of them are between the ages of 70 and 85 years? How many are older than 85 years? How many live alone? How many need assistance with the activities of daily living? What is their income level? What is their level of education? In addition to research pertaining to older clients, the organization will also want to research area families and professionals, the other two target audiences. This demographic information can inform future marketing decisions such as where and how advertising dollars would be most effectively spent.

Developing Community Relationships

Developing and nurturing community relationships with referral sources is important in growing a care management business. The mature geriatric care management organization will have already identified many people with whom to develop relationships and will have initiated these relationships. Marketing professionals can do relationship development, but experience indicates that GCMs employed by the mature organization are perhaps the best candidates for this role.

GCMs may resist understanding their role in developing community relationships and marketing the organization. One technique that may be useful is to provide GCMs with information packets and small gifts to take with them when they are likely to meet another professional in the process of conducting their regular business. For example, an information packet and small gift given to a hospital discharge planner as the GCM is taking a client home from the hospital can result in ongoing referrals. Staff training focusing on how to talk about the services provided by the organization and how to ask for referrals can be very helpful.

Clearly, community relationship building can easily be carried out in the course of daily care management activities. A GCM who accompanies a client to an appointment can educate the physician about geriatric care management in general and the organization's services specifically. The GCM can illustrate the services by talking about how the client's sundown symptoms have been tracked in a logbook that is kept in the client's home or how the GCM is training and supervising the caregiving staff to carry out the physician's instructions. If the GCM works with an attorney on behalf of a client to arrange estate planning, the GCM can again take the opportunity to inform the attorney about the full range of the organization's geriatric care management services. The attorney will encounter other older clients who need the services of a GCM and will refer them, provided he or she understands what geriatric care management is and what services it can involve.

Experience has shown that community relationships take time to evolve. Repeated encounters and firsthand experience with geriatric care management services are often required before other professionals understand the scope of service provided by a comprehensive geriatric care management organization. It takes time for the professional to trust the GCM. In short, relationships are rarely established in one visit. Social workers and many nurses are trained to start any relationship "where the client is." When the desired relationship is with another professional, the principle remains the same. Professionals have a particular point of view: they are trying to accomplish some goal for their client. If geriatric care management organizations can focus on these professionals' goals and learn how to make their work easier for them, the relationships between the care management organizations and other allied professionals will flourish.

Although community relationship building can happen in the course of geriatric care management activities, an approach that combines both organized, concerted efforts and spontaneous encounters will yield the best results. The marketing plan must articulate the targets for community relationship development, who is accountable for developing the relationships, and how these contacts will be tracked. Community relationship activities can be divided by profession (e.g., one GCM is responsible for developing relationships with all the elder-law attorneys in the community). GCMs then attend the association meetings of and network within that one group of professionals. Alternatively, one community relationship development representative can be responsible for a particular neighborhood or geographic area. Within that area, the GCM networks, educates, and develops relationships with physicians, elder-law attorneys, trust officers, hospital discharge planners, assisted living residence administrators, and so forth. How community relationship tasks are divided is not important. What is important is that they are divided in a manner that clearly defines who is responsible for fostering which relationships. For example, a GCM serving a suburban area encounters a supervising trust officer during a routine call to a trust department. The GCM follows up with a letter and an information packet. He or she alerts the person in charge of marketing, who then follows up with a call to the supervising trust officer in the regional office, thereby expanding the company's opportunity to broaden its influence throughout the trust departments in the region.

Advertising

A marketing plan for the mature geriatric care management company must address what advertising will be done. Depending on the local market, different advertising options may be appropriate to achieve the business's marketing objectives. Advertising options for the mature organization include but are not limited to print advertisements, broadcast (television or radio) advertisements, Internet sites and links, billboards, booths at senior health fairs, and sponsorship of community events. Common print advertising options appropriate for geriatric care management organizations include general-interest newspapers (most newspapers have a senior section), senior newspapers, local civic magazines, local business journals, community newsletters, Better Business Bureau consumer guides, elder-care directories, and local professional newsletters. A geriatric care management organization may want to be listed in several categories (i.e., home care, geriatric care management, elder care, senior services) in local directories. The mature organization should have a budget large enough to pay for advertising. Advertising that reaches the most people in the target market at the lowest cost is of course the best choice. For example, is there a radio station that is popular with professionals as they drive to and from work? A timely spot could reach adult children who are professionals as well as professionals serving older people.

Public Relations

The mature geriatric care management organization looking to grow will want to focus on public relations. Major relevant public relations activities can include creating media kits, sending regular press releases, building relationships with media contacts, publishing newsletters, holding open houses, participating in speakers bureaus, attending health fairs, and giving seminars and presentations at conferences. These activities are part of educating the public about the organization's services and building goodwill toward the organization. (See Chapter 10 on marketing.)

The mature geriatric care management organization will want to continue to use media kits to keep the press mindful of the organization's history and aware of information that is in the public interest. Media kits are used to educate media representatives about the organization and to solicit media coverage of the organization's services, activities, and events. Media kits can include the following items: company background/fact sheet; company brochure; appropriate press releases; biographies of the executive team, board of directors, advisory board, and GCMs; client testimonials; reprints of articles on or about the geriatric care management agency or about geriatric care management in general; literature on the National Association of Professional Geriatric Care Managers or Case Management Society of America (CMSA); photos with captions; a sheet of frequently asked questions and their answers; a sheet with common objections and answers or explanations for the objections; newspaper articles about your mature GCM agency; and a narrative of one client's experience with the organization (with the client's name changed for confidentiality).

Press releases can be sent for a variety of reasons: to announce an upcoming event (for inclusion in a newspaper's listing of events), to launch a new service, to announce a new office location, to announce a new contract or affiliation, to announce awards and achievements (awarded to either the company or an employee), or to announce a client's achievements. One organization was able to place a story about a 100-year-old client who flew cross-country to visit her childhood summer home with her caregiver in a feature article in a metropolitan newspaper. (Of course, this type of story requires prior approval from the client.) Press releases should be sent to the following contacts: local press, trade press, business and financial press, investors, and prospective investors. Press releases should be sent on a regular basis by the mature geriatric care management organization because they can build and maintain awareness of the organization. Many organizations providing "home care" are springing up; a good human interest story can highlight the important differences between professional geriatric care managed home care and other approaches to home care.

Relationships with media contacts begin by sending or delivering the company's media kit. Relationships are fostered by sending regular press releases, monitoring editorial calendars for media opportunities, pursuing appropriate opportunities with the media representatives, inviting editors and advertising representatives to visit the company, and working with media representatives on feature articles and interviews. The more these relationships are nurtured, the more often the organization will be mentioned by the local media.

Company newsletters that educate people about geriatric care management can offer a valuable service to the professional community and serve significant public relations functions simultaneously. A well-written, regularly published newsletter, hard copy or e-mail, can establish professional credibility and community presence. Holding open houses to celebrate a new office or a significant anniversary can also serve a public relations function if professional and media contacts are invited.

Inquiries and the Intake Process

Targeted advertising and public relations activities help geriatric care management companies make the public aware of their services. But after an organization does the expensive work of getting people to pay attention, then what? In a marketing (and clinical) model in which relationships are primary, the focus is on educating and creating lasting relationships, not creating instant impressions.

Inquiries are the information-seeking contacts made by family members, older people, or professionals about the organization's services. The intake process is developed to respond to these calls, from the initial greeting at the reception desk to the information exchange, to the point when the caller chooses to work with the organization (as a client, as a relative of a client, or as a source of referrals) or chooses another organization. A critical element of the mature geriatric care management organization's marketing plan is ongoing analysis and improvement of the inquiry and intake processes so that as many inquiries as possible lead to new clients. A monthly summary and analysis of intake calls received, the referral source, and the outcome of the call is a vital management tool. If the research, community relationship building, advertising, and public relations are working, a steady stream of prospective clients will be calling.

These prospects have varying degrees of information about the organization's services. One caller's friend may have heard an ad on the radio. That caller may know nothing about geriatric care management and not be certain that an older aunt wants or needs assistance. Another caller may have heard about the organization from three different respected sources, have done extensive research on how best to provide care for his or her aging parents, and be seeking information about some of the fine points of the services. How does the organization handle these various calls to maximize conversions from callers to clients?

The mature geriatric care management organization has already designed an inquiry and intake process; however, periodic review and analysis are vital to organizational growth. Several elements are involved in designing and refining the inquiry and intake process. These elements include making sure clear information is provided, making sure the information packet is sent on a timely basis, following up on the initial call, referring when appropriate, and refining the intake process itself. Are the first contacts primarily phone calls, e-mail inquiries, written inquiries, or walk-ins? Who fields the first contact? Is it the receptionist? Does he or she convey a good image for the organization? Is he or she warm, inviting, professional, and knowledgeable? This is one of the most important positions in the organization. Does he or she have a script of what to say? Is there an established protocol of how to field inquiries? If not, the organization needs to design a script that includes the initial greeting, the question, "How may we help you?" and the assurance that the intake GCM will respond within the hour if he or she is not immediately available. This initial response tells callers how important they are to the geriatric care management organization. The protocol should include recording of the caller's name and phone number because lost calls are costly.

INFORMATION PACKET

Geriatric care management organizations will need an information packet of materials describing their services. The materials should accurately convey the organization's identity and be of a high quality, to reflect the quality of the services themselves. Remember that relationships are primary and the focus is on educating prospective clients about the organization's services. The material can be as simple as a brochure or as sophisticated as a presentation folder containing multiple pieces (e.g., a brochure, a description of geriatric care management, a sheet of frequently asked questions, a sheet of common objections and answers or explanations for the objections, information about the National Association of Professional Geriatric Care Managers or CMSA, reprints of articles about the organization or about geriatric care management in general, newsletters, and a narrative of a client's experience with the organization).

INTAKE

The intake process itself is very important. This is where the greatest opportunity exists to educate prospective clients and referral sources about the organization's services. The caller is giving the care management organization his or her full attention. The potential to expand the relationship from caller to client is great. It is critical that the intake coordinator keep the caller's full attention. The best intake coordinators have both strong clinical skills and an understanding of and comfort with sales principles. The intake coordinator will want to use a consistent format to find out as much as possible about the caller's situation and needs. Questions to be asked include the following:

- Who is the client?
- What is the caller's relationship to the client?
- How did the caller hear about the organization?
- How is the client's overall health and well-being? Where and with whom does the client live? How independent is the client in caring for him- or herself?
- What was the precipitating event that resulted in the phone call?
- What services does the client want?
- What does the caller know about geriatric care management?
- Does the caller understand the geriatric care management model?

It takes time to educate the caller. While seeking answers to these questions, the intake coordinator must spend ample time listening. It is here, in this sharing of information, that the relationship between the caller and the organization is being formed. Some callers request services immediately, whereas others require a number of follow-up calls before becoming clients, and some are not appropriate for the organization's services at all.

There are many ways to handle these intake/inquiry calls. One person may be the designated intake coordinator, or each GCM working in the organization can be trained to handle intake/inquiry calls. If the organization chooses to use each of their GCMs to handle these calls, it is best to have them scheduled in the office on a regular basis to handle the calls because multiple GCMs with widely varying schedules cannot field incoming inquiries in a consistent manner. The organization that responds most promptly to the inquiry is the most likely to be the chosen service provider when the caller has been given the names of several organizations to call or is calling from a list. Whichever system is put into place, it is vitally important that the intake coordinator/designated GCM intake worker offer information and referrals to callers who are not appropriate for the organization.

The intake worker must be familiar with community resources. Disseminating information and appropriate referrals is an important community service and good public relations. It provides valuable education and builds enormous goodwill in the community toward the organization. In addition, clients who are not a good fit for the organization are weeded out at intake.

Tracking and Learning

The follow-up process is almost as important as the intake process. Intake coordinators at mature geriatric care management organizations can use lulls in the incoming inquiries to follow up on previous calls. A tickler system can be set up to follow up on callers who say no or who are not immediately interested in services. Numerous computer software programs are available to assist in following up on prospects. It is important to know that "no" is not always a final answer in this situation; in fact, marketing experts suggest that it usually means "maybe" or "not just yet."[1] Remember, if people have contacted the organization, they are serious prospects. Organizations that choose to use the intake coordinator model are in a better position to pay special attention to nurturing these relationships because one person is in that position and following up on calls should be included in that person's job description.

The geriatric care management organization, desiring to build equity, must be a learning organization across the board. According to Peter Senge, who developed the concept of the learning organization, a learning organization is a new source of competitive advantage.[2] Nowhere is this learning organization approach more important than in marketing efforts. At a learning organization, people are constantly researching the existing business, tracking every dollar spent on marketing, tracking every response, measuring and analyzing the data, and making modifications to the marketing plan based on those data. Learning organizations continually measure, learn from what they measure, and make changes according to what they learn.

Computer software can make tracking manageable. Some of the information to track will be number of intake calls, number of e-mail contacts, number of inquiries converted into active clients, organizations to which callers are referred, and sources of referrals. This and other information will allow the organization to refine its advertising and public relations plans, community development efforts, and intake process. Adequate tracking is part of the vital feedback loop guiding the marketing plan and the organization as a whole.

■ ORGANIZATIONAL DEVELOPMENT

The information in this section is derived from direct experience building the geriatric care management organization of the original writers of this chapter, the additional experience of the reviser of the chapter, and many discussions with colleagues struggling with the same issues during the course of 20-plus years of providing geriatric care management services. You are encouraged to borrow whatever is useful but ultimately to do whatever works best in your organization. This discussion of organizational development addresses four areas:

1. Defining the organization's identity
2. Assessing and tending the organization's culture
3. Developing leaders and staff members
4. Developing systems

Defining the Organization's Identity

To thrive and grow, a mature organization must have a clearly articulated identity. Organizations can begin the process of defining themselves by focusing on four elements: mission, purpose, values, and culture. (These elements are discussed in the following sections.) Most geriatric care management organizations develop mission and purpose statements early on. As organizations mature and expand, it is useful to revisit these statements, refining them with the participation of the newer members of the organizational team.

Mission

A mission statement tells the community what the organization strives to accomplish through its work. In 2001, the mission statement of Age Concerns, San Diego, California, was "to enhance the quality of life for our clients to the maximum extent possible by fostering the elderly person's health, self-esteem and right to self determination." In 2006, the mission of Stowell Associates SelectStaff, Milwaukee, Wisconsin, "is to maintain the safety, security and independence of our elderly and disabled adult clients by providing the highest quality of professional care management and caregiving services."

Ideally, every employee in the organization helps to craft the mission statement. When employees participate in creating the statement, they are more committed to it than they would be if it were developed by management or the owner only. Once the mission statement is written, it becomes a guide for decision making at all levels of the organization. Placement of this statement on business cards, brochures, and other informational materials serves to remind the staff of their mission and educate the community.

Purpose

Whereas the mission statement speaks to the organization's community, the purpose statement is an internal statement the staff make to themselves about how and why they do their work. According to Collins and Porras, the "core purpose is the organization's reason for being. An effective purpose reflects people's idealistic motivations for doing the company's work. It doesn't just describe the organization's output or target customers; it captures the soul of the organization."[3(p68)] Purpose should not be confused with specific goals or business objectives. The purpose statement answers the question, "Why is what we do important to us?" The purpose statement of the beginning geriatric care management organization may be suitable for the mature geriatric care management organization, but a periodic review of the statement helps staff to maintain focus. As with the mission statement, staff will feel more committed to the purpose statement when they participate in creating it.

A completed purpose statement reminds staff members about how and why they do their work. It can also guide decisions that impact the culture and work environment. Management can ask, "Would implementing this new policy be in keeping with our purpose statement?" In 2001, the purpose statement of Age Concerns was "By serving our clients, their families, and the community, we seek to enhance the quality and meaning of our lives and the lives of those with whom we work. By growing and prospering as an organization, we make a good income for today's needs and have resources and investments for the future. By working together mindfully, respecting and nurturing our unique strengths and talents, we foster growth, a sense of community, and fun." The purpose statement can help management and staff assess how they are doing. Individuals can ask themselves, "Are my unique strengths and talents being nurtured?" "Am I respecting and nurturing the strengths of my fellow workers?"

Values

The third element for the organization to articulate in its process of self-definition is its values. Core values are the essential and enduring tenets of an organization. According to Collins and Porras, "A small set of timeless guiding principles, core values require no external justification; they have intrinsic value and importance to those inside the organization."[3(p66)] These core values are what the organization stands for. The core values of the geriatric care management organization may have been defined and articulated at the start and may have remained unchanged; however, the mature organization will do well to revisit these values as part of new employee orientation and renew them as part of a retreat to remind and refocus all staff. The following questions can be posed to staff to help them define or review the core values of their organization:

- What core values do you personally bring to your work? (These should be so fundamental that you would hold them regardless of whether they were rewarded.)
- What would you tell your children (or grandchildren) are the core values that you hold at work and that you hope they will hold when they become working adults?
- If you awoke tomorrow morning with enough money to retire for the rest of your life, would you continue to live by those core values?
- Can you envision those core values being as valid for you 100 years from now as they are today?
- Would you want to continue holding those core values even if at some point

one or more of them became a competitive disadvantage?
- If you were to start a new organization tomorrow in a different line of work, what core values would you build into the new organization regardless of its industry?[3(p68)]

For a geriatric care management organization, core values might include the centrality of relationships, the belief that clients are best nurtured by staff that are respected and supported, the acceptance of and respect for the uniqueness of every human being, and the acceptance of growth and change as a part of life. Defining values as an organization when it begins is important. To remain effective, the mature geriatric care management organization should revisit its statement of its core values periodically to include new staff in value development, ensure their commitment to these values, and revise its value statements as the organization evolves and changes.

Many successful organizations publicize their values. For example, three core values of the Nordstrom's retail stores are as follows:

1. Service to the customer above all else
2. Hard work and individual productivity
3. Excellence in reputation

Stowell Associates SelectStaff's value statements include "We consider each person—the individual who needs care and those who are part of the caring network." "Our assessments and evaluations are based on understanding your particular needs, as you define them."

Assessing and Tending the Organization's Culture

Work cultures are made up of a variety of elements. These elements, which range from "encouraging innovation" to "maximizing client satisfaction" and "providing secure employment," can be prioritized so that organizations can begin to determine both their current and their ideal cultures. The new organization must assess and define its culture. The mature organization should redefine its culture periodically. The following questions can be helpful in the process:

- What is the overriding strategic intent of the organization? The strategic intent refers to how the organization does what it does. The strategic intent answers such questions as these:
  - What do customers want?
  - How does the organization deliver what the customers want?
  - How is the organization different from other organizations?
- How is the organization structured (e.g., hierarchical, flat)?
- How is work organized (i.e., teams versus individual contributors)? How do teams and individuals interact?
- How are decisions made?
- What behaviors are encouraged? What behaviors are discouraged or prohibited?
- What kind of people work for the organization?
- How do they think?
- How do they act (e.g., in a task-oriented way)?
- How much power do they have?
- How much risk are they allowed—and do they wish—to take?
- How are they selected and developed?
- How are they rewarded?
- How is pay viewed? Is it seen as an investment or merely a cost of doing business?

Once an organization has clearly articulated its mission, purpose, and values and assessed its culture, it can more effectively continue the process of developing. If an honest review of the organization's current reality does not match the desired state, efforts to improve can be planned and implemented. Development is not a one-time event but a continuous process because the point of view being recommended here is that improvement is always possible. Attention must be paid to the organization's culture if the organization is going to remain robust and dynamic. Cultures differ from organization to organization. There is no one right answer. Whatever works is what is "right" for that organization.[4] However, the centrality of relationships appears to be one tenet that is essential to the cultures of geriatric care management organizations.

In the delivery of geriatric care management services, it is the quality of the relationship between the GCM and the client (and the family) that makes this service unique and is a key criterion for success. It is, in part, the absence of human relationships in the nation's bureaucracies, medical system, and elsewhere that creates the need for geriatric care management.

If relationships are the lifeblood of the organization, what is the organization doing to foster them? This element of the culture must be focused on, nurtured, and developed for the organization to continue to mature. It is often said that a child learns what he or she lives. In a sense, we all learn what we live. If management wants the GCM to develop mastery in his or her relationships with clients, managers must develop mastery in their relationships with the GCMs and other staff members. If the organization wants GCMs to nurture their clients, the organization must nurture the GCMs. If the organization wants to support the autonomy and self-determination of older people, it must also support the autonomy and self-determination of its employees. Organizational practices that foster staff autonomy and self-determination include participative management and self-managed teams.[5]

Developing Leaders and Staff Members

Geriatric care management organizations focused on growth must attend to leadership and staff development. Fostering professional development improves individual and team performance, strengthens an organization's effectiveness, creates a more cohesive culture, and encourages staff loyalty. An organization's plan for professional development should be based on an assessment of the organization's needs and the needs of the staff. Leadership and staff development based on an assessment can include training in building teams, conducting meetings, resolving conflicts, supervising, balancing work and life, managing time, making presentations, and handling the inevitable challenges the organization's staff experiences in working with each other, the clients, and their families. Table 8–1 lists different kinds of staff training and their impact on business, leadership, and clinical skills.

A key challenge to the leader of a mature geriatric care management organization is delegating tasks to others. Leaders who are accustomed to being solo practitioners may experience difficulty in delegating and supervising others. For an organization to grow, the leader essentially hires staff to assume roles that she had done herself. A clear job description, well thought out in advance of adding a new position to the organization, helps the leader to clarify what is expected from this new employee. Delegation, to be successful, confers on the new worker the authority to carry out the assigned responsibility. This is a basic tenet, often overlooked as geriatric care management organizations grow. Regular supportive supervision (a set day and time each week) is a way to ensure that the new employee will have opportunities to ask questions and provide feedback. As the numbers of staff increase, it is vital to divide the work into professional/clinical functions and business/support functions, thereby always ensuring that every worker has a supervisor. Adequate delegation frees the GCM for leadership roles. Remember, it is not possible to play all the instruments when one is conducting the orchestra. And delegated tasks create opportunities for staff development.

Caregiver Training

In geriatric care managed caregiving organizations (which is the model adopted by both Age Concerns and Stowell Associates SelectStaff), it is essential to develop orientation and training programs to educate the caregivers in the mission, purpose, and culture of the organization. This training should focus on how to work as a team to foster the client's well-being. It should address these issues and more:

- The caregiver's role and responsibilities
- The organization's guidelines
- Communication skills

Basic caregiving duties must be addressed (e.g., nutrition, hygiene, grooming, exercise, medications). Universal safety training is important to prevent caregiver or client injury. Safety training may include body mechanics (positioning, transfers, lifting), environmental safety (slips, trips, falls), disaster preparedness (earthquake, fire, utility outage), universal precautions (infection control), crime prevention (home security, weapons, theft, loss), and what to do in case of an injury to a client or caregiver. Training that addresses problems of caring for clients suffering from dementia, depression, diabetes, arthritis, Parkinson's, and other conditions helps caregivers to provide excellent care.

Developing Systems

Procedures, policies, processes, and systems must be documented as organizations mature so that institutional wisdom is preserved and processes and procedures become reproducible and transferable. A number of care management–specific computer software programs are available for lease or purchase. Any growing care management organization should be investigating and investing in computer software on an ongoing basis. In addition, the organization should budget for updates of both software and hardware virtually every year to maintain competitiveness in

Table 8-1   Impact of Staff Training on the Development of Business, Leadership, and Clinical Skills

Type of Training	Business Skills	Leadership Skills	Clinical Skills
Team Building	Teaches process skills that enable staff to work together to achieve business objectives.	Teaches leadership skills within the team context. Shared leadership is experienced.	Teaches people to work with family "teams" and caregiver teams.
Conduct of meetings	Teaches business leadership.	Teaches how to get results in teams.	Teaches people to handle family meetings and caregiver team meetings.
Conflict resolution and mediation		Teaches this core leadership competency.	Teaches how conflict resolution skills improve clinical effectiveness with clients, families, caregiving staff, and allied professionals.
Supervisory skills	Teaches communication and relationship skills. Teaches legal responsibility and laws affecting supervision.		
Annual company retreat		Encourages personal and professional renewal.	
Renewal	Anchors individuals in personal values and a sense of purpose. Results in increased motivation and professional commitment.	Encourages personal and professional renewal.	Results in work/life balance and an increased connection to one's sense of purpose
Time management	Improves overall business effectiveness.	Increases the awareness of what is important.	Assists with prioritizing competing client demands. Assists with work/life balance.
Presentation skills	Improves business presentations and professional image and credibility.	Improves communication and leadership skills.	
Countertransference			Increases clinician's awareness of his or her own issues. Teaches strategies for skillful interventions.
Continuing education. Allows staff to customize learning according to personal goals.			

a marketplace that increasingly relies on technology to improve both efficiency and maintain effectiveness.

In addition to using care management software, the agency will need to develop documentation that includes a personnel manual articulating the organization's policies regarding holidays, vacations, sick leave, health insurance, and so forth. The organization must also develop a policies and procedures manual that specifies the tasks of each job function. Growing organizations are not static; therefore, it is vitally important to periodically renew and update policies and procedures manuals. An annual review of the personnel policies should be a part of the human resources function. If there is a human resources manager, this should be part of his or her job description. If human resources is not a separate department, the review and update can be outsourced to a consulting firm. However updating is done, it is imperative that personnel policy manuals reflect current legal requirements. In the mature geriatric care management organization, timely revision of the procedures manual is generally the responsibility of each department head and the overall concern of whoever is in charge of operations.

■ ESTABLISHING WORKING RELATIONSHIPS WITH KEY ORGANIZATIONS IN THE COMMUNITY

The care management organization's CEO serves an extremely important function by being known in many circles in the community and being perceived as a leader. In a larger mature geriatric care management organization with numerous employees, the CEO should make the development of these kinds of relationships a priority. Even in large cities, the CEO can seek to spread her sphere of influence through volunteering with community groups and joining civic organizations.

Often the best way to obtain one's goals is to help others obtain their goals because those who are perceived as helpful can generally build a referral network among allied professionals. Relationships, as previously stated, grow only with time and nurturing. Simple gestures such as sending thank-you notes for referrals and other assistance will help maintain and nurture good relationships.

The CEO of the mature geriatric care management organization may want to consider the following avenues to expand the organization's presence in the community:

- Memberships in service clubs (e.g., Rotary, Kiwanis, Lions). The businesspeople in these groups may not know what care management is, but they often have aging parents. Membership gives one an opportunity to educate and spread the word. From these diverse contacts may come invitations to speak and other opportunities to educate. Referrals of clients often follow from nurturing these types of business relationships.
- A seat on the board of directors of advisory committees and community organizations (e.g., the Better Business Bureau, Community Chest or United Charities, or the YMCA/YWCA). Participation by the CEO on community boards can widen the organization's involvement in the community and enhance the organization's image. Participating in advisory committees for the planning of neighborhood, city, or county services is also an excellent way to extend one's involvement.
- Active involvement in the religious community. Active involvement in the religious community can provide the CEO with opportunities to educate volunteers and clergy working with older people. Religious organizations in every community in the United States are grappling with the problems of serving a rapidly aging population. Older people tend to

look to their religious communities for support. By building a role in the ecumenical conference of churches, synagogues, and other places of worship, one can often educate those who are attempting to guide the efforts of volunteers. By supporting or training volunteers who serve older people, one can contribute to the well-being of many older people. Religious leaders can be a valuable source of referrals of clients who need more services than volunteers can provide.

CEOs may also want to take the following steps:

- **Attend attorneys' community meetings.** A significant group of professionals serving older people are attorneys specializing in wills and probates, estate planning, or other elder-law issues. Elder-law attorneys are becoming aware of the invaluable services GCMs can provide. Educating attorneys by attending their community meetings, providing information on health or psychosocial issues affecting older people, and making referrals to them when appropriate can foster relationships with this group of professionals who can become valuable supporters of a growing care management organization.

- **Call regularly on trust officers, departments, and accounting firms.** These professionals are seeing the number of older people in their practices increase rapidly. Many of them become trusted counselors to their clients, but frequently there comes a time when the client's ability to make safe and sensible personal decisions diminishes or he or she becomes physically dependent and requires more personal care from others. These professionals are not trained in assessment of need, provision, or supervision of home care. The mature care management organization's reputation for cooperation and service can be built by making personal calls, speaking at

group meetings, and providing educational information regarding the role of geriatric care management.

- **Call regularly on senior centers and when possible give presentations or host an event.** In almost every community, senior centers provide education, recreation, and socialization programs vital to the well-being of active older people. The activity directors of these centers are often the first people to see signs of deterioration or disease. Adult day centers providing support and activities for special groups such as people with Alzheimer's or muscular dystrophy serve a very vulnerable group of older people who can often benefit from care management services. Ongoing contact, occasional talks to groups, and sponsorship of special events build awareness and trust of the geriatric care management organization.

- **Maintain contacts with support organizations.** In larger cities there are organizations providing counseling, specialized information, and referrals for older people and their families. These may be regional caregiver resource centers, Alzheimer's associations, or associations organized for the education of people with other diseases and their families. The area agencies on aging provide information and referrals exclusively focused on the needs and issues of older people. Keeping these agencies regularly supplied with printed material describing the care management organization can be an important way to increase awareness of the care management organization expertise. Occasional talks at in-service training programs are also helpful to keep new staff updated about the organization's services.

- **Attend coordinating councils.** In most areas, associations of professionals come together to share information, give mutual support, and network. These are often known as councils on aging or coalitions of elder services. Attendance and participation can foster good relationships with people in a wide circle of related service organizations.

In fact, there seems to be no limit to opportunities for networking with allied professionals. Tracking of referral sources will yield clues to which activities result in the best referrals. Measuring the goodwill engendered by the active participation suggested here is harder to measure. Building community awareness and good relationships is, for the mature care management organization, not only building the business but also building the value of the organization.

■ JOINING ORGANIZATIONS AND NETWORKING NATIONALLY

National organizations dealing with the concerns of aging have grown significantly since the mid-1980s. Many professionals who are still active in the field participated in the formation of these associations. Gerontology is a new field of study, less than 50 years old. The National Association of Professional Geriatric Care Managers celebrated its 20th birthday in 2005, but it is still unknown to many. Media coverage of aging issues in general and care management specifically has increased markedly in the past few years because a growing awareness that the baby boomers are aging is creating new interest among business people, health care providers, and politicians.

Participation and networking in national organizations can inform the growing care management organization of legislative trends in health care, the results of scientific studies, and developments in clinical practices. As geriatric care management develops beyond a specialization of other professions such as nursing and social work into a profession of its own, new knowledge is developing and interaction with colleagues through these national organizations is enriching. Mutual

support and open dialogue can be invaluable. The mature organization has the opportunity to present material to educate and mentor newer colleagues. Opportunities to participate in the development of professional organizations inform efforts to develop the individual geriatric care management organization. Here is a list of some of the leading national organizations of interest to the mature geriatric care management business:

- **National Association of Professional Geriatric Care Managers and CMSA.** Long-term national association (http://www.caremanager.org) and CMSA (http://www.cmsa.org) membership by the mature geriatric care management organization will allow the leader to get involved in the organization's activities and perhaps run for office. This level of participation allows the leader to develop a broader understanding of national trends in aging policy, the policy development necessary to ensure supportive care for older people, and the opportunities for the national organization and its members to strengthen and expand the services that will be needed.
- **The National Council on Aging (NCOA).** NCOA (http://www.ncoa.org), one of the older associations addressing issues relating to aging, focuses on the issues and concerns of service providers, but its scope is much broader than that of organizations focused on provider issues. The needs and concerns of many different groups serving older people, such as home care providers, senior centers, activity programs, or housing projects, to name a few, are addressed. NCOA also provides a legislative advocacy function.
- **The American Association of Retired Persons (AARP).** AARP (http://www.aarp.org) is the largest of all the geriatric associations. Its financial base is insurance and other business ventures. It exerts a strong legislative advocacy presence and ensures the participation of older people

through volunteer groups at the local, state, and national levels. It publishes *Modern Maturity*, a magazine that addresses a wide range of geriatric issues and targets older readers.

- **The National Gerontological Society of America (GSA).** GSA (http://www.geron.org) deals primarily with research and the interests of academia. There are four primary sections: biological, psychological, behavioral, and policy. Emphasis at the annual meetings is on the presentation of research findings.
- **The American Society on Aging (ASA).** ASA (http://www.asaging.org) emphasis is on training at the undergraduate level and sharing information regarding advances in the field. ASA has developed a strong program of seminars, often clustered around annual or regional meetings as pre-conference educational opportunities. The focus is on a wide array of services provided to older people, including care management.
- **The National Association of Elder Law Attorneys (NAELA).** NAELA (http://www.naela.com) is open for membership to attorneys only. NAELA and the National Association of Professional Geriatric Care Managers have held several joint conferences. Opportunities to participate on panels and to promote cooperation between the professions can work to the benefit of both organizations.

Contact information for these seven organizations appears in Appendix A. Other care management organizations are focused on insurance coverage services or hospital/health maintenance organization concerns that may interest growing care management organizations.

The mature geriatric care management organization can benefit from participation in the conferences and activities of numerous national organizations. Choices are clearly necessary. Membership in national organizations can be costly in terms of money, time, and

energy. Establishing priorities for national participation and sampling conferences can help determine the extent to which the mature care management organization involves itself in networking at the national level.

■ ACCREDITATION

Another strategy that mature care management organizations may decide to pursue as part of their strategic planning is to obtain accreditation from a national accrediting organization. Accreditation demonstrates to clients that the organization has achieved a level of national standards that can set the organization apart from its competition. Accreditation can also substitute for state licensing when a client has long-term care insurance—many of these contracts called for state-licensed care providers, but many states do not require any licensure for either care management or the caregiving services provided by many care management companies. In 2006, four national accreditation commissions are in operation. The mature care management organization may want to explore these if it decides to seek national accreditation:

1. Council on Accreditation (COA)
   120 Wall Street, 11th Floor
   New York, New York 10005
   (212) 797-3000
   http://www.coanet.org

The COA was started in 1977 by the Child Welfare League of America and Family Service America. It accredits 38 different services, including care management and home care. COA standards are based on a social service model, consistent with the point of view of care management. Stowell Associates Select-Staff has been accredited by COA since 2000.

2. Joint Commission on Accreditation of Healthcare Organizations (JCAHO)
   One Renaissance Blvd.
   Oakbrook Terrace, IL 60181
   (630) 792-5000
   http://www.jointcommission.org

JCAHO began to accredit health care organizations, primarily hospitals, in 1951. It has expanded its standards to include accreditation of medical equipment, hospices, home care, nursing homes, and other organizations. JCAHO standards are based on a medical model, and most of the home care agencies it accredits are state-licensed organizations that provide Medicare/Medicaid services.

3. Accreditation Commission for Health Care, Inc. (ACHC)
   4700 Falls of Neuse Rd., Suite 280
   Raleigh, NC 27609
   (919) 785-1214
   http://www.achc.org

ACHC began in 1985 in Raleigh, North Carolina, through the efforts of members of the state home care association, and it accredited its first organization in 1987. The company began offering services nationally in 1996. It accredits home care services, as well as other health-related services such as medical equipment and specialty pharmacies. The multistate agency LivHOME, which bought Age Concerns, is accredited by ACHC.

4. Community Health Accreditation Program (CHAP)
   1300 19th Street, NW, Suite 150
   Washington, DC 20036
   (202) 862-3413
   http://www.chapinc.org

CHAP was established in 1965 as a joint venture between the American Public Health Association and the National League for Nursing. In 2001, it became an independent, nonprofit corporation. It accredits 10 services, including home health, private duty services, home care aide services, and supplemental staffing services.

5. Commission on Accreditation of Rehabilitation Facilities (CARF)
   4891 E. Grant Road
   Tucson, AZ 85712
   (520) 325-1044
   http://www.carf.org

CARF was founded in 1966. It is a private, not-for-profit organization that promotes quality rehabilitation services, aging services, child and family services, behavioral health, employment and community services, and medical rehabilitation. It also accredits continuing care communities under the Continuing Care Accreditation Commission.

■ CONCLUSION

As the geriatric care management organization matures, it will revisit many of the steps it undertook in its infancy and take new steps on new pathways. These steps begin with redefining the organization's niche, confirming or changing the model of practice, and strengthening or adjusting its image in the community. The mature organization will need to rethink its marketing program and its strategy for organizational development through ongoing strategic planning. In addition, the organization will need to solidify its working relationships with key organizations in the community and reassess its involvement with national professional organizations. Finally, the mature care management organization may decide to seek national accreditation as a way of distinguishing itself in the marketplace and ensuring it meets the highest quality of national standards.

■ NOTES

1. Taylor W. Permission marketing. *Fast Company*. April–May 1998;198–212.
2. Senge P. *The Fifth Discipline: The Art and Practice of the Learning Organization*. New York: Doubleday; 1990.
3. Collins J, Porras J. Building your company's vision. *Harvard Bus Rev*. 1996;74:65–77.
4. Wheatley M, Kellner-Rogers M. *A Simpler Way*. San Francisco, CA: Berrett-Koehler Publishers; 1996.
5. Anderson B. *Pathways to Partnership*. Whitehouse, OH: Soulworks; 1998.

Chapter 9

Fee-for-Service Care Management in Not-for-Profit Settings

Stephne Lencioni and Kathleen McConnell

■ INTRODUCTION

The growth rate of the world's older adult population represents the most dramatic demographic shift in history. Projections are that in 2030, more than 20% of Americans will be 65 of age or older, with the fastest-growing segment being the "oldest old," those 85 years and older. Increased longevity can produce an array of specialized needs, ranging from services such as health care, housing, home care, and nursing facilities to opportunities for recreation, leisure time activities, and education. Older adults may face health, cognitive, financial, legal, and housing problems with little or no idea of where to get help. Family members who care for older relatives also struggle with these same issues. To address these unique needs a senior services industry has developed that has become big business and has enormous potential for profit.

One of the important components of the aging business is care management. Many older adults and their families are willing—and able—to pay for assistance with care planning and service selection. The growth of for-profit care management business has demonstrated the fact that there are customers to purchase these services. Picking up on this trend, the presence of fee-for-service (FFS) care management in the not-for-profit (NFP) agency has been slowly but steadily growing.

Probable reasons for the slow growth lie in both philosophical and operational issues. As NFPs have considered adding FFS services, agency leaders have found themselves in debates about their organizations' missions. Some struggle with what they see as conflicting goals. Traditionally, NFPs focus on service and meeting community needs, whereas the for-profit culture often measures success in terms of profitability. Others resist the new emphasis on the market. However, many large NFPs have taken the position that if there is no profit margin, they cannot continue their primary mission of serving people in need. The debate is not a simple one nor has it been resolved.

Contrary to the past, today NFPs and government agencies are no longer the only trusted providers of services for older people. Quality services are now found in the for-profit sector as well. As funding sources shrink, NFPs are at risk of being left to serve only the poor and to operate at a deficit. Thus, to expand the client base and to offset the expenses of serving those who cannot pay, many NFPs are competing with private for-profit entities for clients who can afford to pay for service.

Initial interest in establishing FFS case management programs within NFP agencies was twofold: to develop the capacity to meet the needs of multiple income groups and to generate revenue. FFS case management evolved very slowly within NFP agencies during the mid- to late 1980s, and then picked up during the 1990s. Knutson and Langer, in a survey of geriatric care management practice, found that by 1997, NFPs made up 16% of the membership of the National Association of Professional Geriatric Care Managers, an organization formerly accepting only for-profit practices as members.[1]

This chapter explores the development of FFS case management programs in NFP settings. It draws on the experiences of three agencies that have successfully implemented such programs: the Council of Jewish Elderly (CJE) in Chicago, Illinois; Huntington Hospital Senior Care Network (SCN) in Pasadena, California; and Older Adults Care Management (OACM), a division of the Institute on Aging (IOA), in Palo Alto, California. CJE, a large NFP agency, has always provided some form of case management services. FFS care management was started in 1995 to address the need for producing revenue from services to offset budget deficits. By the late 1990s, FFS care management was a part of CJE's continuum and a self-supporting service. SCN developed FFS case management in response to a clear need; namely, people with higher incomes had no access to case management services even though they experienced the same problems as people with lower incomes. Another objective was to generate revenue. The program grew from one to six care managers and incorporated a variety of care management services, including long-term care insurance underwriting and claims assessments, elder care services for employed caregivers, and other fee-based contract services. In contrast, OACM began as a for-profit agency in 1982 and only later became an NFP after being gifted to the nonprofit IOA in 1999. OACM was originally conceived as a case management business but soon added a licensed home care component to meet the identified need for hands-on assistance to elderly clients. Its history as a for-profit agency along with the coexistence of care management and home care services created both opportunities and challenges for OACM.

■ TERMINOLOGY AND DEFINITION

Historically, social workers were "caseworkers." The term *case management*, which implies that people are "cases" with their lives to be "managed," has come to seem both negative and paternalistic. Despite numerous potential alternatives (e.g., "care coordination," "service management," "service coordination"), *case management* continues to be a commonly used term. However, *care management* is gradually becoming the preferred terminology, especially among FFS professionals. But, as pointed out by Bodie Gross and Holt, "from a consumer's perspective, there is no difference between a care and case manager. The sole standard of judgment is one of satisfaction with the services being delivered."[2(p23)]

For the purposes of this chapter, *care management* is most frequently used, especially when referring to fee-based services. However, *case management* may be used when referring to a particular program or where that is the common terminology.

Just as no one name or title is used for case management, there is no single agreed-upon definition of case management or scope of services. However, there is consensus on the key tasks performed by the case manager: assessment, care planning, coordination, follow-up (including monitoring of client status and service delivery), reassessment, and termination or case closure. Although the focus here is on care management for older people and their families, it is important to note that care management is used in a wide range of settings for a variety of populations.[3]

■ BRIEF HISTORY OF CASE MANAGEMENT

It is difficult to trace the beginnings of case management definitively because many disciplines lay claim to inventing at least some element of it.[4] Its principles can be found as early as the turn of the 20th century in the social work settlement movement, but public nursing, mental health, disability, and other fields can all point to historical beginnings of case management within their own discipline. Clearly, identifying and solving problems by assessing needs, linking people to needed resources, and coordinating the delivery of services are central themes of case management throughout the history of human services.

Geriatric case management grew popular as a means of reducing public costs of long-term care. Case management programs of the 1970s and early 1980s largely were funded with public dollars—specifically through the Medicaid program—and targeted the low-income, frail elderly population at risk of institutionalization. The goal of case management was to decrease the utilization and expense of nursing home care by keeping individuals at home with supportive services. Through these and other national demonstration projects, case management became an important part of long-term care programs.[5] Many of these projects were implemented in NFP agencies as part of a continuum of services provided for older people. They all used case management, which rapidly became a popular approach to linking clients with needed resources.

By the mid-1990s, some form of case management could be found in virtually every service setting: geriatric care management was delivered in public government agencies; in private not-for-profit settings that used a combination of public funds, fund-raising, grants, and FFS dollars; and in FFS private practice. In fact, the private practice business was enjoying enough success that professionals and paraprofessionals from a wide range of educational and disciplinary backgrounds were opening FFS care management businesses catering to families of means. This trend continues and is expected to grow.

■ THE DEVELOPMENT OF FEE-FOR-SERVICE CARE MANAGEMENT

With the proliferation of publicly funded case management programs that focused on low-income populations, private FFS care management was a logical development. The need for help with solving problems associated with aging is not linked to income. Families at all income levels share the same sense of helplessness when crises occur, and often lack knowledge of available resources. Parker delineates the reasons why families hire care managers:

The need for a professional assessment
The need for an objective opinion regarding service options
Help with the feeling of being overwhelmed
The inability to resolve family conflicts
Help in transitioning a relative to a nursing home
Long-distance caregiving issues
The need for respite care
Help with filling out forms[6(pp4-5)]

Higher-income families ineligible for income-based case management programs provided the ideal market for the for-profit care management business. These families had the means and the willingness to pay for services they wanted.

■ PUBLIC NOT-FOR-PROFIT AND PRIVATE SETTINGS

Geriatric care management has similarities that are independent of the setting in which it is provided. The same tasks are performed with regard to assessment, care planning, referral, service coordination, and monitoring. Care managers must have the educational background, professional skills, and training to handle the challenges they will encounter when called into difficult and complicated situations. There must be some provision for after-hours emergencies. Caseload numbers are limited to enhance the quality of service delivery. Forms, procedures, and billing may be similar in both NFP and private agencies; however, the NFPs may have federal, state, or local regulations; external funding requirements; and/or internal policies and guidelines because of their nonprofit status that may affect their practice and procedures.

Overall, FFS practice has the major advantage of being free of constraints, thus enabling a customized, intensive, and personal relationship that is important to clients looking for a surrogate family member. This may be even more true for a FFS private practice as opposed to a FFS program within an NFP setting. Parker explains how FFS private practice is different from public and NFP geriatric care management:

- **Eligibility.** Whereas there are strict eligibility requirements to participate in a publicly funded program, the ability to pay a fee is usually the only criteria for becoming an FFS client.
- **Availability.** Private practitioners will typically be on call or actually available 24 hours a day and on weekends.
- **Staff turnover.** Unlike the public agency with higher caseloads and more frequent staff turnover, the private care manager is more likely to be able to offer a more stable, long-term relationship.
- **Conflicts.** There appear to be fewer conflicts about providing direct services in addition to care management, including home aides and companions.[6(pp4–5)]

■ FEE-FOR-SERVICE IN A NOT-FOR-PROFIT SETTING

The FFS geriatric care management program within an NFP agency offers different kinds of advantages. Many NFPs provide other services in addition to care management, giving clients served by the agency more choices and an opportunity for more closely coordinated services. NFPs often employ a multidisciplinary staff, enabling cross-training and collaboration that may result in a better-quality product for the client. A case in point is the OACM client who chooses to take advantage of both the case management and home care programs. The client will receive coordinated care by a team consisting of the care manager, a nurse, a home care coordinator/scheduler, and a home care aide. Additional services of the parent IOA NFP may also be considered and coordinated. A well-established NFP can also offer greater fiscal security to a fledgling FFS care management program. Unlike many of the smaller for-profit companies, a well-funded NFP is more financially secure and therefore able to support the care management program in times of slower business.

Another advantage of the NFP is its standing and perception in the community. Through its established community relationships and reputation, the NFP brings immediate credibility to the geriatric care management program and can help it grow. Many potential referral sources come from social service settings with cultures that are more comfortable with NFP programs than with private for-profits. Geriatric care managers (GCMs) have an entire agency behind them and great support in the beginning of the program when many crises are to be faced and much is still to be learned.

In addition to positives, Vocker discusses some negatives of integrating FFS geriatric care management into an NFP agency.[7]

Many NFPs receive case management funding through the Older Americans Act (OAA) and are thereby subject to certain requirements and criteria. To be a recipient of OAA-funded case management services, a client must be at least 60 years old and live in the geographic area served by the agency. OAA also requires that the agency be open 8 hours each weekday and never closed for 4 or more consecutive days. When the agency is closed, alternative assistance must be offered. This could include access to staff pager numbers or arrangements with police and fire departments. In addition, the agency must meet the needs of non-English-speaking and physically challenged clients. Other types of requirements cover case assignments, care plans, and supervision.

Geriatric care management is an around-the-clock business, and it can be hard to get staff to participate in after-hours service. Also, because of its time-intensive nature, FFS geriatric care management typically means smaller caseloads; thus, keeping track of client caseloads is especially important. In some NFP settings, FFS clients are not the only clients served by any one care manager in the agency, so it is important to monitor the GCM's ability to respond to the intensive expectations of FFS clients.

If the NFP offers both publicly funded and FFS case management programs with separate staffing, friction may arise between the different care managers. Because geriatric care management is so labor-intensive, staff in the public program, invariably working with a low-income population with fewer available resources, may feel that they are "in the trenches" doing the hard work and may resent the disproportionate amount of time spent with the paying clients. It is critical that an NFP create an internal culture that is mutually respectful of both case management programs.

■ NOT-FOR-PROFIT FFS PROGRAM DEVELOPMENT CHALLENGES

In making the decision to implement FFS care management, NFP boards and staff address many questions. Will FFS alter our commitment to serve those most in need? Will revenue-seeking activities compromise other social service involvement? If building the business means selling services, how can client interests come first? Are we being driven by profit motives? Should services be different if people are paying? What would it mean to have a two-tiered system? How can we work with demanding customers when we went into this to help the needy and vulnerable? Will we be asked and have to do things that seem unprofessional yet are therapeutically appropriate and within the scope of case management such as escorting someone to the opera?

NFPs continue to struggle with these fundamental questions as they develop FFS programs and must consider and resolve them if programs are to succeed. Among the biggest hurdles is overcoming the reluctance to charge fees. Other major challenges include developing a customer orientation and marketing FFS care management services.

Overcoming the Reluctance to Charge Fees

Charging fees in exchange for services remains one of the most difficult challenges in developing FFS care management in an NFP setting. Generally, charging for services has been considered inappropriate for the NFP sector. The reluctance to charge for services most likely stems from traditional attitudes that the NFP sector's mission is to provide access to those who are unable to pay or to meet other criteria such as need, status, condition, location, race, ethnicity, or religion. In many cases, services are given to clients who are not eligible for public sector case management or prefer not to use it. But decreasing opportunities to acquire public dollars and private donations for direct care have led more NFPs to generate revenues through fees.

Although there are clinical as well as fiscal and operational reasons to collect fees, there has been significant resistance within NFPs to implementing FFS programs. This resistance has come from all groups: staff, volunteers, administrators, and clients who have been receiving free services for many years.

Many human service professionals who have worked in publicly funded social services and the NFP sector appear to suffer from a type of "fee phobia." For example, when SCN first developed its FFS program in 1985, it was difficult to find professionals who were comfortable with charging for care management. These professionals felt that social services should be free to clients and that clients would not pay or would refuse help if they were charged. The professionals were inexperienced in setting rates and did not feel confident about negotiating fees. Many of them objected to the idea of "selling" services, stating that they did not choose to become a social worker (or nurse or other human services professional) to work as a "salesperson."

CJE struggled with many of these same issues. CJE began its FFS private geriatric care management service with a few interested staff members who took on cases. The intake worker who responded to initial inquiries played a significant role in engaging callers to view the service as viable. An after-hours call system was developed, and only supervisory staff responded, to protect staff time. As the number of cases grew, the staff became excited, particularly by the positive feedback they received from clients. CJE staff members were soon sold on the idea and requested beepers so they could respond to their own after-hours calls. The few specialists' enthusi-

asm was infectious, and other staff members became interested in providing care management services.

Most practitioners who provide care management in NFPs have backgrounds in helping professions in which revenue is not discussed. Many of these practitioners believe that older adults have no disposable income and should be taken care of because they are needy and frail. It is difficult for these practitioners to see their services as products and think that older people should pay a fee for those services. The OACM experience was different in that they did not encounter "fee resistance" from the case management staff. The OACM model used clinical supervision from a licensed clinical social worker (LCSW) in private practice who was used to "selling" services. One of the case managers also had a background with a large assisted living chain and was quite comfortable with marketing activities. These two factors combined with the fact that OACM has been in the business of selling home care services for many years created a culture where fee-for-service was the norm.

Early in SCN's FFS program, staff noticed that clients also created barriers to "selling" care management as a service. Many clients said that they should not have to and could not afford to pay for this kind of service. Others thought that because they had already donated to the organization, they were entitled to get free services. Still others believed that if they did pay for both case management and a service provider, they would spend more money than necessary.

In his study of nontraditional in-home services, Hereford reports that older people did not see case management as a distinct product worthy of a fee.[8] Prior to implementing its FFS care management program, CJE conducted market research that reinforced this perspective. CJE found that fees of $50 to $100 per hour were considered too high; a few older adults would pay $20 per hour, but most wanted to pay nothing. Family members, on the other hand, supported the concept of paying fees for this service.

Many of today's older adults still have what is known as "Depression-era" thinking—the desire to preserve every penny to save for a "rainy day." Many services to seniors have been based on entitlement, and consequently, many seniors expect services to be provided for them. Older adults also find it distasteful to pay for something they could previously do for themselves. Others resist outside involvement by a professional because they fear a greater loss of control than they already experience as a result of aging. The OACM experience has found that it is easier to deliver quality service when the bill paying is done by someone other than the older adult (i.e., an adult relative, a bank, a trustee, a conservator, etc.).

A reorientation of practice philosophy is necessary to shift staff members' thinking about charging fees for these services. An NFP needs to help staff see the need for revenue to offset deficits and survive in a time of more limited resources. Full-paying clients are needed so the agency can continue to serve those who cannot afford to pay.

Sales training sessions, sessions to increase understanding of NFP funding mechanisms, and sessions teaching about marketing and appreciating the value of care management as a professional service were all held for FFS staff at SCN. Letting staff members articulate their objections and do role-playing helped

them be comfortable with charging fees. SCN care management program managers focused on establishing a business mentality, paying attention to changing attitudes as well as language. Figure 9-1 shows an example of training materials used to help achieve this shift.

In response to similar issues, CJE spent considerable time defining care management so that staff could comfortably articulate the benefits of the service. Then staff could better help older adults and families understand the value and necessity of care management when it was indicated. Staff worked on increasing their comfort with fees through outlining and challenging staff biases and paternalistic views about what older people could understand and afford. Discussions were held with private practice GCMs about their views, which helped staff members realize the value of their services in the marketplace. Role-playing was used to increase everyone's comfort level. Once again, OACM's experience was different in that the hourly rate was set at $100, charging for visits, phone calls, and e-mails. The client was told of this up front, and a contract was signed. The main challenge that OACM faced was getting its care managers to keep careful track of billable time. A weekly time sheet was developed that motivated staff to keep better track of time spent. In addition, a monthly revenue report is done where the case managers can see how much they billed both in regards to individual clients and also in relationship to their coworkers.

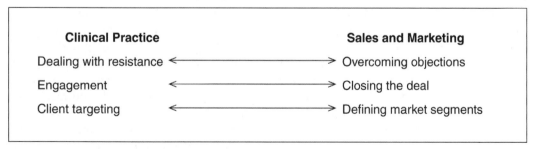

Figure 9–1   Clinical Practice with Sales and Marketing

Source: Reprinted with permission by Lynn Hackstaff, LCSW, Downey Kaiser Permanente, Orchard MOB Family Medicine & Orchard Urgent Care HealthCenter (OUCH).

This type of a practitioner paradigm shift takes time. The reality is that some care managers have an easier time with charging fees than other care managers do. To integrate a private care management philosophy into NFP structures, an organization needs to allow for some anxiety and sadness about the change. It is important, wherever possible, to create mechanisms for staff input into the development of the service. One way to begin is to identify staff who are comfortable with fees and create specialist positions. They can then act as champions as the program develops. The organization's leaders should think about similar changes from the organization's past and what helped ensure staff commitment as those changes were taking place.

Developing a Customer Orientation

Care management, for a fee, provides many of the case management services traditionally offered by senior and social services agencies at no cost to clients. When an NFP decides to develop an FFS care management model, it must also develop a customer orientation rather than the traditional client orientation. Customers expect to have choices and to be treated in a special way, with privacy, flexibility, control, quality, and a personal touch. The client should be involved in the decision-making process whenever it is feasible.

In traditional case management, the case manager identifies what he or she thinks the client needs, and then tries to ration services to meet those needs, when possible still relying on the support of family members, neighbors, and other people in the client's life. This is very different from the "surrogate child" or "substitute family member" model associated with private geriatric care management. Private GCMs are available weekends and evenings to provide the personalized touch that accommodates requests above and beyond just client need.

At CJE every effort was made to develop an FFS geriatric care management business that

reflected an integrated practice model. This model balances customer wishes with assessed needs and priorities to maximize independence, reduce risk, and strengthen family support. For both paying and non-paying older people, the values and goals were similar.

A major goal at SCN was to develop a true care management continuum with a full range of opportunities for older people to receive services regardless of income or condition. Centered on a triage model with professional telephone screening, consultation, information, and referral, SCN established case management programs with several public and private funding sources. The addition of FFS care management made the service available to virtually anyone. It also created a customer service approach that eventually permeated the other programs. Although OACM provides strictly fee-for-service care management, its parent organization, IOA, provides services to those who cannot pay.

Marketing

A critical factor in creating an FFS geriatric care management business in an NFP is the image of the organization. A marketing plan needs to be developed that communicates that the agency is broadening its program. To seek services from an organization viewed as serving lower-income clients, FFS customers must realize that FFS services are being offered and trust the organization to provide high-quality services. Conversely, residents of the community may well be drawn to the NFP's care management program because they view the NFP as having no profit motive. Outreach and marketing staff must be prepared to deal with both perspectives. In either case, the reputation and credibility of the NFP organization are the most important factors in the success of the new program.

Marketing of FFS care management is rarely focused directly on the person who will receive the service. Rather, it is aimed at adult children and other individuals (e.g., attorneys, physicians, financial planners) who help older people make decisions. Different marketing strategies are needed to reach these different audiences. An NFP can look to the for-profit business sector to learn about successful marketing and, at the same time, build on the NFP's history and tradition of service to set itself apart from the for-profit business sector.

Before developing FFS care management, an NFP's leaders must consider whether there are enough potential customers in the community. The leaders should also consider whether the community already has enough organizations providing these services. The OACM experience was able to capitalize on the strong reputation of the agency as a home care agency. This level of respect fostered respect for the case management program based on reputation.

The success of the services will depend on a network of trusted, caring service providers committed to quality and open to suggestions for improvement. A trusted provider network is an important part of what is being sold. The case manager continually needs to be marketing. Key referral sources need to be reminded frequently of the services. Marketing of case management services isn't a one-step process, but rather needs to be ongoing and is a series of collaborative activities. Helping an assisted living facility with a talk or health fair is more effective than giving a fancy holiday gift. Marketing for case managers involves developing long-term relationships with referral sources and always delivering excellent services.

■ COSTS, RATES, AND BILLING

One of the first questions typically asked by potential clients is, "How much will it cost?"

Setting rates takes a good understanding of direct and indirect agency expenses. Profits can be built in but must be reasonable, keeping prices competitive with those of similar service providers in the community. Many NFPs are able to keep their prices somewhat lower than those of for-profit businesses because of their size and funding from other programs. However, FFS care management fees are billed by the task or hour; thus, staff productivity becomes an important element in the program.

Productivity in an FFS program most commonly means the number of hours each care manager can bill. This is a strange concept to those unaccustomed to billing and requires training and experience to become second nature. As noted by Bellucci and her colleagues, productivity can be raised through methods such as objective feedback.[9] A study in an NFP's FFS case management program serving human immunodeficiency virus/acquired immune deficiency syndrome clients showed a 13.4% increase in billable hours after an expected number of billable hours and weekly reports were provided to each team of case managers. These findings show the importance of good supervision, target setting, and ongoing staff development.

■ CONCLUSION

Many decisions must be made prior to implementing an FFS care management program in an NFP setting. Choices must be made about the program's purpose, staffing, structure, rates, relationship to other programs, and marketing strategies. In the years to come, there will probably be more questions than answers as NFPs further develop for-profit enterprises. These debates will help ensure that the mission and values of NFPs can be maintained while paying customers are accommodated. Moving into the FFS world will enable NFPs to survive and to serve a broader range of people.

■ NOTES

1. Knutson K, Langer S. Geriatric care managers: a survey in long-term/chronic care. *GCM J.* 1998;8:9.

2. Bodie Gross E, Holt E. Care and case management summit—the white paper. *GCM J.* 1998;8:22–24.

3. White M. Case management. In: Maddox GL, ed. *The Encyclopedia of Aging.* 3rd ed. New York: Springer; in press.

4. White M, Gundrum G. Case management. In: Evashwick C, ed. *The Continuum of Long-Term Care: An Integrated Systems Approach.* 2nd ed. Albany, NY: Delmar Publishers; 2000.

5. Austin CD, McClelland RW, eds. *Perspectives on Case Management Practice.* Milwaukee, WI: Families International; 1996.

6. Parker M. Positioning care management for future health care trends. *GCM J.* 1998;8:4–8.

7. Vocker M. Care management from the perspective of a not-for-profit agency. *GCM J.* 1996;6:11–15.

8. Hereford RW. Private-pay case management: let the seller beware. *Caring.* 1990;9:8–12.

9. Bellucci M, Tonges MC, Kopelman R. Doing well by doing good: the case for objective feedback in case management. *J Case Manage.* 1998;7:161–166.

Chapter 10

Marketing Geriatric Care Management

Merrily Orsini

■ OVERVIEW: MARKETING TO THE GERIATRIC CARE POPULATION

Although the concept of marketing may initially seem complex for the average geriatric care manager (GCM), an understanding of marketing communications is an important component of building a thriving practice. Taking the time and resources to understand basic marketing strategy and to develop and implement a strategic marketing plan helps the GCM to increase visibility, credibility, and knowledge of services.

Because geriatric care management is an "at-need" service that consumers seek only when the need arises, it requires a specific approach to marketing. The key to marketing for a GCM is to first educate consumers about what a GCM is and does, and then to get the increased knowledge of the company/GCM name known so when a potential client has a need, he or she will inquire, and then a request for service will hopefully follow.

According to traditional definitions, *marketing communications mix* is described as follows: "Marketing communications sometimes referred to as '*promotions*' involve marketer initiated techniques directed to target audiences in an attempt to influence attitudes and behaviors."[1(p375)] Together, advertising, public relations (PR), sales promotions, personal selling, and direct marketing communications constitute the marketing communica-

tions mix, often referred to as the promotional mix. The three major objectives of marketing communications are these:

- To inform
- To persuade
- To remind marketer's audience"[1(p375)]

Understanding the marketing communications mix can assist the GCM in deciding what to do when, how to budget for marketing, and how best to reach desired targets. Overall marketing strategy is necessary to understand how best to use which tactics and for the best usage of resources, time, and money. Marketing is the overall strategy used and is based on thoughtful understanding of the environment, competition, and services provided. Sales are activities that are used to actually get clients to sign up for services. Public relations strategy influences public perceptions, whether in face-to-face communications or through targeted media relations, whether in articles, radio/TV spots, or on the Internet. Advertisements are paid and placed in relevant media outlets.

Beginning GCMs might have less money to spend on marketing activities, yet marketing is essential to starting and growing a business. A seasoned GCM still needs to use marketing strategy to grow the business, but the tactics are different because the GCM has a client base and is better known in the community.

Being a salesperson for oneself is not intuitive, and only practice and experience make sales a comfortable practice for the GCM.

Consumers have many choices to make when they already know about available products and when they use products on an ongoing basis. Consumers may not know about geriatric care management and the differences between providers. Because using a GCM is usually based on a specific triggered need or an event, education becomes an important part of marketing. Understanding the marketing mix and how to use education as a large part in the sales, marketing, and PR efforts is not unique to care management, but it is incredibly important.

In regards to marketing and sales, note that most GCMs are uncomfortable with the idea that profitability is positive. The concept that a profitable business is a healthy business, and only a healthy business can survive and grow, is crucial for the GCM to comprehend and embrace. Understanding and getting better at sales and marketing are key ways to make a business healthy.

■ CREATING A MARKETING STRATEGY AS THE BASIS FOR SPENDING MARKETING DOLLARS (BEGINNING/MATURE)

Before the business can start generating revenue, a marketing strategy and sales techniques must be in place. The message communicated to the public about the business is of primary importance. Geriatric care management sells solutions to aging and end-of-life issues: assistance with decisions for housing and medical and personal care, and support that family members cannot provide and on a level that a non-GCM cannot provide.

Geriatric care management is better known today than when the profession got its start in the mid-1980s. In some areas, there is even fierce competition between providers. Reaching the elderly themselves, their trusted advisors, and their family takes a combination of education, careful design of marketing materials, a targeted database of potential referral sources, and lots of positive public relations. Inherent to business success is that the GCM is educated, experienced, and truly provides a value-added service to clients and/or their families and loved ones.

Potential clients must have the ability to pay for geriatric care management services, and thus are a very small segment of the general population. Furthermore, they must have a need that family, friends, physicians, and trusted advisors are not meeting.

For the seasoned GCM as well as the beginner, most new clients will come from referrals, both personal and professional. The marketing strategy must revolve around positioning the GCM for reaching potential referral sources and educating contacts about the benefits that a GCM brings to a complicated or underresourced situation. How the GCM presents services and how clients are managed and serviced are critical to the GCM's ongoing success.

When creating marketing strategy and material, the following messages resonate with clients and referral sources: security and comfort, peace of mind, solutions, appropriate care, choices in care providers, and access to resources. The other component of marketing strategy is the educational component of what a GCM can bring to the table related to aging and care needs. Educating the consumer as to when care at home is appropriate, what one can expect from certain diseases common to aging, and which resources are available along the spectrum of care also place a GCM in the consumer's mind when the need arises for services relating to aging or health issues.

■ DEVELOPING A STRATEGIC MARKETING PLAN

When it comes to distinguishing a geriatric care management business, nothing compares to a solid and well-thought-out marketing plan. A strategic and successfully executed marketing plan has the power to shape a geriatric care management business and how it is to be perceived by current and potential customers. It forces the GCM to take the time to define the values and unique benefits offered and available and to develop various, affordable (time and money) ways to communicate those things to a specifically defined target audience.

The long-term benefits of marketing are obvious. A GCM can have the best product or service imaginable, but if no one knows about it or buys it, no business is generated. It's wise to invest time and resources in creating and implementing a results-driven marketing plan.

The classic 4 Ps of marketing (product, price, place, and promotion) have been updated for the 21st century to include the 4 As:

- **Accountability.** Marketing must prove its contribution to the business and be accountable for measurable results, that is, new clients.
- **Analysis.** Marketing requires both art and science, and analysis must no longer be an afterthought; instead, measurable results will drive strategy; that is, if it works, do more of it.
- **Accuracy.** Performance metrics must be consistently and accurately measured across all marketing initiatives, that is, tracking results.
- **Action.** Optimization is successful only when it's an ongoing process of leveraging your analysis to take decisive actions toward improving results; that is, change tactics to do more of what is working.[2]

Focusing primarily on opportunities that bring face-to-face interaction, whether one on one or in a group setting, is the best marketing strategy for the GCM, but also the most time-consuming. This tactic also allows for the education component to be a primary factor in the marketing effort.

A strategic marketing plan should include descriptions of the following:

- **Target audience.** Prioritize who is most receptive to your services and keep track of those who use your services. This measurement will enable you to refine your target audience as the business progresses.
- **Sales and marketing objectives.** How many clients can a geriatric care management practice handle and how many new referral sources does it take to generate enough business? What gets measured gets managed, so setting objectives and measuring against them is one sure way to achieve success.
- **Product benefit overview.** What benefits do you and your geriatric care management practice bring to the clients and your target audience? This is the crux of why clients would want to use your services and what problem you are solving for them. Understanding this is crucial to selling services.
- **Positioning strategy.** How do your business model or service offerings differ from the competition's? Is your background or experience different from other GCMs'? Are you specific about that and why a client would choose you over someone else?
- **Lead sources.** Who do you know now? Where can you meet others that you need to know to get more business?
- **Selling and lead generation tactics.** What can *you* do that will start you on the road to (1) selling your services and (2) making certain that you are always gaining more information on those to which you can present information to start the selling cycle?
- **Communication strategy.** How will you reach these leads? Phone calls, follow-up letters, visits, seminars?
- **Creative/promotion strategy.** What collateral materials are you using that work with your positioning strategy and that also "speak" to your target audience?

- **Recommended activity.** This includes the one, two, or three activities that you do today, tomorrow, weekly, monthly, quarterly, and annually to achieve the business you want to achieve.

■ UNDERSTANDING BRANDING AND BRAND DEVELOPMENT

What is a brand? "A product is made in a factory; a brand is made in the mind," says branding expert Walter Landor, founder, Landor Associates. Taking the time to understand branding and how it is important to your success can mean big rewards for you and your geriatric care management business. Although often associated with just advertising, branding is essential to everything a company puts in front of current and potential clients: business cards, brochures, Web site, trade show booth, letterhead, and so forth.

Branding is about managing people's image of a company and making sure that image is one that is in line with your company values and the benefits your company provides. By taking the time to manage expectations and build positive gut feelings about your company, you establish yourself as a trusted leader in your market.[3]

Your brand identity is built upon your key messages and position, the unique customer benefits that you provide, and the expectations you set for your target audience. By consistently delivering the same symbols, messages, and design, you are reinforcing those messages, creating a link to your brand, and building an identity for your business that people will remember. You want to create a consistent look and feel for everything related to you and your business.

Logo creation is the single most important part of the design branding process. The logo sets the stage for colors and for the overall look and feel of your specific identity and marketing collateral. When developing a logo, let your key messages guide the design.

Develop a stand-out image that plays on the benefits and messages that you want to communicate to your potential clients. Keep in mind that a logo must be easy to see and interpret on the smallest intended usage, such as a give-away pen, and on the largest, such as a business sign or trade show banner.

Through consistent use of the same logo, tag line, even company colors, you'll create a cohesive identity for your business and help drive home the messages that you want people to know about you and the business.

For example, if your tag line is "Understanding Care Needs; Delivering Options," then use it whenever you send anything to anyone. If it is "Resources for Aging," use that tag line on all materials. If you are specializing in some aspect of information, such as Alzheimer's disease, note that on all correspondence. Keep it simple and repeat it. You want people to remember the one thing you do best and for them to make a connection with it.

■ TARGETED AUDIENCES

The primary key target audiences on which geriatric care management marketing should focus range across personal, group, and networking contacts. The geriatric care management market is a very narrow market because only those who can afford to pay can access services, and the client must be at a point in life to need assistance with some aging- or disease-related issue but might not necessarily be ill or injured. Some clients come out of rehabilitation facilities, hospitals, or nursing homes, but many simply have gotten to a point in their aging process where they really do not know where to go for assistance. They may need housekeeping, meal preparation, or assistance with walking and not falling. They may need 24-hour supervision, but not hands-on care. They may simply need someone to provide balanced meals, medication monitoring, and assistance with money management. Although the range of needs can be broad, the primary requirement is assistance with determining resource allocation for assistance to maintain the quality of life that they desire and can afford.

Thus, geriatric care management marketing targets those who may buy services for themselves or a loved one, as well as anyone along the spectrum of care services who works with seniors and could be a referral source: seniors themselves, adult children of aging/frail or demented parents, trust officers, certified public accountants (CPAs), elder-law attorneys, trust and estate attorneys, hospice nurses or volunteers, long-term care (LTC) insurance agents, home care and home health care agencies, retirement communities, assisted living facilities, hospitals, and rehabilitation facilities, to name a few.

Additional referral sources and audiences to educate about geriatric care management services include Alzheimer's Association personnel and volunteers, clergy, and any community and/or disease groups/associations serving seniors. In short, the target market for geriatric care management services is anyone who has a care need or anyone who knows or works with seniors and can provide referrals. The following section describes specific strategies for reaching these targets.

Reaching Desired Target Audiences

Because there usually isn't any specific way to identify the adult children of aging/frail or demented parents, the placement of news articles and focusing media attention on aging and related issues are probably the best, and should be the first, usages of time and resources. Finding a spot on an early-morning or a noon talk show as an expert in elder care, using senior centers as a place to give talks, sponsoring events (if finances allow), and generally getting your name out as a resource and expert on aging or disability issues are the most effective ways to reach the masses. The

use of public relations is simply the best way to reach the general consumer successfully and build third-party credibility for a geriatric care management business.

Trust officers can be targeted with direct mail. Updating the list of trust officers regularly and sending them information on geriatric care management issues can introduce the GCM name to banks. Asking to present to a bank to discuss using a GCM for planning of care for bank clients can also get the GCM name recognized. Establishing a relationship with a trust department can be the best referral source available to a GCM for long-term clients. Mining those relationships, keeping in constant contact, and keeping the GCM name in front of them in a variety of ways are the best marketing tactics for this group.

Reaching the CPA as a referral source may be more difficult because the target audience is wider. It might be helpful to see whether there is a division of the local association for CPAs that deals with elderly or aging persons or trusts and estates. Apply the same tactics as used for trust departments to this select group. Getting the GCM name in front of this group is the key. Education is one way to do this, in addition to direct mail. The CPA group is not known as a good source for referrals for GCMs because they are not "trusted advisors" as attorneys are to a family and given the annual or quarterly nature of tax work, as opposed to regular, ongoing contact for legal issues. However, if a GCM does some good work in relationship building, CPAs can become referral sources in the GCM's informal network as well.

You can easily obtain a list of LTC agents in an area by finding out all local agents for all companies that provide LTC. These agents will need a referral source for their clients who have questions about which services they need for their LTC needs. Also, insurance agents may have clients who do not qualify to buy LTC insurance, have an elimination period, or do not want to use their benefits unwisely. Find the local chapter of the National Association of Insurance and Financial Advisors and ask to be a speaker. This group is usually very interested in continuing education, and most agents do not understand the differences in the care their policies cover. Giving a presentation is the key to getting in front of this audience.

The key to all referrals is to never take on a client unless you can provide assistance in solving that person's problem. Keep all of these referral source lists updated and communicate with contacts regularly. Let your contacts know when you are presenting somewhere so they can provide your name and engagement as a useful resource for their clients.

Educating the home care and home health care agencies about the value a GCM brings to elder care enables these agencies to work with you and establish an ongoing relationship. As the care manager, you can supervise a difficult case and alleviate time/cost that is not reimbursable for the agency. Plus, they can learn a lot from a GCM relating to elder care and aging issues. You can also offer to co-present with quality agencies for more public exposure.

Hospital discharge planners are a fluid group. Continually update this list of contacts so it is always current. One strategy to introduce yourself to a new set of clients is to provide community resource guides stamped with your logo and contact information to discharge planners to be disbursed to patients with geriatric care management needs when they are being discharged from the hospital. When a call to assist following patient discharge does come in, follow up with the social worker or nursing case manager. Try to take this contact to lunch; the time and expense is usually worth it. Offer to do in-service presentations on the spectrum of care, how a GCM's services fit into other services available, and when it is appropriate to make a referral to you. Educating the discharge team as to when GCM intervention is appropriate creates a trust level that turns into referrals.

Estate and trust attorneys need to understand the services and advantages a GCM brings to clients when care/resource needs become apparent. Clients of these attorneys are usually long term because a responsible family member may not be available to provide any care or ongoing support that frail elderly persons so often need. Also, clients usually are financially well-off and have the potential of becoming long-term clients. Many times, estate and trust attorneys remain as a point of contact in addition to the GCM when problems arise. Making an attorney's life easier on weekends and holidays is just one additional value a GCM brings to the situation. When a relationship is established with an attorney, try to do a joint seminar so both of you can promote your businesses and educate potential clients.

Many times, physicians truly do not understand appropriate resources and options for care. They are programmed to refer to skilled care and Medicare. The best way to get the information about geriatric care management services to a physician is either to form a relationship with the doctor's nurse or to accompany a client to physician appointments and discuss with the doctor the geriatric care management services available and how the client benefits from them. Always send an introductory letter to a client's physician introducing yourself as a part of a care team. Offer to educate physicians on geriatric care management services and the spectrum of care available to their patients. Physician relationships and referrals are worth their weight in gold. If the doctor "orders" it, then patients usually will comply.

The assisted living and retirement community population sometimes has clients with needs that cannot be met in these nonmedical, non-one-on-one living arrangements. Establishing rapport with the administrative staff can be accomplished by offering to hold special events or other kinds of activities with the facility personnel. Offering to educate on aging-related topics and activities can also provide an entree into the facility. Consistent visits and participation in activities, such as health fairs, are essential.

Rehabilitation centers also discharge patients back to their home, and sometimes the patient is not ready for 100% self-care. To get referrals, try to get to know the therapists and keep them apprised of the geriatric care management business and how you can assist their patients upon discharge, or while patients are in therapy and trying to make decisions about living arrangements when they are discharged.

A Medicare-certified agency may be willing to refer clients to you when a need arises, if it understands what a GCM does and how a GCM can assist clients. The agency may want a referral agreement in place so all skilled care is referred to them, that is, when the client is hospitalized and then discharged with home health. As a part of the care team, it is possible for you to influence the selection of Medicare-certified agency upon discharge.

Joining the Alzheimer's Association or other associations dealing with chronic diseases is one way to spread the word about your geriatric care management services. In addition to joining and working on committees, you can sponsor events, write for the newsletter, and present at educational conferences.

Dementia is one of the leading issues faced by the elderly population. Specializing in the best options in care for persons with dementia can position a GCM as a leader, and referrals will come. Consider providing training on how to work with dementia patients and assistance to the home care agencies to help them understand what staff characteristics are best: patience and kindness.

Keeping the GCM name out in front of trusted advisors is one way to get referrals. Pastoral counselors oftentimes have access to families and need more in-depth resources when their congregation has needs. Also community groups serving seniors can be a source of referrals.

Using a Web Site for Marketing

A must for the 21st century is having a Web site that is easily found, informative, and easy to use. When it comes to designing a Web site, navigation is key, and then comes content. Understand that the Internet is a fluid medium, interactive and fast. Users must be able to find what they want quickly, get the information they seek, and be able to find the site again and return to the site while involved in a search.

Start with a good site design that matches your other marketing material. Make it uncluttered and easily navigable, and use only relevant content. Give the customers what they want:

- Information, including the specifics
- Resources that are helpful
- How they can contact you

Web site text should *not* be traditional marketing brochure content. The information must be concise and easily readable in a short time. All pages should have headers and bullets. The content has to be conversational and engage the user. Content has to be current. Make certain to maintain and update regularly, adding any articles written and any information that is new and pertinent. And use established conventions for Web site design so there is nothing unusual or odd about your site.[3]

■ SALES AND MARKETING OBJECTIVES

Starting a geriatric care management business starts with one client. Sales and marketing objectives will vary depending on your location and the population density. The keys to growth are continuous learning, updating of resources and options, keeping clients happy, and serving them beyond their expectations.

Benchmarking business growth and tracking where business is coming from are essential for a start-up GCM as well as for seasoned professionals. Keeping monthly track of referrals, who made them, and which kinds of clients turn out to be longer term can enable a geriatric care management business to set realistic sales and marketing objectives.

Marketing tasks should be divided into passive tasks (advertising, direct mail, birthday cards) and active tasks (visits, presentations, thank-you and follow-up notes). Objectives need to be set based on a budget as to how many tasks are done daily, weekly, and monthly.

Sales is the conversion of demand into orders.[4] The sales process is sometimes called a sales cycle. There are definite steps in this cycle:

- Prospecting (lead generation)
- Cold calling (by phone or face to face)
- Initial questioning (can be phone inquiry)
- Sales meetings (face to face)
- Rapport building (face to face or by phone)
- Needs analysis (strategic and tactical questioning, usually using an inquiry form)
- Solution presentation (positioning, what the GCM can do to solve the problem or meet the need)
- Closing (signing on a new client or referral source)

These steps are described in the following paragraphs.

Prospecting, or lead generation, is the act and process of actually collecting names and contact information of those people or businesses who would make a good target for services or for referring for services. It is logical that, to make sales, you must know to whom you could possibly sell. The more names on this prospecting list, the better the chances of making a sale.

Cold calling is making a call, either on the phone or in person, to someone you do not know, but who is a good target person for using geriatric care management services or for making a referral for services. Sometimes a cold call can be made to someone you already know, but who is not aware of your business and what you could do for them.

Initial questioning of a potential target is not unlike performing a needs assessment on a client. You question the target to see what need the person has that you can fill. Because a GCM offers a wide range of services, different people will want to use different components of what you offer. For example, a physician may want assistance with resource listings and appropriate placements so her patients have to move only once when they leave their homes. A bank trust officer may want assistance with transportation to doctors' appointments for a frail client. Only by questioning potential clients or referral sources will you know which services you offer that fit their need.

A sales meeting is best if it is face to face so you can establish credibility and a relationship. It is best not to call this encounter a sales meeting, and for the GCM who is "salesperson phobic," it is best to think of this as a relationship-building meeting. You are presenting yourself and your services to a potential customer or referral source. If you were selling widgets, you would have some various sizes of widgets to show. Because you are selling geriatric care management services provided by you, it is good to know what your audience is interested in (you have questioned targets already and know this information), so you can take this wonderful face-to-face opportunity to focus on the services this particular target wants to know more about or wants to purchase.

Building rapport is a natural outgrowth of the face-to-face sales meeting process, and it will continue by phone (as you follow up when a referral is received), e-mail, and face-to-face meetings.

The needs analysis is a more in-depth questioning about ways you can assist. It is an extension of the inquiry process and simply occurs during the natural evolution of a relationship as the client uses services and wants to learn more about other services you provide.

You can present the solutions you can offer to meet the specific needs expressed by the target verbally and with marketing collateral materials. Usually, testimonials, case studies, and real-life examples are the best way to present geriatric care management services to the public and to interested referral sources. For example, describe a real-life scenario similar to the target's situation in which you had a positive impact. Geriatric care management services are not understood by many, so presenting real-life examples is a wonderful way to explain what you bring to the situation and to present yourself as a useful component in the relationship.

Closing the sale is when you get the contract signed, accept the initial payment, and start to work. Simply presenting and talking with a potential client does not bring money in the door; you must close the sale with a specific plan of action in place. And, as Peter Drucker was fond of saying, there is no business until money changes hands.

GCMs traditionally might be shy about performing all the sales steps. However, understanding that a needs assessment and a phone inquiry are natural parts of the sales cycle and that the genuine assistance that a GCM brings to a family in need should help new GCMs get over any fears of the sales cycle.

One well-known theory of persuasion—the Elaboration Likelihood Model—can work for the GCM and should help in the sales process. "Specifically, when consumer motivation and ability are high, persuasive message arguments are more thoroughly processed, and the strength of the arguments influences persuasion in what is termed 'the central route' to persuasion."[1(p409)]

Because geriatric care management services are sought after at-need for the client, the likelihood of the client being receptive to your sales approach is greater if the person inquires about services. The National Association of Professional Geriatric Care Managers sells a forms book that contains several initial inquiry and assessment forms that make the inquiry process less painful as a sales technique.

When someone inquires about what you as a GCM do, the main point to remember is to ask the question, "What is it you are looking for?" Then, clarify what it is the person is looking for and tailor your response to fit that person's specific need. As a GCM, you can either meet the need or make a referral to someone else. That way, you meet people's needs and also build referral relationships.[5]

Product Benefit Overview

Identifying key benefits of service helps shape communications. Generally, geriatric care management businesses benefit the client by assistance in choosing arrangements, including best living choices, in what can be thought of as "frailty to the grave" care.

Peace of mind that results from contracting for professional geriatric care management services benefits the older person's family and support system. Frailty is usually unplanned and often occurs when family members do not have the time to learn all they need to know about care and aging issues. It's important for an older person's support system to understand there are options for care, that some are better than others, and that each person has individual needs and resources available to meet those needs. The downside to geriatric care management services is that most options for care are private pay and cost the consumer. The benefits of care management must outweigh the costs, so GCMs must continue to show ongoing benefits to clients and referral bases.

■ POSITIONING STRATEGY

A positioning strategy is simply a statement of how the GCM should be viewed (i.e., caring, intelligent, hard-working). The positioning strategy essentially defines the GCM's personality and how the clients, prospects, and referral sources can perceive services offered. Usually, it is based on the personal nature of the relationship between the GCM and the client.

A positioning statement should be brief and emphasize one or two points. Your positioning statement will help guide the direction of your marketing material. For instance, this is a positioning statement: Specializing in Alzheimer's Care. This positioning informs the consumer that the GCM understands dementia, the demands made on the family and care staff of Alzheimer's patients, and that care will be taken to match and train care personnel used or to assist with placement in a facility where dementia care is the specialization.

■ LEAD SOURCES

As identified earlier, the geriatric care management market has three key target audiences: individual clients who need care, referral sources, and children of aging parents. Following are some key ideas for lead sources for individual prospects and referral sources. The source of existing customer leads will come directly from clients.

Use a contact management database. ACT and GoldMine are the best known, but a Microsoft Office Excel spreadsheet also works. Get as much contact information as possible to insert in the database. If you use Excel, make certain that you use separate columns for last name, first name, street address, city, state, zip code, phone number, fax number, e-mail address, type of business, source of inquiry or identification, notes, and dates for follow-up. Track all inquiries by getting at least the person's mailing address, e-mail address, and phone number. Note when a person calls and for what reason he or she is calling. Follow up on a regular basis with those who have not yet become clients.

Referral sources should also be tracked in a contact management database system. Additional items to add for referral sources are the numbers of calls received and the numbers of referrals actually received, plus the types.

■ SELLING AND LEAD GENERATION TACTICS

This section provides details on selling strategies and tactics for reaching client goals. Creating an actual written plan for sales and lead generation tactics can ensure success. Table 10–1 shows an example of a suggested format. Break down tasks into weekly, monthly, and quarterly activities.

Lead Generation

Lead generation is finding new targets for business. Example: You are at a luncheon for the Chamber of Commerce and meet an attorney who works with estate and trust clients. Get the person's business card, add the attorney to your database, and include the attorney in your regular communication. Or while you are driving, you see that a physical therapist has set up a new office. Stop in, get the name of the manager, and make certain the staff know that you provide assistance to the frail elderly so that when they see a client who is in for therapy you can become a resource. Add the manager's name and information to your database and keep in contact with the office through regular communication.

Tactics for lead generation include the following:

- Record all inquiries/calls for assistance coming into the office.
- Keep a contact management database of all inquiries, and follow up at set intervals.
- Respond immediately with information via a direct letter and other marketing information.
- Send a hand-written thank-you note to those with whom you have had meetings.
- Follow up monthly with articles of interest or news on the business.
- Optimize your Web site so it can easily be found by interested searchers.
- Submit aging-related articles to targeted print and online publications.

- Use all communications to drive traffic to your Web site.
- Do volunteer work with local senior, aging-related, or chronic illness organizations.
- Join local elder-law, guardianship, and trust department groups.
- Develop a seminar series that discusses choosing care options, caring for an aged parent, or the "sandwich" generation.
- Hold seminars at churches, hospitals, and community organizations.
- Hold seminars at various times of the day and evening to capture all potential prospects.

Consider Strategic Alliances

Strategic alliances are mutually beneficial alliances; for instance, consider aligning with Alzheimer's Association staff and volunteers. Other ideas for strategic alliances include these:

- **Form partnerships with other businesses related to yours.** Home care and home health agencies are a natural fit. Most need geriatric care management services and do not provide them. These agencies can be wonderful cross-referral sources because they need clients also. Durable Medical Equipment stores also

---

Table 10–1   Quarterly Activity Tracker

Objective	Description	Getting It Done
One seminar focused on dementia.	Create a 20-minute lecture focused on care needs for those with dementia. Offer this seminar to bank trust departments and senior centers. Goal: 15 attendees (keeping it small enough so individuals get attention but large enough so they don't feel singled out).	Use some outside assistance in planning and communication of the event.
One article written for the aging network newsletter.	Use a "case study" example to showcase how a GCM can assist a family in need. Write one 1500-word article to be submitted to appropriate publications.	Contact and send to all aging network newsletters in area, one at a time, and follow up with a call to ensure publication. First come, first published.
Send reprinted article to referral sources on contact management list.	Reprinted article to use as educational tool for referral sources and keep name in front of them on a regular basis.	Mail merge contact list with a cover letter stating this reprint can be used for educational purposes.
Referral source appreciation luncheon.	Have at least one referral source appreciation luncheon each quarter to serve as a cross networking event for aging related referral sources.	Find an inexpensive but quiet place to offer a lunch and ask each referral source to describe his or her business to all in attendance.
Community involvement.	Promote or attend at least one aging or care continuum related community event.	GCM responsible for selecting and attending.

have clients with geriatric care management needs and could use a referral source for assessments. Elder-law attorneys can find a GCM partner incredibly helpful when trying to determine next steps with frail clients.

- **Work with universities.** Use students from nursing or social work programs as interns.
- **Identify one or two Web presences.** Chronic disease associations all have Web sites, some with local chapters. Having your Web link as a referral source and cross-linking from your site to theirs can bring you credibility and also serve as an educational resource for clients visiting your site. Home care companies with whom you have referral relationships can also serve as good reciprocal links.
- **Partner with school groups or community service groups.** This is a way to offer something to the community. Perhaps you can partner with a group to host a fund-raiser that will benefit seniors in your community.

Don't Forget Your Current Customers

Frequent and useful communications with customers are essential to maintaining and growing your business. With the variety of communications vehicles available today, not only do clients (and prospects) expect immediate answers—they expect them to arrive in many different ways.

Use e-mail effectively for those who like to communicate this way. Possibly once every month, send clients brief communications with a link to an interesting article or with the status of their account.

Consider creating a quarterly newsletter delivered via e-mail and regular mail that keeps clients up-to-date on what's happening with recent home care legislation and care options, and provides answers to frequently asked questions and information on other pertinent topics. This can also be used as an

"opt-in" tactic to communicate with prospects on a regular basis. Plus, "teasers" to articles can be included in the newsletter with full text appearing on your Web site. This format also can easily be turned into a print newsletter for general prospecting for those who prefer to receive a hard copy.

Don't underestimate the power of taking the time to recognize holidays, birthdays, anniversaries, and so forth. This helps show your clients that they really are your priority.

■ COMMUNICATIONS STRATEGY

Your communications strategy provides a clear guide to be used when developing all communications. It lists key messages that need to be considered in everything from collateral materials, to e-mail, to Web site copy.

A communications strategy can help you create consistency among your key messages. You can then create a connection with potential customers and referrals by reiterating those messages again and again to your target audiences.

■ CREATIVE/PROMOTION STRATEGY

To maintain a consistent look and image for a geriatric care management business, it is important to define and document creative guidelines, including graphic and copy standards. This helps keep anyone who works on your creative materials informed of the specifications to be used in creative development and keeps your business looking professional and consistent to the public.

Develop graphic standards for your business that require use of the same images, font colors, and typefaces for every communication. Standards provide clear directions on when and how to use your logo and messages to anyone who may be working to promote your business. Carefully consider which fonts, colors, and styles to use and how your look might be interpreted by the public. Fonts with seraphs (little feet on them) are more pleasing and easier for older people to read. Red text is easier for the older eye to read. Large print size, at least 12 points, is also easier to read.

In an industry such as the aging needs industry with many messages competing for notice, the use of a consistent logo and tagline on all materials is a must. This helps drive home those messages you want to communicate, creates a personal connection, and helps set you apart from the competition. Contact information on *every* page of communication is a must. You are striving for recognition and development of subliminal relationships that show that you are in the business of providing information and resources to frail elderly persons, and you are the best available at providing these services. Consistent communications and design state this without many words.

■ MEET YOUR MARKETING GOALS: RECOMMENDED ACTIVITY

Marketing goals need to be specific and measurable. Include specific weekly, monthly, and quarterly activities that you will ultimately use to meet the goals set forth in your marketing plan. Constantly watch for client demand; then, talk about it with your core staff. Listen to what the client needs and meet that need. The marketing plan should prioritize lead generation tactics and face-to-face opportunities and include the best local and national organizations to join to increase business. I found that the local Rotary Club is a great organization with which to be involved because the membership is older and because members are community leaders who have accumulated some wealth. Not only did our local rotary club use our geriatric care management service, but they recommended us to others.

When considering which media to use to reach potential targets and referral sources, use every "channel" available and affordable: Internet, mail, phone message on hold, media, e-mail tag line, stationery, signage, and so forth.

Every contact needs to be a positive contact. If you have staff, consider using a "mystery shopper" service to perform regular checks on your staff's customer service performance. Answering the phone is probably the most important sales tool because the call may be an initial inquiry from an interested party. Excellent customer service and engaging the inquirer with questions about his or her situation and needs can lead to a new client. Always ask if you can send the caller information. If yes, send it *that day*. As always, record the contact in the database. One caution is not to solve the problem in one phone call. Decide on a time frame—15 minutes is suggested—for listening and responding to the caller. Also, explain that geriatric care management services are professional services for which there is a fee, just like for the services of an attorney or an accountant.

Measure referrals and client sources and assess monthly where business is being generated. Track referrals to identify those who refer repeatedly. Each caller should be asked, "How did you hear about us?" Send thank-you cards to every referral source, or at least make a phone call to thank them. Ask previous clients if you can use them as references.

Make the most of current referral prospects. Use note cards and give out business cards. Send press clippings to interested people. Use a contact management tool such as Gold-Mine, Act!, Outlook, or Microsoft Access. An Excel spreadsheet of contacts can work in a pinch if the file is set up correctly to capture the necessary information.

When it comes to media interest, make sure that you respond immediately if you receive a call from a reporter. Be clear about the services you offer and use your key messages and positioning statements to guide how you describe your business. Add reporters to your contact management tool, and code them as media for type of group.

A Yellow Pages listing is also a source for phone inquiries. List small ads under several sections rather than using one large ad. Because sometimes there is not an established category for care management, people will search for assistance under the categories of "geriatric consulting," "nursing," "sitters," "companions," "home health," and "senior services," to name a few. Also use Yellow-Pages.com listings so families from afar can find your service.

■ SETTING YOURSELF APART FROM COMPETITION

With so many aging resources available, the key to success is to use a specific strategy to decide on which messages, targets, and specific goals will accomplish the business growth you desire. Setting your business apart from the competition occurs only after you have assessed the competition and implemented a strategic plan that includes providing an excellent service, good customer relations, good referral relations, and using contact management tools effectively to set your business apart.

Mystery shopping is a term used to describe the act of surveying the competition while acting as a consumer making an inquiry. Conducting this type of competition survey is one way to look at the competition and find out what they are doing that is different, better or worse, and to use that information to your benefit.

First, you need to create a mystery shopping scenario. Your first step toward completing a competition analysis for your business is to create a scenario for mystery shopping. For example, you pretend your aunt is going to need some help because she is confused. You do not know what to do for her at this point. You are checking options available and are responsible for reporting back to the other family members.

Make a list of the competitors who do business in your area and include their phone numbers and Web site information.

Then, make the calls to the competition. Use your predetermined mystery shopping scenario, ask the following questions, and track the answers as you go. Make certain to ask that a brochure or any other marketing information be mailed to you. In this way, you can compare not only what services are provided and the prices, but also how your inquiry is handled and the time it takes the business to respond.

Finally, take all of the information you have compiled and summarize it, along with your comments regarding the information your competitors sent to you:

Name of Agency
Phone number:
Web site?
Spoke with?
How long in business?
Services offered:
Cost?
Advance notice needed to begin service?
Can they send information?
How did the staff person handle the call?
    (1 = excellent service, 5 = poor service)
How well did the staff person meet your needs
    about the information you requested?
Did the staff person present the company
    appropriately?
Overall impression:
Date material received:
Comments on materials:

Secrets of Marketing Success

The number one secret for marketing success is being where the customer can find you when he or she has a need. A close second is listening to customers when they do find you and providing excellent service. Setting very high standards for responsiveness can also contribute to success.

A very good resource for information on marketing and public relations for the GCM is "Public Relations/Marketing Tips for Professional Geriatric Care Managers" that is offered on the National Association of Professional Geriatric Care Managers Web site in the GCM Store. Also, use the checklist in Table 10–2 as a tool for helping you implement a successful marketing program for your business.

Table 10–2 Start-up GCM PR/Marketing Checklist		
Description	**Services Needed to Complete**	**Done?**
Brand Identity, including logo design and collateral material design	Research competition, develop key differentiating factor, develop "brand positioning" statement, develop business name, graphic design for logo, colors for business communication	
Business Identity (i.e. coordinated business cards, letterhead, envelopes, note cards, and folders)	Graphic design, printing, and delivery	
Product Sheets and/or Brochure	Copywriting, graphic design, printing, and delivery	
Testimonials captured in usable format	Identify procedures for obtaining testimonials	
Targeted Referral Sources	Plan, design, and develop a system; data maintenance/administration; fulfillment	
Web Site	Obtain URL, establish hosting account; develop content; maintain updated site	
Desktop & Industry Reminders (promotional items sporting the GCM's logo, brand image, and contact information)	Brainstorm and select items to be used, decide how to "brand" item with product logo, when to distribute	
Internet Newsletter	Design format, write content, publish on a regular basis; create system for obtaining e-mail addresses and updating data	
Regular Newsletter	Design format, write content, publish on a regular, established basis	
Charitable and Volunteer Work	Research for a match with key marketing factors; use publicity and seminars	
Seminars and/or Workshop Presentations	Create text and PPT and use publicity; create evaluation form; use system for retrieval of attendees for marketing purposes	
Methods of Feedback/Measurement	Interviews, surveys, research, development of measurement methods	
Current/Former Referral Communications	Client/referral communication, follow-up phone calls	
Web Site Integration (all press releases, newsletters, and publicity posted on web site)	Web site content updates/maintenance	

■ CONCLUSION

The most important thing to remember about marketing a geriatric care management business is that services of a GCM are "at-need" and consumers seek a GCM only when the need arises. Being where the client or referral source is looking when the need arises is the goal. Secondarily, the GCM must, in many cases, educate consumers about what a GCM is and does. Projecting a professional image and a well-designed and well-thought-out message that resonates with the consumer is necessary to deliver your message to at-need consumers and turn them into clients.

■ NOTES

1. Bearden WO, Ingram TN, LaForge R. *Marketing Principles and Perspectives.* 4th ed. New York: McGraw-Hill/Irwin; 2003.

2. Orsini M. Marketing private-duty home care services. *Home Health Care Manage Prac.* February 2006; 18(2):114–123.

3. Orsini M. Branded! Use branding to cement image, gain referrals. *Success in Home Care.* July/August 2005; 9(4).

4. Kotler P. *According to Kotler; The World's Foremost Authority on Marketing Answers to Your Questions.* AMACOM: 2005:90.

5. Orsini M. *Private Duty Business Manual.* Marketing Module. Available at: http://www.markethomecare.com/business.html#. Accessed July 1, 2006.

Chapter 11

Private Revenue Sources for the Fee-Based Care Manager

Robert E. O'Toole

The independent professional practice of geriatric care management has continued its steady growth since 2001, when the first edition of this book was published. Private care management, however, remains a relatively young and developing sector of the larger long-term health care industry. Prior to taking the bold step of developing an entrepreneurial, fee-based alternative to the largely third-party financed long-term-care service delivery system, most geriatric care managers (GCMs) worked in non-fee-based settings, such as private hospitals or health care systems, nonprofit agencies funded by grants or the United Way, church-supported organizations, or tax-supported public or quasi-public agencies. Regardless of the care setting, the money to pay for the services provided to frail elders usually did not come directly from the recipient of the service. Neither did family members of the care recipients make financial contributions of any significance in most cases. In hospitals, outpatient health clinics, certified home health agencies, or nursing homes, the primary source of funding was likely to be various forms of third-party insurance, most likely from a federal insurance program such as Medicare or the joint state and federal insurance program known as Medicaid.

■ DECLINING PUBLIC FUNDING AVAILABLE TO PAY FOR ELDERCARE: A CRISIS OR ESTABLISHED PUBLIC POLICY?

The first of two "age waves" is about to crest. The size and impact of our rapidly aging nation is like two tidal waves, one very close to shore, and the other visible, but far off in the distance.

The first tidal wave is about to crest with the unprecedented number of people living into their 80s and 90s. (See Figure 11–1.) Currently, people age 85 years and older are almost six times more likely to need chronic, ongoing health and social services than those in their 60s.[1]

This first age wave is already taxing the resources set in place to meet the demand. Medicaid, the joint federal and state-funded health program for the poor, is now the largest and fastest-growing segment of most state budgets. The largest portion of Medicaid budgets pays for nursing home bills for both poor and middle-class persons who are ill prepared for the staggering costs of care.

The other major government health care program for frail older people is the Medicare program. The Congressional Budget Office (CBO) has warned that, unless we increase financing or reduce Medicare services, in the

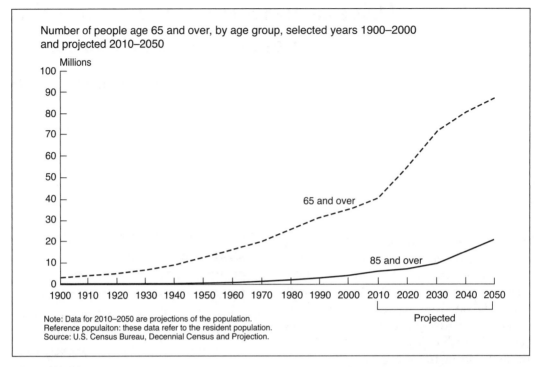

Figure 11–1   Age Wave

coming decades the nation will face consider-able growth of federal deficits that are already at historic levels.[2]

> Diagnosing the problem for Medicare is much easier than finding viable solu-tions. As is well known, 78 million baby boomers will start to turn 65 in 2011. They will continue reaching retirement age over the next 20 years, doubling the population covered by Medicare. More-over, these boomers will live longer than their predecessors. And almost as impor-tant, their generation is followed by the unusually small "baby-bust" generation. [3]

The response by state and federal govern-ments to this growing demand for long-term health care, so far, has been to reduce the amount of care available and require

elders to pay for more out-of-pocket expenses for long-term illnesses. If elders don't have sufficient funds to pay for the added expenses, increasingly they will need to rely on their baby boomer offspring to help them pay the bills.

The second age wave will make the first wave look like only a ripple by comparison. The large number of baby boomers, who will begin to reach age 65 in 2006, will swell the ranks of the elderly because life expectancy is expected to continue to increase in the 21st century. The baby boomers are likely to live longer than their parents did. Seventy-six million people were born during the postwar years of 1946 to 1964. Add the number of aging baby boomers to their long-living parents and the age 85-plus population will grow by nearly 150% by the year 2030. (See Figure 11–2.)

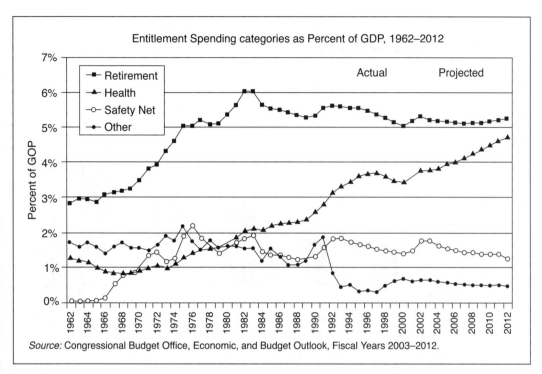

Figure 11–2   Entitlement Spending Categories

■ IS THERE A "CRISIS" IN ELDERCARE SERVICES IN THE UNITED STATES?

Many Americans, including elected officials, public policy analysts, and journalists, have begun to refer to the gap between available public funding and the aging of the U.S. population as a "crisis." [3,4]

At the end of 2005, *USA Today* declared

As 1,200 national delegates, policymakers and advocates for the elderly converge on Washington, D.C., this week for the fifth White House Conference on Aging, many come with mixed feelings of hope and frustration that, though they've been sounding the alarm for years about a looming crisis in caregiving resources, Washington still doesn't seem to be listening.

The list of concerns includes an increase in Alzheimer's disease, expected to strike up to 16 million Americans by 2025; major shortages of family and professional caregivers; lack of proper housing and transportation for seniors; and shortages of geriatric physicians. [5]

Author and elder-law attorney Dallas Atkins writes, "If you are providing care to incapacitated 70- to 100-year-old parents, you already know the bitter taste of the long-term care crisis of the 21st century, a crisis scheduled to explode when the Boomers reach retirement age. An unfathomable number of elders will face a critical lack of care providers and facilities, and too few wage earners to support a tax basis for providing care to the multitude." [6]

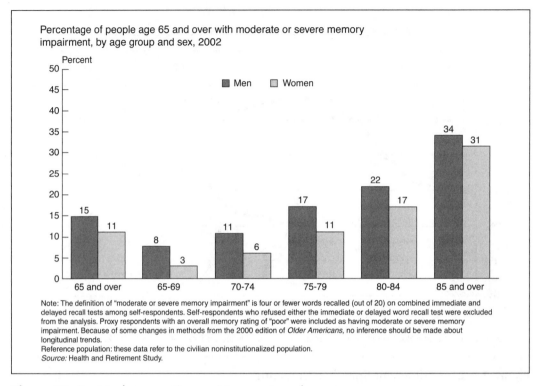

Percentage of people age 65 and over with moderate or severe memory impairment, by age group and sex, 2002

Note: The definition of "moderate or severe memory impairment" is four or fewer words recalled (out of 20) on combined immediate and delayed recall tests among self-respondents. Self-respondents who refused either the immediate or delayed word recall test were excluded from the analysis. Proxy respondents with an overall memory rating of "poor" were included as having moderate or severe memory impairment. Because of some changes in methods from the 2000 edition of *Older Americans*, no inference should be made about longitudinal trends.
Reference population: these data refer to the civilian noninstitutionalized population.
Source: Health and Retirement Study.

Figure 11–3   Moderate or Severe Memory Impairment

■ A SERIOUS PROBLEM BUT HARDLY A CRISIS

It can be hard to believe that it has been nearly a quarter century, since the early 1980s, when the "crisis of an aging America" first began to be forecast by political leaders such as Republican President Ronald Reagan and House Speaker Democrat Tip O'Neil. Public policy analysts and experts also tried to raise awareness of this growing problem.

In a radio address to the nation in 1981, President Reagan said: "Some 30 years ago, there were 16 people working and paying the social security payroll tax for every 1 retiree. Today that ratio has changed to only 3.2 workers paying in for each beneficiary. For many years, we've known that an actuarial imbalance existed and that the program faced an unfunded liability of several trillion dollars."[7]

Now, the short range problem is much closer than that. The social security retirement fund has been paying billions of dollars more each year than it takes in, and it could run out of money unless something is done. The president said that some in Congress had suggested borrowing from the Medicare surplus that was growing at that time, to pay for the current costs. In 1982, Stephen Crystal, in his book *America's Old Age Crisis: Public Policy and the Two Worlds of Aging*, wrote:

> In many ways, aging policy has become a major dilemma for our society. Benefits for the aged command an increasingly large share of the budget, putting the squeeze on other programs. Yet many elderly suffer severe deprivation, and the "social safety net" fails to catch them. Despite fast-escalating costs, our benefit system is neither equitable nor efficient.

Why do we seem to be spending more now but getting less for it?

Deciding what to do is all the more difficult because we are not clear about the nature of the problem or about our own objectives. There is little understanding of how existing programs actually operate, what they cost, and who benefits.[8]

More than a decade later, in 1994, gerontologist and author Carrol Estes and her colleagues at the University of California described the inadequacies of public funding for eldercare services as "alarming." "What happens when efforts to contain spiraling costs collide with health and social services delivery in a competitive market? The unintended results can be alarming." Estes described the situation at that time as an "insidious relationship between recent transformations in hospital care financing and the manner in which older Americans now receive—or, more accurately, do not receive—health and social services in the community," and she called it the "No Care Zone."[9]

Still another decade passed. The conditions grew even worse and the warnings ever more dire. Senator John Breaux (D-La.), chairman of the Senate Special Committee on Aging, urged Congress to consider a comprehensive long-term-care system and warned that the burgeoning pressures of long-term-care services and escalating Medicaid costs might soon overwhelm state budgets.

"Our nation is sorely in need of a comprehensive long-term care system," said Senator Breaux. "The current system costs billions of dollars yet fails to deliver the services we expect or to provide seniors with the essentials they need for daily life. With 77 million baby boomers approaching retirement, this crisis must be addressed now to preserve our fiscal solvency and ensure state budgets are not completely overrun."[10]

Senator Breaux's comments came at an Aging Committee hearing examining how the failure to establish a national long-term-care system will harm the nation's fiscal stability. With Medicaid and long-term-care costs skyrocketing, Senator Breaux and the witnesses urged federal, state, and local legislators to look at Medicaid and long-term care alongside Medicare and Social Security as the final component of any entitlement reform effort.

"Everyone has a plan, but everyone's second option is always to do nothing," says Stuart Altman, an economist specializing in federal health policy and a presidential appointee to the Bipartisan Committee on the Future of Medicare.[11]

A former deputy assistant for planning and evaluation at the Department of Health, Education and Welfare, Altman retraced the history of Medicare and Medicaid, emphasizing the lack of planning that went into the Medicaid law when it was originally developed. He indicated that many of the problems associated with the program, including the transfer of assets to qualify for benefits, stemmed from its having been created as a footnote to Medicare. No one ever imagined, says Altman, "that almost overnight, Medicaid would become long-term care insurance."[11]

On February 8, 2006, President George W. Bush signed the Deficit Reduction Act of 2005 (DRA) into law. According to the CBO, the Act is expected to reduce federal Medicaid spending by $11.5 billion over a 5-year period and by $43.2 billion over the next 10 years. Currently, Medicaid pays the nursing home bills of 12 million elderly and disabled people.

For many families, the law drastically and suddenly changes the way that long-term care, especially nursing home care, will be paid for. The National Academy of Elder Law Attorneys (NAELA) issued a statement saying that the DRA creates "a health care crisis of unprecedented magnitude for our most vulnerable citizens."[12]

According to NAELA attorney Jeffrey A. Marshall, elders will have to cope with provisions that attempt to shift more of the financial burden of nursing home care onto families and nursing facilities. "Few seniors have insurance that covers long term care and most nursing home residents rely on Medicaid to cover part of the cost of their care. The new law will make it more difficult for these residents to obtain this financial aid."[12]

The devastation to the city of New Orleans caused by Hurricane Katrina was a crisis. The 2004 Indian Ocean earthquake that triggered a series of destructive tsunamis that inundated coastal communities across South and Southeast Asia and that killed more than 275,000 was a crisis. Can a quarter century of worsening conditions in public programs for elders still be considered a crisis, or should the nation finally recognize that the underfunding of eldercare services is an established public policy? (See Figure 11–4.)

■ IS THE DEMAND FOR ELDERCARE LARGE ENOUGH TO SUPPORT FEE-BASED ELDERCARE PROFESSIONALS?

One response to decades of declining public funding for elder services has been the emergence of a private sector alternative. It is not unreasonable, after all, to think that elders and family caregivers who can't get the services they need from state and federal sources would seek to obtain them elsewhere, using their own resources.

When the first edition of this book was published, geriatric care management was still a young and developing sector of a larger and rapidly growing "eldercare industry." The vast majority of the profession's membership consisted of either solo practices, or very

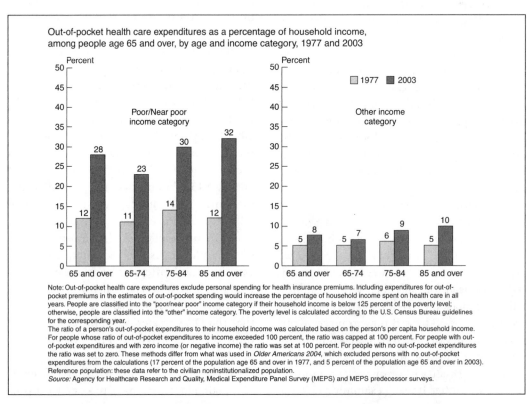

Figure 11–4   Out-of-Pocket Health Care Expenditures

small business ventures with only a few owners and employees.

While growth in this profession has increased steadily, the increased number of private, for-profit elder care enterprises has been modest, when compared with the growth of the aging population.

Why is it that, in a nation that is aging rapidly with unprecedented numbers of people living into their 80s and 90s, fee-based, geriatric care management is still a "cottage industry?"

When we look at research and demographic data published in dozens of studies funded by the American Association of Retired Persons (AARP), and the MetLife Mature Market Institute among others, we see a well-documented need for the services provided by private care managers. These studies report that "25.8 million family caregivers provide personal assistance to adults with a disability or chronic illness" and that "nearly one of every four households is involved in caregiving to persons aged 50+" and "by the year 2007, the number of caregiving households in the United States for persons aged 50+ could reach 39 million."[13,14]

■ "NEED" VS. "DEMAND" FOR GERIATRIC CARE MANAGEMENT SERVICES

If we see the potential market for our geriatric care management services the almost 40 million households, it's tempting to base an elder-care business model on this growing need and expect it to keep GCMs busy and profitable. After all, isn't the basic formula for building a successful business "find a need and fill it?"

Although "find a need and fill it" looks good on one of those ubiquitous and inspirational posters, it is not a sound revenue model for an eldercare business. It's clear that the need for services is huge, but to survive as independent business owners we GCMs must look more closely at the data and embrace a more realistic philosophy. "Need" doesn't pay the bills, "demand" does. Only those with sufficient financial resources can pay privately for home care at home, assisted living facilities, continuing care retirement communities, and other expensive discretionary health and preventive services, which are generally not paid for with public funds.

The tradition of having most long-term care paid for by third parties has created an expectation that has become firmly established in the American psyche; the prevailing attitude about the payment for long-term care services, whether provided in a facility or in the community, has been that long-term care should be paid for by somebody else, regardless of the family's income. According to Jane Bryant Quinn, personal finance columnist for *Newsweek* magazine, "As the population ages, Medicaid spending on nursing homes could easily lurch out of control. That is, unless it's limited to the people who really need it. . . . Medicaid is supposed to provide support for poor persons. But, increasingly, it's being exploited by the well-to-do. Instead of buying nursing home insurance or using their personal savings, they're getting the government to cover their bills."[15]

The resistance to paying privately for care has been so strong in this country that often even those with income and assets that place them in the middle and upper economic classes have used laws designed to help the poor to avoid paying for their care or the care of a family member. This deeply ingrained entitlement mentality, coupled with the legal process that supports and encourages this attitude, makes the move to become an independent provider of long-term-care services by nurses, social workers, and other eldercare professionals a risky business venture.

The target market of any fee-based eldercare business is not the 39 million families who need geriatric care management services, but the much smaller subset of those families who can afford to hire a GCM, are willing to pay for the services GCMs provide, and can actually find their way to the GCM's door (or voice mail, e-mail, or Web site). Those with their own resources to pay for care can afford to hire a private care manager. Often, care managers can save caregivers and care recipients money by using their skills and knowledge of how to find the best care and how to use that care in the most cost-effective way.

Those who can afford to pay privately for care management, home care, and care in the best facilities actually represent a small percentage of those who need the services. A recent report by the Brookings Institution confirms this. "Despite the estimated cost of paying for LTC [long term care] services and the strain it puts on retirement savings, very few people in or approaching retirement have private resources or sufficient public benefits to protect them from long-term care costs."[16]

In addition, another barrier to setting up a geriatric care management services business that relies on care recipients to pay for services from private resources is the existence of a "mythology of long-term care," which consists of the following beliefs:

1. **The "entitlement" mentality: Medicare will pay for long-term care.** The tradition of having most health-care-related services paid for by an employer during a person's working years and then by Medicare when the person retires has created an expectation that has become firmly established in the American psyche. The prevailing attitude toward the payment of long-term-care services, whether provided in a facility or in the community, is that "long-term care should be paid for by somebody else regardless of the family's income and assets."

   A 2001 survey sponsored by Care-Quest found that 4 in 10 Americans age 65 and older believe that Medicare, or Medicare supplemental insurance (Medigap), would pay for long-term care. The reality, of course, is that Medicare will pay for up to 100 days of "short-term" nursing home care in qualifying circumstances, but it will not pay for long-term custodial care.

2. **"I'm not old enough to worry about that now."** The need for long-term care can occur at any age. An accident, a chronic illness, or an injury can result in the need for long-term care. According to the National Center for Health Statistics, nearly half of the population in the United States will need some type of long-term care. Forty percent of the population of people with disabilities who need long-term care are working-age adults. Unfortunate events that prevent a person from working can happen at any age, not just in old age.

3. **"It will never happen to me."** Demand for long-term care is on the rise. Already, 60% to 70% of Americans who live to age 65 require long-term care assistance at some point in their lives, according to research by the CBO.[17]

   Paul Hodge, director of the Generations Policy Institute at the Kennedy School, writes in the debut edition of the *Harvard Generations Policy Journal*, a publication exploring age-related policy issues, "And even though many of those long-lived people will remain healthy for most of the additional decades of their lives, others will require years of assistance."[18]

4. **"My family will take care of me."** Until a few decades ago, women traditionally cared for their aging parents and other relatives. With the rise of the two-income household, working women can no longer serve as full-time caregivers. Many women start families later, meaning they're busy raising their own children just as their elders need help; in

addition, elders often live hundreds or thousands of miles away from potential family caregivers.

5. **"I have enough in savings."** According to the American Council of Life Insurance (ACLI), in about 40 years, a two-year nursing home stay could cost about $500,000. Therefore, a 45-year-old would have to save about $3,500 per year for 40 years and achieve a 7% annual return to fund the expense at age 85.[19]

In contrast, an annual long-term care insurance premium of $2000 for a 45-year-old paid over the same 40-year period would create an immediate benefits pool of $365,000. The benefits will grow at a five percent compounded rate to more than $2 million. In other words, by paying a long-term care insurance premium that costs a little over half of the amount in the ACLI example, the same individual would accumulate four times as much and be able to pay for care for 8 years instead of 2. Long-term care insurance, if purchased when a large number of Americans can afford it, would substantially increase the demand pool for professional geriatric care management services.

As long as most Americans continue to embrace the prevailing mythology of long-term care, these myths will continue to create a barrier to operating a profitable eldercare service business that is based on fees paid by the care recipient or a family member.

As eldercare professionals who provide services largely paid for from private funds, GCMs have a vested interest in raising the level of awareness of the U.S. public about the various private funding resources available to pay for geriatric care management services, the importance of planning ahead before a crisis occurs, and the undesirable consequences that await if people continue to hold on to the mythology of long-term care.

■ BASING A PRIVATE ELDERCARE BUSINESS MODEL ON DEMOGRAPHICS: THE REALITY OF A NEED- VS. DEMAND-BASED REVENUE MODEL

We've all seen the data: America is growing older. The population of persons age 85 years and older is the largest in history and will keep growing for the foreseeable future. There is also those 78 to 80 million baby boomers, the oldest of whom started turning 60 in 2004. Many eldercare entrepreneurs enter the private, fee-only market with a business plan that is based on these demographic projections.

It is tempting to base a business plan to serve elders in need on the demographic projections of an aging society. However, as noted earlier in this chapter, such naive thinking must be tempered by the harsh reality of many who have ventured into the private market and failed. Those who build an eldercare business model based on the number of elders who need care will sooner or later go out of business.

The preceding warning is simply another version of the first basic principle taught in Economics 101. Economists call it supply and demand. If you're in the business of providing eldercare that is paid for by your client's/customer's private resources, you'd better focus on the fact that a much smaller percentage of those in need of elder services can afford—or are willing—to pay for those services. That smaller group is the "demand" segment of the growing population of elders.

Because the vast majority of GCMs come to the private sector of eldercare services from a human services health or educational background, the fact that many of those who seek out geriatric care management services can't afford to pay for them is often hard to accept. But to stay in business GCMs simply can't afford to provide services to those in need; only those who can pay the fees can keep GCMs in business.

No longer supported by the third-party-funded infrastructure that provided them with an office, a predictable—if often modest—salary, supplies, and overhead costs such as reimbursement for travel, independent practice professionals learn very quickly that they must charge fees to those whom they provide services. The fees must be paid out of the pocket of the consumer rather than from a third-party source.

Even many of those who can afford geriatric care management services and who aren't eligible for subsidized services resist paying GCMs out of their own funds. Probably more than any other factor, the private fee-based nature of independent geriatric care management practice, in the context of a widely held attitude opposed to paying directly for such services, is a barrier to operating a profitable business.

In developing a business plan for a fee-based eldercare service business such as geriatric care management, it's important for GCMs to have a basic understanding of all likely sources of income, private and public, that are available to pay for the expanding range of long-term care services.

State and federal government officials are proposing Medicaid cuts that will further limit care options for those who rely on public funding for their care. Also, the pool of workers in the labor-intensive, long-term care industry will continue to shrink as the numbers of frail and disabled elderly steadily grow at an ever-increasing pace.

The future of long-term care funding will not only be shaped by the past 25 years of public policy victories of political conservatives, but by more moderate political voices who now recognize that a high-quality publicly funded long-term care system will never become a reality in the United States. Former U.S. Senator and Secretary of Defense William Cohen of Maine, a prominent moderate political voice, declared, "The U.S. must not create any new, unrestrained, non-means tested programs for long-term care." Cohen, who sup-ported many progressive social programs in his long senate career, calls for the encouragement of "personal responsibility among middle and upper income Americans to prepare for their own long-term care needs."[20]

To plan for their future long-term care needs properly, Americans must understand that the quality of care and the options available depend on whether they can pay the bill from private funds or rely on government funding to pay for care. The evidence is overwhelming and undeniable: the choices and the quality of care provided to those who rely on public funding are very limited and will only become more so as the aging population grows.

Those who are dependent on Medicaid and other sources of public funding receive poor care, very little care, or no care at all. It is a well-documented fact that nursing homes that rely on Medicaid funding are seriously understaffed, and their personnel are often poorly trained. And the situation is expected to worsen, not get better.

Many needy elders and other disabled adults languish for months on waiting lists for publicly funded community care programs, even when they meet the eligibility guidelines. When service finally becomes available, it is typically much less than is needed. The publicly funded case manager is likely to be someone with little training or experience, carrying a caseload of 75, 80, and in many cases more than 90 people with complicated needs and few resources.

It sometimes seems that the general public isn't paying attention to the growing crisis in long-term care for the elderly, but the press cannot be blamed for not trying to get the message out. It seems that almost daily newspapers and other national and local media outlets publish articles that highlight the growing severity of what has already become one of the major problems facing an aging America in the 21st century. In October 2005, *USA Today* reported, "Each year from 2000 through 2004, three of five nursing homes were cited for at least one violation of state or federal fire safety standards. Many of those violations involved relatively minor problems. But about 10%, on average, involved more serious problems, characterized by regulators as those that can cause patients actual harm or put them in immediate jeopardy."[21]

Also, around that same time, Leon Kass, president of the President's Council on Bioethics, wrote the following in the *Washington Post*:

> A crisis in long-term care will soon be upon us. The shortage of caregivers is made worse by our cultural refusal to honor the need for care. As a society, we have preferred to place our hopes in programs that promote healthy aging and in scientific research seeking remedies for incapacitating diseases. We offer little communal support to the millions of Americans—more each decade—who give demanding daily care to aged parents or spouses. Our society has embraced living wills, through which individuals specify how they wish to be treated should they become incapacitated. We are encouraged to believe that if only we execute the proper documents, we can remain in control of our future and avoid unseemly dependencies and indignities. But this ignores our unavoidable need for human presence and care, especially when we can no longer take care of ourselves. Written directives cannot substitute for reliable and responsible caregivers devoted to the daily welfare of the incapacitated.[22]

■ UNDERSTANDING THE FUNDING SOURCES TO PAY FOR LONG-TERM CARE

There are nine basic sources of funding to pay for long-term care services:

1. Medicare
2. Medicaid
3. Private savings and other liquid assets (including funds from adult children)
4. Private long-term care insurance (LTCI)
5. "Blended" life/LTCI policies
6. Long-term care annuities
7. Life settlements
8. Reverse mortgages
9. Investor-owned life insurance for those older than age 75

These revenue sources are reviewed in the following sections along with a discussion of the still small but growing demand for services from employers who are beginning to recognize the need for caregiver support for their aging work force.

Medicare and Medicaid

As already noted, probably the most erroneous belief about paying for long-term care held by both elders and family caregivers is that "when an older person needs long-term care, the government will pay for it." Despite the fact that this has never been true, the availability of universal coverage for acute care needs under the Medicare program fosters this myth even today.

GCMs know that *long-term care* refers specifically to a person's need for assistance with the activities of daily living (ADLs). These ADLs include six specific functional needs: assistance—hands on or through cueing—of another person with bathing, dressing, feeding, transferring from a bed or chair, ambulation, and bowel or bladder incontinence. Assistance with ADLs is not considered by Medicare to be a "skilled" service. Because Medicare only pays for skilled services, most long-term care needs will not be paid for by Medicare. Following is what Medicare *will* pay for:

Medicare in a Nursing Facility

Medicare covers some skilled care in an approved skilled nursing facility.

A minimum 3-day prior hospital stay is required.

The patient must enter a facility within 30 days after discharge from a hospital.

The patient must continue to show improvement.

Medicare in a Home Setting

The patient must be confined to home and under a doctor's care.

Covers part-time skilled nursing care or physical therapy, speech-language therapy, and home health aid services.

The patient's condition must continually improve.

Examples of skilled care under Medicare include the following:

Short-term intravenous lines or tubing
Physical or speech therapy
Dressing bedsores

Even when the skilled care requirement is met, Medicare funding is often limited. For example, once a Medicare-eligible patient is in a skilled nursing facility, the maximum amount of time Medicare will pay for care is 100 days. If it is determined that the patient can no longer benefit from skilled services such as physical therapy after 30 or 60 days, payment for care ceases.

Consumer Confusion about Medicare vs. Medicaid

Because both programs have similar sounding names and operate with public funds, elders and family caregivers frequently confuse the two programs. Despite their similar names, Medicaid and Medicare are two completely separate—and very different—programs.

Medicare provides certain health benefits only to Americans who are at least 65 years old. It is completely administered by the federal government. On the other hand, Medicaid is a health care assistance program for poor Americans of all ages. Funding comes from both the federal government and state governments. Within limits, the federal government allows the states some degree of leeway in how they run their own Medicaid programs. Medicaid payments can be used to cover the cost of nursing home care. With a federal waiver, Medicaid funds can also be used to pay for

home health care. However, in reality, the availability of Medicaid-funded home care services is severely limited. While there have been recent moves to shift more Medicaid spending in several states, the overwhelming share of Medicaid payments for long-term care goes to fund care in nursing homes.

Age has nothing to do with whether a person can qualify to receive Medicaid benefits. Instead, each state, within broad federal guidelines, sets its own eligibility requirements. There are limits on the maximum amount of income a person can have and the amount of assets the person is allowed to keep. In addition, Medicaid requires a 5-year "look-back" assessment to prevent people from giving away assets ahead of time so they can meet the Medicaid eligibility requirements.

Private Savings and Funds from Family Members

Despite the fact that the costs of long-term care pose a substantial financial risk to most Americans, most will be required to pay for these costs from personal savings or other family resources until they have exhausted income and assets and become eligible for the Medicaid program. The average cost of long-term care in nursing homes and assisted living facilities continues to increase faster than the rate of inflation. Assisted living and in-home costs are rising more sharply than nursing home care costs, according to a study published in March 2006.[23] The average annual cost for a private one-bedroom unit in an assisted living facility rose 7% to $32,294 since the 2005 survey, while the combined average hourly rate for a home health aide spiked 13% to $25.32 per hour. The average annual cost for a private room in a nursing home rose modestly by 2% to $70,912.

The Genworth study reports that "as the first wave of America's 77 million baby boomers head into retirement it becomes more critical for Americans to seriously evaluate how they will maintain their lifestyles as we live well into our 80's, 90's and beyond. . . . The fact remains that most American households remain unprotected from the costly health challenges that come with greater longevity.

According to a national survey by Public Opinion Strategies, 65% of Americans admit to having made no long-term care plans. The poll also revealed that most individuals recognize the need to prepare for the cost of long-term care, but were largely unprepared.[23]

Private Long-Term Care Insurance

The LTCI industry began in the late 1980s when policies consisted mainly of nursing home coverage marketed to consumers in their late 60s, 70s, or 80s. Today, comprehensive coverage is most widely sold to protect against the high costs of nursing home or assisted living residence and in-home care. Due to slower than expected sales and a substantial consolidation of carriers in the mid to late 1990s, the number of companies selling this insurance declined sharply during the 1990s and has dwindled to fewer than a dozen major carriers.

The target market for this product is now the preretired baby boomer that is looking at LTCI as a retirement planning element rather than as a financial product to add to his or her retirement portfolio.

Still, LTCI has been a hard sell. Only an estimated 8% of the potential market of eligible consumers has been penetrated. In a 2003 Roper study conducted for the American Society on Aging, 71% of respondents said they believe it is very important to have some type of private or government coverage for long-term care. However, only 17% said they have specific LTCI to pay for the costs.[24]

Consumers just don't understand what LTCI is and what it covers. They also have difficulty making an informed choice from an array of options, and they may be in denial about becoming dependent and needing this type of insurance, according to a report from the Center on an Aging Society at Georgetown University.[25] A majority of the respondents in the survey had misconceptions about who provides long-term care coverage or the conditions under which it is offered.

"Blended" Life/LTCI Policies

One reason many consumers give for not buying LTCI is the fact that, if they die and never need to use the benefits, they will not receive a refund of the premiums they paid. Of course, millions of Americans pay premiums for 50 years or more to insure their homes and automobiles with no expectation of a refund if they never make a claim. This is the fundamental insurance principle of "pooled risk," with many paying insurance premiums with relatively few ever filing claims. No matter the logic behind this reluctance to purchase LTCI, several insurers have recently announced a new approach to insure the costs of long-term care that provides a payment to survivors if the insurance isn't used to pay for care.

Genworth Life Insurance Company, Nationwide Financial Services, Lincoln Financial, and others now offer a more comprehensive insurance solution that merges features of universal life insurance and LTCI into a single product. This approach helps consumers control their assets, protect their beneficiaries, and have access to long-term care benefits.

These new, so-called blended insurance products provide benefits such as the following:

- Policies can provide a death benefit or payment of benefits for long-term care expenses—or a combination of both. By choosing a single insurance product to meet multiple needs, customers can free assets for other uses.
- The complete return of the initial premium is another potentially accessible

feature if the policy is terminated by the customer in the first 15 policy years.

- A limited death benefit that is payable even if the entire benefit amount has been allocated to a customer's covered long-term care expenses.
- Inflation protection options to help the customer keep pace with the rising cost of long-term care.
- A comprehensive set of benefit options, including a lifetime coverage option.

Long-Term Care Annuities

This approach to financing the costs of long-term care uses a single premium deferred annuity to address the "what if I pay premiums and never file a claim" concern and also to provide a vehicle for those who are declined coverage for LTCI because of health problems. Consumers can set aside a specified amount of money to pay for long-term care expenses if needed. A higher interest rate is credited to funds if withdrawn for this purpose. Because the annuitant is, in effect, self-funding a portion of his or her long-term care risk, it becomes the equivalent of a very large deductible. As a result, the insurer is able to take a more liberal approach to underwriting and the consumer is able to obtain coverage for which he or she otherwise might not be eligible. If the funds in the annuity are not needed to pay for care, they are passed on to the beneficiary.

Life Settlements

Some geriatric care clients likely purchased life insurance policies many years ago that no longer meet their needs. When clients arrive at this conclusion, the common response is for them to stop paying the annual premium, terminate the policy, and recover any cash value that may have built up. What they—and typically their financial advisor—may not realize is that they can recover significantly more cash by selling the policy to third-party investors.

The National Association of Insurance Commissioners estimates that every year nearly $1.5 trillion face amount of life insurance policies expire, lapse, or are canceled by policyholders; each policy could have been converted to a resource to pay for long-term care costs had the owner sold it on the secondary market.

The growth in the secondary market for life insurance policies has soared over the last decade. According to A. M. Best Company, life settlement purchases have climbed from approximately $2.5 billion in 2003 to more than $10 billion in 2005 based on face amounts.[26]

Life settlement firms target policyholders with impaired health but not terminal illnesses. This typically includes seniors 70 years or older with no-lapse universal life insurance policies with face values of $250,000 or higher.

Examples of Life Settlement Transactions

Example 1. Joe, 70 years old, decides he no longer wants his $1 million universal life insurance policy. His health may have worsened, his beneficiaries may have died, or he simply can no longer afford the premiums. Prior to the emergence of the life settlements market, Joe would have had two choices: (1) accept the insurer's contractually agreed-upon surrender value, which is well below the policy's fair market value, or (2) let the policy lapse and receive nothing. That's an easy decision!

On the other hand, in the life settlements market, Joe could sell his policy to a life settlement company for up to three times its cash surrender value. The life settlement firm will pay future premiums on the policy and receive the $1 million death benefit upon Joe's death.

Example 2. A 76-year-old man owned a policy with an $8 million face amount and a $795,000 cash surrender value. He sold the policy for $2.3 million rather than letting it lapse, canceling it, or taking the cash value.

Had he not sold it, he would have left at least $1.5 million on the table.[27-29]

Reverse Mortgages

According to an AARP housing survey, the most important issue facing those who need long-term care is remaining in one's home. Yet the costs of staying in one's home can be overwhelming. Many older Americans are trying to meet those costs with limited income and assets.

Until recently, many older homeowners were faced with selling the home they had worked hard for because they could not afford to live there any longer or could not afford the daily cost of home health care, which is often more expensive than nursing home care. But a new type of loan, called a reverse mortgage, has given homeowners the option of keeping their home and solving their financial dilemma.

A reverse mortgage is a special type of loan for homeowners over the age of 62. The loan does not have to be repaid for as long as the homeowner continues to live in the home. Reverse mortgage income may be used to finance living expenses, home improvements, home care costs, or any other need. As the name suggests, with this type of loan, the payment stream is reversed: the lender makes payments to the borrower, rather than the borrower making monthly payments to the lender. And, unlike traditional mortgage loans, there are no income or credit requirements for a reverse mortgage.

The amount of money for which a borrower can qualify is based primarily on age (the older the homeowner, the more funds available). Interest rates and lending limits can also affect this calculation. Because the federal government insures reverse mortgages, under no circumstances will the borrower (or the borrower's estate) ever have to repay more than the value of the home, which is the sole source of repayment for this type of loan. Lenders cannot force borrowers to leave the home if they lend them more money than the home is worth. Nor can lenders lay claim to other assets or the assets of the borrower's heirs.

Elders and their caregivers need to be aware of other benefits of reverse mortgages. All payments received from a reverse mortgage are tax free, and the proceeds from a reverse mortgage do not affect eligibility for Social Security or Medicare. Also, most of the closing costs associated with a reverse mortgage can be financed, thereby limiting the amount of cash required from a borrower.

The two largest reverse mortgage programs are administered by the U.S. Department of Housing and Urban Development (HUD) and by Fannie Mae. HUD's reverse mortgage loan is called the Home Equity Conversion Mortgage and was established in 1989. Fannie Mae's product, called the Home Keeper, was first introduced in 1995.

One of the consumer protections built into these programs is a requirement that borrowers attend an approved financial education session before they can even fill out an application for a reverse mortgage loan. During this no-cost session, the counselor—an objective third party—advises the senior on the suitability of the product to his or her needs, outlines the costs involved, and frequently dispels any misconceptions the client may have. It is advised that seniors have a trustworthy individual (such as a caregiver) accompany them throughout this process.

A study by the National Council on Aging, funded by the Centers for Medicare and Medicaid Services and the Robert Wood Johnson Foundation, shows that more than 13 million Americans can use reverse mortgages to pay for long-term care expenses at home. In this way, many can stay independent and live in their homes longer.

For example, a 75-year-old with a home worth $100,000 could receive a reverse mortgage loan that could pay $500 a month for almost 12 years. The extra cash could go a long way to help with family caregiving and other long-term care expenses.[30]

Investor-Owned Life Insurance for Those Older Than Age 75

Another trend of interest to healthy elders over age 75 is the leveraged purchase of life insurance policies initiated by investors. This new insurance strategy can provide substantial funds for a healthy elder who faces an expensive and stressful caregiving situation as a result of the poor health of a spouse. This approach does not require any payments from the insurable elder. Instead, investor groups (similar to those who purchase life settlements) pay the full premium. If the insured dies within the first 2 years that the policy is in force, all of the death benefit is paid to the beneficiaries. After the 2-year period, the investors become the beneficiary.

Funds to pay for the long-term care of a spouse are provided by the investors who also provide the insured a large, up-front cash settlement in addition to paying the otherwise unaffordable premium on the policy.

Long-Term Care Carriers Recognize the Value of GCMs

Insurance companies began to utilize care managers early on in the development of these policies. During the initial application, or underwriting stage, care managers have been used to help determine whether an applicant is an acceptable risk. Nurses and social workers with experience in long-term care have been retained, on a fee-for-service basis, to conduct interviews with selected applicants, usually those over age 70. Using a variety of functional assessment instruments, case managers help underwriters get a picture of how independent a potential insured is prior to approving the application.

When claims are filed, insurers use case managers to expedite the claims process. A GCM is retained to go to the home or the facility where the claimant is receiving care. Using ADL-based functional assessment tools, the care manager prepares a report that helps claims specialists confirm that the claim is valid.

GCM roles in LTCI will continue to expand. Most major insurance carriers now see care managers as a cost-effective, value-added benefit for policyholders as care coordinators. As policyholders age and claims activity of insurance companies grows, the care management/care coordination role will grow steadily.

The services of GCMs are also used to help policyholders develop a plan of care that makes the best use of their policy benefits. The care coordination benefit was initially offered as an option for which the insured paid an additional premium. Today, newer LTCI products include care coordination as part of the basic benefit package at no additional cost.

Some insurers require that the case manager must be a participating member of that insurer's preferred providers network. Increasingly, the option to choose a GCM is left up to the policyholder or the family caregivers.

Most LTCI policies are issued with a deductible or limitation period. This limitation period, during which no benefits are paid, typically ranges from 20 to 100 days, a choice the insured makes when the policy is purchased. More policies now waive the elimination period for care coordination benefits and allow payment to the care coordinator as soon as the claim is approved.

Geriatric Care Managers As a Resource for Working Caregivers and Their Employers

One potential source of fee-based income for care managers is the workplace. Because of the aging work force and the increasing percentage of workers with aging parents, some employers now provide support services for working caregivers. These services have been around for more than 20 years but, as yet, have not resulted in a significant source of business for most care managers.

In 2003, the National Association of Professional Geriatric Care Managers entered into a contract with a national work-life benefits provider that raised hopes that care managers would be called upon by private industry to provide assessment, information and referral, and care management to their employees. This has not yet resulted in much new business for care managers but still has significant potential for the future. According to a study conducted by the MetLife Mature Market Institute, there is substantial evidence that caregiving for older family members creates significant stress for many employees and has an impact on the profits of caregivers' employers.[14] Several studies have documented the costs of caregiving to business in lost productivity on the part of the employed caregiver as well as management and administrative costs based on the time supervisors spend on issues of employed caregivers. According to one study, caregiving costs individuals upward of $659,000 over their lifetimes in lost wages, lost social security and pension contributions because of time off taken, loss of job entirely, or compromised opportunities for training, promotions, and "plum" assignments.

According to Sandra Timmermann, a gerontologist and director of MetLife's Mature Market Institute:

> It is a staggering figure for the 22.4 million U.S. families who provide care. . . . Of the caregivers we studied, 84 percent made adjustments to their work schedules by doing at least one of the following: taking sick leave or vacation time, decreasing work hours, taking a leave of absence, switching from full to part time employment, resigning or retiring. Very few of their employers provided programs or resources to support their caregiving

efforts. Only recently have policy-makers and business leaders begun to recognize the sacrifices and contributions made by working caregivers.[31,32]

■ TARGETING SPECIFIC GROUPS AND RESOURCES TO GROW A PROFESSIONAL PRACTICE

One way private care managers have found to reach those in need and those who can benefit from their services is to target specific groups. Private practice professionals have found, for instance, elder law and estate planning attorneys, bank trust officers, and financial advisors who manage the resources of affluent clients can be excellent sources of referrals that can help GCMs build an independent practice.

To succeed the private care manager must spread a message with three important components:

1. Eventually, you or a member of your family may need specialized professional attention because of aging or disability. Finding the services needed to help can be difficult, time-consuming, and frustrating, so planning ahead is a good idea.
2. A high-quality alternative to the publicly funded long-term care delivery system is available if you want to pay for it.
3. The services of a geriatric care manager are well worth the price.

If GCMs fail to get this message across to consumers, it will be difficult for them to operate a profitable business. GCMs must be diligent and effective in spreading this message and raising awareness about geriatric care management as an effective alternative to the chaotic and underfunded public long-term care system. Otherwise, the consumer, who has been conditioned to expect that most if not all long-term care services will be covered by Medicaid or private charity, is likely to balk at having to pay fees for geriatric care management services.

A variety of ways exist in which GCMs can be paid for their services. One way is to seek reimbursement from private LTCI policies. At intake, care managers should ask whether the client owns a LTCI policy. The care manager should review any insurance policies to determine exactly what benefits in regards to long-term care may be available. If necessary, the GCM can contact the insurance carrier or third-party administrator who manages the coordination and payment of claims. Since the mid-1990s, the inclusion of specific clauses in privately purchased LTCI policies that provide for the services of a care coordinator (also referred to as the "personal care specialist," "case management agency," or "personal care advocate" in various policies) have become the norm. Older policies may not contain a specific clause providing for reimbursement of the care coordinator, but it is worth calling the company that issued the policy and asking whether the services of a care manager can be reimbursed under the policy. Even if the services of a care manager are not specifically defined as reimbursable, a phone call to the benefits administrator explaining how care management services may be cost-effective can elicit a response that may result in payment of at least some services. In some cases, having the insured's family member contact the claims administrator and request compensation for care management services can be more effective.

An encouraging newer trend is the growth of toll-free caregiver support services provided by LTCI carriers for all their policyholders. Similar services are offered by some, mostly larger employers for working caregivers who are trying to balance their job responsibilities with caring for an aging family member. Although the services are currently provided by only a handful of national work-life companies, as the work force ages and employers realize the significant impact caregiving has on their bottom line, it is likely they will turn to local and regional care management networks to provide the services.

Because the sale of LTCI policies has yet to achieve the market penetration expected for these products, insurance carriers are looking for new ways to raise awareness and visibility of their LTCI products. One way to achieve this is for insurance carriers proactively to offer care manager information and referral services or on-site educational seminars on caring for aging parents combined with a LTCI employee benefit.

The most significant growth in the sales of new long-term care products over the last 5 years has been from employer-sponsored policies. Although in some cases the employer contributes a portion of the long-term care policy premium, in the great majority of cases LTCI is offered as a voluntary, employee-pay-all benefit. In some cases, employees can buy policies through their employer at a discounted rate or obtain coverage they might otherwise not qualify for because of the more liberal underwriting rules of group policies.

GCMs can also form joint ventures and alliances with other eldercare professionals to grow their practices. The appeal of operating one's own business, free of the restrictions and compromises imposed by working for highly regulated wholly funded public or nonprofit agencies, is very seductive for the independent-minded professional. But the development of a small business is never as easy as it appears. Becoming an independent health care professional is no exception—the hard realities of managing and growing a small business soon become evident. Getting the message out about the availability of a GCM's services requires mounting a marketing and networking campaign that can be both expensive and time-consuming, and it is difficult for newer businesses to compete with other companies that have more capital. Many independent professionals first starting out find that the resources of both money and time are in short supply.

After realizing that an individual or small group practice has its limitations, some care managers have begun to explore the idea of developing affiliations with other eldercare professionals in what are sometimes referred to as "virtual" partnerships. Care managers who are solo or small businesses can consider experimenting with such ideas as pooling their resources or banding together with related professionals to launch a cooperative marketing effort. Elder-law attorneys, independent home care providers, LTCI companies, or financial advisors are natural alliances for private care managers to cultivate. Each member of the group can maintain an independent business while jointly developing marketing materials, Web sites, and Internet marketing campaigns and planning and cosponsoring joint educational programs in the community.

■ CONCLUSION

This chapter discusses a variety of ways care managers in the private marketplace·can fund and grow their businesses while providing prospective clients more attractive alternatives to care management than can be provided by publicly funded sources.

Despite the growing awareness of the crisis that is looming in the nation's long-term care service delivery system GCMs have had difficulty educating the public about the fact that a private-sector alternative exists and can be far more effective and desirable. Even 20 years after the formation of the National Association of Professional Geriatric Care Managers, most consumers are still unaware that this alternative exists.

Paying privately for highly skilled professional services is nothing new in the American marketplace. When consumers seek the services of an attorney and architect and accountant or a financial advisor or even a carpenter or plumber, they are well aware that they will be expected to pay for services rendered. Because of the well-established precedent of eldercare services being paid for by tax payers, charities, or third-party insurance sources, consumers have different expectations about eldercare services than they do about other fee-based services in the marketplace.

Care management entrepreneurs who stay abreast of the constant changes in the marketplace, especially changes that can directly or indirectly affect revenue and referral sources, have a far better chance of being successful than those who don't. Care managers who continue to believe that the revenue base will always be growing because the aging population is growing are likely to miss out on the real private eldercare marketplace, which is a much smaller subset of the aging demographics.

■ NOTES

1. Administration on Aging. A Profile of Older Americans. U.S. Dept. of Health and Human Services, Administration on Aging. Washington, DC: 2003.

2. The 2004 Annual Report of the Board of Trustees of the Federal Old-Age and Survivors Insurance and Disability Insurance Trust Funds. Available at http://www.aoa.gov/prof/Statistics/profile/2003/profiles2003.asp Accessed March 23, 2004.

3. Kempthorne, D. Confronting America's Aging Crisis. National Governors Association. Washington, DC: July 19, 2004.

4. White House Conference on Aging. U.S. Dept. of Health and Human Services, Administration on Aging. Washington, DC: Dec 11–14, 2005.

5. Kornblum, J. Crisis in Elder Care Foreseen. *USAToday.* Available at http://www.usatoday.com. Accessed December, 11, 2005.

6. Atkins D. Ready Yourself Now for Crisis in Elder Care. Associated Students Legal Resource Center. April 1, 2002;12(13).

7. Reagan R. Address to the Nation on the Program for Economic Recovery, September 24, 1981. Social Security Online. Available at: http://www.ssa.gov/history/reaganstmts.html#state. Accessed September 5, 2006.

8. Crystal S. *America's Old Age Crisis: Public Policy and the Two Worlds of Aging.* New York: Basic Books; 1982.

9. Estes CL. *The Long Term Care Crisis: Elders Trapped in the No-Care Zone.* Thousand Oaks, CA: Sage Publications; 1994.

10. U.S. Senate Aging Committee, March 21, 2002.

11. Institute for Socioeconomic Studies and Manhattanville College Conference on Long-Term Care; April 24, 2002.

12. National Academy of Elder Law Attorneys (NAELA). Medicaid reforms threaten long-term care insurance industry. *Eye On Elder Issues.* February 2006;3(1).

13. Novelli WD. How Aging Boomers Will Impact American Business, *AARP.* Presented at Meeting of The Harvard Club, New York: February 21, 2002.

14. The National Alliance for Caregiving with Zogby International. Miles Away: The Metlife Study of Long-Distance Caregiving, July 2004.

15. Quinn JB. Medicaid abuse by wealthy jeopardizes program health. *Los Angeles Business Journal.* June 4, 2001.

16. Ahlstrom A, Tumlinson A, Lambrew J. Linking Reverse Mortgages and Long-Term Care Insurance. Brookings Institution. March 2004.

17. Holtz-Eakin D. The Cost and Financing of Long-Term Care Services Presented at the Committee on Energy and Commerce, U.S. House of Representatives. April 27, 2005.

18. Hodge P. Aging Population Will Transform Society. *Harvard Generations Policy Journal*, February 23, 2004.

19. American Council of Life Insurers. Long-Term Care Insurance or Medicaid: Who Will Pay for Baby Boomers' Long-Term Care?, Washington, DC: December 5, 2005.

20. General Accounting Office. Long-Term Care: Current Issues and Future Directions. Report to the Special Committee on Aging. Washington, DC: April 1995.

21. Analysis finds clusters of nursing home violations. *USAToday.* Available at http://www.usatoday.com/news/health/2003-05-19-nursing-home-analysis_x.htm - 63k.

22. Kass LR. Lingering Longer: Who Will Care?, *Washington Post.* September 29, 2005; 23.

23. Genworth Financial. Yearly Long Term Care Costs Move Above $70,000 in 2006. Richmond, Va: Genworth Financial; March 27, 2006.

24. American Society on Aging. Americans fail to act on long-term care protection. San Francisco, CA: May 23, 2003.

25. Georgetown University Center on an Aging Society. Choosing a Long-Term Care Insurance Policy: Understanding and Improving the Process. October 2004.

26. General Accounting Office. Long-Term Care: Current Issues and Future Directions. Washington, DC: April 1995.

27. National Association of Insurance Commissioners. Viatical Settlements Model Act, § 2(L). 2005.

28. Life settlements enter the mainstream. *National Underwriter, Life and Health/Financial Services.* September 19, 2005(20).

29. Life Insurance Settlement Association. January 2006.

30. National Council on the Aging. Use Your Home to Stay at Home. September 2003.

31. MetLife Mature Market Institute. *Americans Pay a Staggering Price in Lost Wages and Other Costs to Care for Elderly Relatives and Friends.* New York: December 1, 1999.

32. Brock F. Who'll sit in the boomers' desks? *New York Times.* October 12, 2003.

Chapter 12

Care Management Credentialing

Monika White and Cheryl M. Whitman

■ INTRODUCTION

Care management continues to play a major role in the complex health and social services delivery systems. Advances in medical technology, drugs, and other interventions have increased the numbers and types of consumers who need care management services. Older people, people with developmental disabilities, people with chronic mental illness, and others benefit from care management. Furthermore, care management has been increasingly encouraged by legislative and funding actions that have included it as a means of addressing the demographic, medical, and social challenges that create the need for ongoing, multiple services. For example, care management was a specific component of the Developmental Disabilities Act of 1975. During the 1980s, care management became a prominent feature of the Medicaid waiver programs and in workers' compensation. Private practice care managers also emerged as resources for older adults and their caregivers. The growth of managed care in the 1990s and the emergence of long-term care insurance further established the need for care management.

In the late 1980s and early 1990s, numerous professional associations—including the National Association of Professional Geriatric Care Managers, the National Council on Aging, the National Association of Social Workers (NASW), and the Case Management Society of America—began to promote standards for care manager practice. Funded by a grant from the Robert Wood Johnson Foundation, Connecticut Community Care, Inc. (CCCI), established and convened the National Advisory Committee on Long-Term Care Case Management. The work of these national experts culminated in the 1994 publication *Guidelines for Case Management Practice Across the Long-Term Care Continuum*. Finally, efforts to certify individual care managers began in the early 1990s as the demand for care management staff expanded prior to the development of academically based curricula. In 1999, the American Accreditation Health-Care Commission/URAC (Utilization Review, Accreditation and Certification) established standards for care management organizations.

All of these developments demonstrate a broad-based consensus that care management has become a useful and important component of the health and social services delivery systems. Despite apparent agreement on the value of care management, there is little to guide individual or corporate purchasers about who should do it, under what circumstances, for whom, and through which funding mechanisms. This has created confusion among consumers, funders, policymakers, and even personnel.

Many professions use credentialing to establish criteria for quality and competent services. *Credentialing is a form of recognition or acknowledgment that a standard body of knowledge and the skill set has been met.* Because care management has evolved as a transdisciplinary field, it is important to delineate the functions, roles, values, and ethical perspectives of a competent care manager that may or may not correspond with the standards of the "parent" profession.

Rehabilitation, managed care, acute care, long-term care insurance, and chronic care increasingly request or require care management certification as a condition of employment, and health care professionals in these settings are obtaining certification by the thousands. At the same time, there has been little demand for care management certification in nonmedical settings. Many care managers from the proprietary and nonprofit community-based service and long-term care arena rely on their educational degrees and professional licenses and do not perceive a need to add another credential. Yet interest in credentialing programs continues to grow, as does the number of programs offering certifications.

This chapter discusses credentialing in general, and for care managers specifically. After a section discussing the motivations behind and history of care management credentialing, the chapter provides an overview of selected credentialing and certification organizations. A discussion of some current and future issues concludes the chapter.

■ WHAT IS CREDENTIALING?

According to the National Organization for Competency Assurance (NOCA), *credentialing is the umbrella term that includes the concepts of accreditation, licensure, registration, and professional certification. Credentialing is used by an entity to acknowledge that a standard has been met; that is, the body of knowledge and the skill set that enable the practitioner to perform the job tasks of a specific field of practice.* Credentialing confers an occupational identity and serves a number of purposes such as the following:

- Protecting the public
- Establishing standards for professional knowledge, skills, and practice
- Meeting the requirements of government regulators
- Assuring consumers that professionals have met specific standards of practice
- Regulating a profession
- Assisting employers, insurers, practitioners, and the public in identifying individuals with certain knowledge and skills
- Advancing the profession
- Acknowledging the attainment of knowledge and skills by a professional
- Providing the certificant with a sense of pride and professional accomplishment
- Demonstrating a person's commitment to the profession and lifelong learning

NOCA describes professional certification as the "voluntary process by which a nongovernmental entity grants a time-limited recognition and use of a credential to an individual after verifying that it has met predetermined and standardized criteria."[1(pp 4–5)]

■ MOTIVATION

In addition to validating education and experience, people are motivated to earn care management certification for several reasons. Among them are the following:

- Informed consumer choice
- Consumer protection
- Marketing
- Insurability
- Education
- Research
- Self-regulation
- History

The following sections discuss each rationale.

Informed Consumer Choice

One of the primary reasons for the development of a credential is to enable the consumer to make a discriminating choice of the type of care manager who should be hired for a given circumstance. For example, an acute medical setting might warrant the employ of a nurse or other clinical technician with in-depth experience with a particular diagnosis. In a community-based setting, a care manager with a background in social work, psychology, or mental health might better serve the client, such as a grieving widow or individual with chronic mental illness. In other situations, an expert with a background in both medical and psychosocial fields might be most appropriate. There might also be differentiating circumstances based upon the specific population whose needs are to be met. A care manager with a gerontological background might better serve an older adult, just as an individual with human immunodeficiency virus/acquired immune deficiency syndrome would need the expertise of someone knowledgeable about this specific disease process, treatment, services, and emotional impact. Rosen and colleagues note that certification could provide some consensus about expectations for service delivery.[2]

Consumer Protection

The consumer also needs protection from an individual who might call him- or herself a care manager but who has neither training in the care management process, roles, and functions nor an understanding of health and social services systems and psychosocial dynamics. Because no licensing or other regulation currently exists, the consumer has no guidelines with which to "shop" for services. The professional certifications, then, are very important mechanisms for guiding the consumer. They provide protection for other well-trained, appropriately experienced care managers who are competing, perhaps unfairly, with individuals of lesser capacity, who charge lower fees often for inferior services.

Marketing

Most health care and social services providers today seek a competitive advantage in the individual, corporate, and nonprofit markets. Credentialing of individual employees on the basis of their competency becomes a selling point, especially when providers are looking to broaden their markets and when there is a likelihood of passing along risk. Network providers of all types look to affiliate with organizations and individuals that meet industry standards for practice. Care managers can use the professional certification as a marketing tool to distinguish themselves from those who are not certified and as proof of core competency for network affiliation or membership.

Insurability

Another rationale for credentialing is the ability to be covered by malpractice insurance and to receive payments from third-party insurers and other reimbursement sources. Although reimbursement for care management is still limited, it is expected to increase as care management is more fully recognized and funded, especially in the social services arena. An insurer that is considering a malpractice policy for care managers or care management organizations needs to be able to identify whom it is insuring, for which job functions, in which settings, for what populations, and with what decision-making or fiduciary responsibilities. Without this knowledge, it would be impossible for an insurance company to develop such a liability policy. As of 1999, there were three insurance companies offering care managers malpractice insurance. With the growth of care management networks that require insurance coverage, there are indications that certification may become the norm in the future.

Education

Educating care managers in a defined body of knowledge is another rationale for providing a credentialing process. As previously stated, care management did not evolve from an academic program within the nation's college or university systems but developed in response to consumer need. For a field of practice or a discipline to become professionalized, there must be a defined and determinate body of knowledge so that it can be taught with uniformity and consistency.

Care management degrees and certificate programs are being offered or are under development in a number of universities. Many schools of nursing and social work have well-developed care management courses, specialty areas, or clinical tracts. Courses in care management can also be found in gerontology schools, undergraduate human services departments, and continuing education programs. In the last 5+ years, the number of certificate programs at colleges, large companies, and online have increased significantly. Knowledge-based, curriculum-based, and attendance-based certificate programs are training programs focused on a specific topic such as care management. They typically require completion of course work and may require demonstrated attainment of course objectives. A credential is not usually given at the end of a certificate program.

Research

Credentialing of care managers enables research that defines specific outcomes and accountabilities as a result of the process of providing care. Outcomes need to relate to health status, quality of care, cost of care, and efficient use of systems to coordinate services. Outcomes must also be defined in terms of client goals. Such goals might include quality of life, knowledge about needs, increased ability to participate in or maintain care, ability to better use systems of care to meet needs, and better social/emotional functioning of the consumer and the consumer's support system. Again, most outcome measures currently in use come

from medical settings. In psychosocial areas, outcomes tend to be anecdotal. Their value is limited because they are self-reported and self-selected by the provider organization.

Limited empirical research exists in these areas, especially in consumer-defined outcomes, but the body of research is growing. For example, Geron and colleagues have developed client satisfaction measures to determine consumer perceptions of home care and care management services. These measures are already in use by several states and agency programs and provide hope that the quality and success of care management will be more easily quantified in the future.[3]

Self-Regulation

Self-regulation is an essential aspect of any professional field. Just as it is in the best interest of consumers to be involved in defining and creating the systems that work for them, it is in the best interest of care managers to be involved in defining appropriate regulation for their work. Only in this way will accurate expectations for the individual practitioner or system be developed. Government-imposed guidelines often miss the essential ingredients of the value system, nature, and realities of the profession. It is important for care managers to participate in development and implementation of standards and guidelines, in research studies, in legislative or policy activities, and in available and relevant professional associations.

History

The disability movement of the 1970s spurred the development of several professional organizations focused on the rehabilitation needs of individuals. The more specific move toward credentialing of care managers began to gain momentum in the late 1980s and early 1990s with the emergence of a number of professional organizations focused on care management services to various populations in diverse settings. These organizations recognized that they had both competing and mutual interests that could best be served by moving toward a consensus in the role played by care managers in the evolving health and social services environments.

A meeting of these organizations was held in 1991 and resulted in the formation of a National Case Management Task Force, which appointed a steering committee to address the issues of philosophy, definition, and existing standards of practice. There were 29 organizations involved in this task force. In 1992, the steering committee proposed the development of a voluntary care management credential.

An Interim Commission was incorporated as an independent credentialing organization and in July 1995 was renamed the Commission for Case Manager Certification (CCMC). The CCMC continues to be responsible for the Certified Case Manager (CCM) credentialing process. The CCM eligibility required that an applicant: "Hold an acceptable license or certification (see the CCM Certification Guide) based on a post-secondary degree program in a field that promotes the psychosocial or vocational well being of the persons being served."[4] This means that the CCM is effectively an advanced practice credential.

Although the Interim Commission included representation from the Certification of Insurance Rehabilitation Specialists Commission, later renamed the Certification of Disability Management Specialists Commission (CDMS), it is important to note that this group maintained its individual identity. It was instrumental in creating the new certification, and there was apparently no sense that this was a further fragmentation of the care management field.

In 1993, two other organizations began a second set of discussions about credentialing care managers: The National Association of Professional Geriatric Care Managers and the Case Management Institute of CCCI. Both viewed the CCM as medically oriented and focused primarily on rehabilitation and acute care management. Furthermore, the eligibility criteria for the CCM excluded most of the staff employed in the home- and community-based, long-term care, and social services programs serving clients through various nonprofit and publicly sponsored programs. It left out many of the front-line staff who provide direct client services through the Area Agencies on Aging, vocational and rehabilitation services, substance abuse programs, peer counseling programs, and other grassroots organizations. Such organizations rely upon both formally and informally trained and supervised staff, including those with many years of hands-on care management experience.

For these reasons, an independent credentialing organization was formed in 1994 called the National Academy of Certified Care Managers (NACCM). The credential, offered since 1996, is the Care Manager Certified, given subsequent to meeting education and experience requirements and the successful completion of a standardized, validated examination that tests the skills, knowledge, and practice ethics need to serve consumers. The NACCM exam is focused on the core care management functions of comprehensive face-to-face assessment, care planning, care implementation, monitoring/management, reassessment, termination, and professional issues and ethics.

Throughout the field's history, there have been formal discussions held between the various stakeholders in care management. In 1992–1993, six professional organizations came together as the National Coalition of Associations for the Advancement of Case Management. These associations represented more than 20,000 health and social services professionals and were hoping to influence the health care reforms that were part of the President's Task Force on National Health

Care Reform, chaired by Hillary Rodham Clinton. A variety of organizations met throughout the 1990s and began the process of developing consensus about the definitions of the process of care management and the role of care management in ensuring quality care and making efficient use of resources. This process also began to point the direction for the future role of care management in defining needs and solutions and acting as a change agent within the system. In fact, in a 1994 paper published by the Foundation for Rehabilitation Certification, Education, and Research, Michael J. Leahy found that the most frequent settings in which surveyed CCMs worked were:

> independent case management companies (23.8%), followed by hospitals (11.7%), independent rehabilitation/insurance affiliates (11.0%), and health insurance companies (8.0%). The most frequent job titles of respondents include case manager (45.9%), registered nurse (19.8%), rehabilitation counselor (10.9%), and administrator/manager (7.6%).[5]

Two important meetings were held in 1997 and 1999 under the auspices of the Foundation for Rehabilitation Education and Research and the National Association of Professional Geriatric Care Managers. These meetings were identified as the Care and Case Management Summits I and II. Sixteen associations and organizations participated in discussions about care management definitions, existing credentialing options and their ethical standards, and knowledge domains of the various definitions and options. According to the Summit II minutes, participants expressed interest in forming a coalition to continue discussions.[6] Although this particular group did not meet again, many of its members participated in the establishment of the Case Management Leadership Coalition in the early 2000s. This coalition met in 2002 and 2004 and continues to be active (see

http://www.cmlc.org for more information). Membership is predominantly in the medical and rehabilitation arenas.

■ OVERVIEW OF SELECTED CREDENTIALING AND CERTIFICATION ORGANIZATIONS

There are many credentialing and certification organizations, and they each offer something slightly different. The number of programs has grown since the initial publication of this book. Care managers must be aware of the variety of programs, the difference between credentialing and certificate programs, and what will be most appropriate for their practice setting. Table 12–1 describes the credentials recognized by the National Association of Professional Geriatric Care Managers. Some of the other credentials that professionals may earn are listed in Table 12–2. These credentials are associated with nursing and rehabilitation and are institution oriented.

Commission for Certified Care Managers

The Commission for Certified Care Managers has defined case management as "a collaborative process that assesses, plans, implements, coordinates, monitors, and evaluates the options and services required to meet an individual's health needs, using communication and available resources to promote quality, cost-effective outcomes."[7] The Commission considers case management as an advanced practice area within an already licensed or certified profession. Hence the following experience criteria: 12 months of acceptable full-time case management employment or its equivalent under the supervision of a CCM for the 12 months; or 24 months of acceptable full-time case management employment or its equivalent, without supervision by a CCM; or 12 months of acceptable full-time case management employment or its equivalent as a supervisor, supervising the activities of individuals who provide *direct* case

Table 12–1 Overview of Eligibility Criteria and Examinations for Credentials Recognized by National Association of Professional Geriatric Care Managers

	Education	Experience	Prerequisite (license or other)	Exam Content (partial list)	Recertification
Commission for Case Management Certification Certified Case Manager (CCM), (847) 818-0292 http://www.ccmcertification.org	Postsecondary program in physical, psychosocial, and vocational well-being	12–24 months full time as case manager or supervisor, 12 months under CCM or 24 without CCM	Valid license or certification	Coordination, service delivery, physical and psychological factors, benefit systems, case management concepts, community resources	Every 5 years 80 CEUs total
National Academy of Certified Care Managers, Care Manager, Certified (CMC) (800) 962-2260 http://www.naccm.net	1. Master's (field related to care management) 2. Bachelor's (field related to care management) 3. Postsecondary degree unrelated to care management, diploma for RN, LPN, or LVN	1. 2 years as supervised care manager 2. 2 years as supervised care manager + 2 years direct client care in human services fields 3. 2 years as supervised care manager + 4 years direct client care in human services fields	NA	Comprehensive assessment, care plan development, coordination, service delivery systems, monitoring, termination, ethical and legal issues	Every 3 years 1,500 hours practice + 45 CEUs total
National Association of Social Workers Certified Advanced Social Work Case Manager (C-ASWCM)	Master's in Social Work (MSW)	One year supervised, post MSW, direct case management	ACSW or DCSW or state SW license or passing score on ASWB exam and NASW membership	No exam	Every 2 years 20 CEUs total Maintain ACSW-, DCSW-, or MSW-level state licensure and NASW membership
Certified Social Work Case Manager (C-SWCM)	Bachelor's in Social Work (BSW)	One year supervised, post BSW, direct case management	ACBSW or current BSW level state license and NASW membership	No exam	Every 2 years 20 CEUs total Maintain ACBSW- or current BSW-level state licensure and NASW membership

CEU, continuing education unit; RN, registered nurse; LPN, licensed practical nurse; LVN, licensed vocational nurse; ACSW, Academy of Certified Social Workers; DCSW, Diplomate in Clinical Social Work; ASWB, Association of Social Work Boards; NASW, National Association of Social Workers.

Table 12-2   Additional Credentialing Organization (alphabetical order)

	Education	Experience	Prerequisite	Exam Content	Recertification
American Institute of Outcome CM, *Case Manager Certified (CMC)*	1. BA, MA, PhD 2. Associate or Diploma RN	1. 36–60 months full-time 2. + professional license	1. License at Associate Level	1. Clinical, customer service, management/supervision, quality improvement, risk aspects, payer, and resources	1. Every 2 years 2. Contact hours based on scores
Certification of Disability Management Specialists Commission, *Certified Disability Management Specialist (CDMS)*	1. RN or CRC 2. MA or PhD 3. BA 4. Any degree, BA or higher, in other field	1. 12 month full-time 2. 24–36 months 3. 36 months 4. 60 months	1. License at Level 1	1. Job placement, vocational assessment, case management and disabilities, rehabilitation services and care, and forensic rehabilitation	1. Every 5 years 2. 80 contact hours
Commission on Rehabilitation Counselor Certification, *Certification Rehabilitation Counselor (CRC)*	1. MA or PhD in rehabilitation counseling or related field (including 600 hours of an internship)	1. 0–5 years depending on status of requirements, as well as, 12 months of supervision under a CRC	1. NA	1. Focus on medical, psychosocial service coordination, client assessment, and planning for individuals with disabilities	1. Every 5 years 2. 80 contact hours
National Board for Certification in Continuity of Care, *Continuity of Care Certification, Advanced (A-CCC)*	1. Bachelor's Degree	1. 2 years full-time	1. NA	1. Continuity of care process, health delivery system, clinical, legal, reimbursement, and professional issues	1. Every 5 hours 2. 50 contact hours or retake the exam
Rehabilitation Nursing Certification Board, *Certified Rehabilitation Registered Nurse (CCRN)*	1. RN	1. 2 years in rehabilitation	1. RN license	1. Rehabilitation, rehabilitation nursing models	1. Every 5 years 2. 60 contact hours

RN, registered nurse; CRC, certified rehabilitation counselor management services. The CCM designation has been available since 1993.

National Academy of Certified Care Managers

The NACCM defines care management as "a service that links and coordinates assistance from both paid service providers and unpaid help from family and friends to enable consumers with functional limitations to obtain the highest level of independence consistent with their capacity and preferences for care."[8] Eligibility criteria reflect a biopsychosocial approach to care management in long-term, chronic, community-based, health, social, and mental health settings. The higher the educational level of the candidate, the fewer years of care management experience are required. (See Table 12–1.)

Care management experience must include face-to-face interviewing, comprehensive assessment, care plan development, implementation and monitoring, problem solving, reassessment, and quality evaluation. Supervision is individual, group, or peer review of performance, use of clinical skills and core care manager functions, record review, peer consultation, case review and/or case conference in the amount of 50 hrs/yr. These criteria are more inclusive and reflective of the experience of care managers in the social services system, as differentiated from the health delivery system. The CMC designation has been offered since 1996 following a two-year process creating a standardized, valid, and reliable examination.

National Association of Social Workers

The NASW Credentialing Center establishes and promotes credentials, specialty certifications, and continuing education approval program required for excellence in the practice of social work. NASW specialty certifications and other professional credentials provide recognition to those who have met national standards for higher levels of experi-

ence and knowledge, and they are not a substitute for required state licenses or certifications. The C-ASWCM (MSW level) and the C-SWCM (BSW level) both require one year of supervised direct care management experience. Additional prerequisites and supervision are tied directly to NASW membership and designations as well as state-specific social work licenses. See Table 12–1.

National Board for Certification in Continuity of Care

The NBCCC administers the Continuity of Care Certification, Advanced. This certification is open to people from multiple disciplines, including nurses, social workers, therapists, dietitians, and physicians. The candidate must have a bachelor's degree plus 2 years of full-time experience within the last 5 years in continuity of care, or equivalent part-time experience (4,000 hours) within the past 5 years. This certification evolved from the area of discharge planning within a number of institutional settings.

Rehabilitation Nursing Certification Board

The Rehabilitation Nursing Certification Board administers the Certified Rehabilitation Registered Nurse certification. This certification is solely for those who have an "unrestricted RN license plus at least two years of practice as registered professional nurse in rehabilitation nursing within the last five years."[9]

This process then is limited to those within the nursing profession and does not address the inter- and transdisciplinary nature of care management.

Certification of Disability Management Specialists Commission

The CDMS Commission administers the CDMS certification. This commission was originally developed in 1984 as the Certification of Insurance Rehabilitation Specialists Commission and was changed to the current name in 1996. This certification has four different categories within which a candidate may qualify. Here again, the emphasis appears to be on the nursing profession; however, the more advanced degrees do allow for other training as long as they include specific courses in disability, vocational/occupational information, counseling, and other direct service training criteria.

Commission on Rehabilitation Counselor Certification (CRCC)

The CRCC, mentioned earlier in the chapter, administers the Certified Rehabilitation Counselor certification. This certification also allows people multiple ways of meeting the eligibility requirements. There are at least 10 categories and several subcategories, seven of which have very specific course requirements. The reader is referred to the Commission for more specific details. This credential defines care management as an advanced practice field, making the credential similar to the CCM.

Contact information for these certifying entities is shown in Exhibit 12–1.

■ CURRENT AND FUTURE ISSUES

To date, there is no unified approach to care management; there remain diverse views and even controversy in a number of areas. This section highlights some of the major issues that continue to be discussed:

- Philosophical approach
- Training and multiple disciplines

Exhibit 12–1 Contact Information for Selected Certification Entities

1. Certification of Disability Management Specialists Commission
   www.cdms.org
   (847)-944-1335

2. Commission for Certified Care Managers
   www.ccmcertification.org
   (847)-944-1330

3. Commission on Rehabilitation Counselor Certification
   www.crccertification.com
   (847)-818-0292

4. National Academy of Certified Care Managers
   www.NACCM.net
   (800)-962-2260

5. National Association of Social Workers
   www.socialworkers.org/credentials/default.asp
   (202)-408-8600

6. National Board for Certification in Continuity of Care
   www.nbccc.net
   (888)-776-2023

7. Rehabilitation Nursing Certification Board
   www.rehabnurse.org
   (800)-229-7530

- Supervision
- Specialty credentials and levels of credentials
- Organizational versus individual credentialing
- Implications for policy development and reimbursement

Philosophical Approach

Many philosophical questions are related to care management. Several are posed here.

Is care management a social, medical, integrated, or coordinated service model? Traditionally, the social and medical models have been considered separate largely because of the diverse funding sources for each. In addition to reimbursement and funding differences, the fragmentation in legislation, authority, and standards in health, mental health, and social services programs have made it nearly impossible to develop a unified holistic or integrated model of care. There is increasing recognition on both health and psychosocial sides of the debate that there is a need for greater crossover and flexibility to allow the integration of these components. However, the structural and financial issues have yet to be resolved. Ideally, future public policymakers will look at the total needs of the population and provide funds to be used for any social service, mental health, or medical service needed by an individual or family at any given moment. Private insurance policies might likewise be integrated. The role of care managers would be to triage clients to help determine the most appropriate level of intervention and to monitor client status and service delivery.

Does the care management process cut across the continuum of care or can it be performed within a single setting? There is growing consensus that care management services cut across settings as evidenced by a modification in the CCM eligibility criteria requiring provision of services across a continuum of care that addresses the ongoing needs of the individual being served by the case management process.

This does not change the fact that funding remains tied to particular settings and is not typically portable to other parts of the continuum of care. Long-term care insurance policies that include services beyond skilled nursing care often offer care management services as an integral part of the benefit or as an additional rider to the policy.

Is there a value to maintaining an individual at a level of functioning, or is the goal rehabilitation? There is a growing sense that there is value in ensuring that a level of functioning is maintained. Perry's study concluded that delaying institutional care through a program of maintenance would save the government $5 billion in health care and custodial costs in just 1 month.[10] Other studies suggest similar savings. The National Alzheimer's Association estimated that the annual cost of Alzheimer's to U.S. businesses is at least $33 billion. Families and people with Alzheimer's pay an estimated $3.7 billion to $6.5 billion for the medical costs of Alzheimer's.[11] These costs are not borne by the general public. The implications for empowering caregivers and focusing on the quality of life are enormous.

Is care management considered a profession, a practice field within a primary profession, or a role that does not require professional status? In 1964, Carr-Sanders and Wilson provided a model of professionalization that includes the following:

Attracting practitioners on a full-time basis;
Having acquired support from foundations and large governmental sponsors;
Having a growing body of literature supported by academic journals;
Having numerous university training programs;
Having accreditation of academic programs;
Practitioners receiving a fee for services;
Being successful in influencing public policy;

Having a professional association with conditions for entrance; and

Having registration or licensure requirements for practice.[12]

According to this definition, care management has not quite reached professional status because of the lack of accredited educational programs to prepare individuals for practice and the lack of regulation to govern the field. Care management has been added to the curricula of many education programs such as nursing, social work, and continuing education departments.

Is the role of the care manager inherently that of a gatekeeper and resource allocator? The care manager's approach to service provision is best addressed in light of the practice setting. There are major differences in the ability to authorize, distribute, or utilize resources in a health maintenance organization, a state waiver program, and a private practice. Although all aspects of care management include some resource allocation, resource allocation is not always the role of the gatekeeper. Furthermore, in times of scarcity, use of resources becomes an ethical matter regardless of the source of funding or reimbursement. It is clear, however, that the way a care manager views this role will affect other decisions.

Training and Multiple Disciplines

Who should do care management and what core knowledge is needed to perform the essential tasks and activities within a given setting or specific population have long been topics of debate and discussion. Because the practice of care management developed from within the field rather than from an academic program, there is little consensus about the required body of knowledge nor is there a unified set of core skills for care managers. Further complicating this issue is the lack of common standards for continuing education

of care managers. The various credentialing organizations listed in Table 12-1 have different criteria for what continuing education credits will be accepted, what those credits should consist of, and who should have provided those credits.

There is great disparity as well among practicing care managers about what their core training should be. The backgrounds and training of social workers, nurses, psychologists, gerontologists, counselors, and therapists vary widely. Increasingly, practitioners are also coming into care management from other fields because of changes in demographics, corporate downsizing, midlife career decisions, and technology. Some come into care management as a result of their own experience in dealing with an aging loved one or other person with a catastrophic or chronic illness. Others enter from such diverse venues as the long-term care insurance field, law, financial planning, life planning, retirement planning, accounting, and recreation. This great diversity helps explain why some of the credentialing organizations require a prior license or certification.

Supervision

As Table 12-1 and the preceding text make clear, several credentialing organizations require an individual to have been supervised. An individual care manager's professional training and degree may already include or require supervision to practice at the independent level. Supervision is one of many tools the professional has to ensure the quality of service delivery. The purpose of supervision includes but is not limited to the following:

- Ensuring compliance with internal and external policies and regulations
- Enhancing professional practice skills
- Ensuring the quality of service delivery to consumers

- Ensuring client outcomes
- Providing objective feedback and fresh ideas for interventions
- Complying with professional practice standards
- Clarifying ethical issues

Supervision/consultation is particularly important in care management because care managers work within the constantly changing health and social service delivery systems and with the intensely diverse dynamics of each family system often with complex needs, preferences, values, faith traditions, and resources. Although a sophisticated practitioner may be experienced in working with a multitude of these complex systems, the specific details of each case remain unique. This challenging array of factors affects care management practice and necessitates periodic review to ensure high-quality and ethical service delivery.

This raises the question of who is qualified to provide supervision. The desire for supervision in the work setting is largely a result of the lack of practicum experience focused on care management, the lack of availability of credentialed supervisors, and the desire to ensure that the knowledge base of the care manager has been successfully transferred to direct client contact. For some credentialing organizations, the supervisor must be an individual who already holds the care management credential. Other organizations have a broader interpretation to include anyone in a supervisory capacity that can attest to the candidate's successful performance of care management functions. Even the most experienced independent practitioner benefits from a supervisory/consultative process. For the solo practitioner, burnout is a particular hazard. The opportunity for consultation/supervision in solo practice can be essential for maintaining an objective approach, working out ethical issues, and staying up-to-date with new interventions and services.

Specialty Credentials and Levels of Credentials

Another distinction that might be made among the various credentials is a determination of the level of practice and an area of specialization. The credentialing bodies that require another license or certificate might characterize the care management credential as a form of advanced or specialty practice. Several of the credentialing organizations that do not have such prerequisites might also consider this a specialty credential but not an advanced credential. NACCM, for example, characterizes its examination as a test of "core" knowledge of the care management process and anticipates that workers will specialize based upon their work with a specific population or setting. The specialty or advanced credential requires the differentiation of knowledge, skills, interventions, and outcomes from those of the general or nonadvanced credential. This is a controversial area and one that is only now beginning to come to the forefront of credentialing activities.

Organizational versus Individual Credentialing

With the recent publication of the American Accreditation HealthCare Commission/URAC standards for credentialing care management organizations, a new question appears: Should organizations, individuals, or both be credentialed? As provider organizations have carved out service specialties and the incidence of risk sharing has increased, credentialing of organizations has become important as part of risk management protocols. The question remains whether this credentialing has a tangible impact on quality or is just an additional cost to providers with little or no benefit to the consumer. It would be premature to speculate on the answer at this early stage. However, the burden imposed and the potential for positive outcomes should be carefully examined as organizational credentialing becomes more widespread.

Implications for Policy Development and Reimbursement

The failed attempts to reconfigure the health care delivery system in the early 1990s demonstrated how difficult it is to make revolutionary changes in an established set of services where so many individuals appear to have conflicting interests. Over the past decade, there have been dramatic changes in the health care delivery system because of a combination of administrative changes, regulatory modifications, economic changes, and the growing recognition of the needs of populations with chronic conditions. Typically, change has continued to be incremental and, therefore, fragmented. This has hampered the ability to integrate or coordinate the funding and delivery of health, mental health, and social services. Although a fully integrated system is a distant vision that may not be shared by the majority of policymakers, it will be necessary to address many emerging issues such as the following:

- How care management will be funded
- Under what auspices care management will be provided
- Who the care managers will be
- How the impact of particular programs goals will be measured
- Which people will be served by care management, how long they will be served, and what level of service they will receive

In addressing these issues, policymakers will need to be cognizant of different approaches and philosophies so that programs can be sculpted to meet the particular needs of each setting and population. This potentially means that there is a need for recognition of different skill sets in different environments that still come within the commonly defined process of care management. It also means that all funded programs need to have a research component so that outcome data can be obtained to answer these questions. Research design will be critically important if it is to enable comparison of different care management models across programs and professions.

■ CONCLUSION

The growth of care management over the past few decades has been significant. Virtually every human services setting in the country provides some form of care management regardless of the population served. The growth of geriatric care management has also been noteworthy, especially in the private practice arena. The move toward credentialing is an effort to control quality by requiring those who want to do the work to meet established criteria and standards and to set some agreed-upon level of consumer and professional expectations. Geriatric care managers can play an important role in both developing credential mechanisms and by becoming certified themselves.

Because there are many types of care or case management, individuals seeking credentialing need to determine which type of certification to obtain and which certifying entity is the best fit. This decision should be based not only on background and discipline, but also on the focus of current or planned practice in terms of population, setting, or specific condition.*

---

* For a good discussion of types of care and case management, please see White, M. Case management. In: Evashwick, C., ed. *The Continuum of Long-Term Care: An Integrated Systems Approach.* 3rd ed. Clifton Park, NY: Thomson Delmar Learning; 2005.

■ NOTES

1. Durley CC. *The NOCA Guide to Understanding Credentialing Concepts*. Washington, DC: National Organization for Competency Assurance; 2005. Available at: http://www.noca.org/publications/publications.htm. Accessed September 18, 2006.

2. Rosen AL, Bodie-Gross E, Young E, Smolenski M, Howe D. To be or not to be? Case/care management credentialing. In: Applebaum R, White M, eds. *Key Issues in Case Management Around the Globe*. San Francisco, CA: American Society on Aging; 2000.

3. Geron SM. Measuring the quality and success of care management: developments and issues in the United States, England and other countries. In: Applebaum R, White M, eds. *Key Issues in Case Management Around the Globe*. San Francisco, CA: American Society on Aging; 2000.

4. Commission for Case Manager Certification. *CCM Certification Guide*. Schaumburg, IL: Commission for Case Manager Certification; 2006. Available at: http://www.ccmcertification.org/pages/12frame_set.html. Accessed September 18, 2006.

5. Leahy MJ. *Validation of Essential Knowledge Dimensions in Case Management*. Rolling Meadows, IL: Foundation for Rehabilitation and Research; 1994. Technical report.

6. National Association of Professional Geriatric Care Managers. *Care/Case Management Summit II Minutes*. Tucson, AZ: National Association of Professional Geriatric Care Managers; March 1999.

7. Commission for Case Manager Certification. Definition of case management. Available at: http://www.ccmcertification.org/pages/13frame_set.html. Accessed September 18, 2006.

8. Geron SM, Chassler D. *Guidelines for Case Management Practice Across the Long-Term Continuum*. Bristol, CT: Connecticut Community Care, Inc.; 1994.

9. Perry D. Aging research: keeping older Americans healthy. *Health Aging*. 1977.

10. Association of Rehabilitation Nurses. CRRN eligibility criteria. 2006. Available at: http://www.rehabnurse.org/certification. Accessed September 18, 2006.

11. Koppel R. Alzheimer's disease costs business $33 billion a year in caregiver loss, medical expenses. Presented at: Washington National Press Club for the Alzheimer's Association; September 1998; Washington, DC.

12. Peterson DA, Wendt PF. *A Draft Proposal for the Certification of Professionals in Gerontology*. University of Southern California; September 1992; unpublished paper.

Chapter 13

Preparing for Emergencies

Erica Karp and Angela Koenig

■ AN OVERVIEW

No one wants to imagine horrible things happening to people, but "bad things happen to good people." Hurricanes, tornadoes, terrorist attacks, epidemics, earthquakes: the list of possible disasters is overwhelming. Neither are disasters the only emergencies that can befall a professional geriatric care management agency. The absence of key personnel can also occur suddenly for a variety of reasons. Nevertheless, we can prepare ourselves and our agencies to negotiate safely through an emergency. The key is to plan, plan, and plan some more. Our colleagues who experienced sudden illness, 9/11, or one of the recent hurricanes have taught us much about what did work, as well as what should have and what could have been done to make a bad situation better.

We also know that, in any emergency, the geriatric client is particularly at risk. Preparing a professional geriatric care management agency for a disaster means having twin primary concerns; one is for the agency and the other is for the clients. These concerns are inextricably tied together. This chapter begins by addressing the survival concerns of the agency, and then proceeds to address how to prepare clients for disasters. In this chapter, we consider a number of emergency scenarios as well as practical guidelines, checklists, procedures, and resources to

enable care managers to develop useful emergency care plans for their businesses and their clients. Exhibit 13–1 is provided as a guide to help you become familiar with what should be done before, during, and after an emergency.

■ PREPARING THE AGENCY: ABSENCE OF KEY PERSONNEL

The ability of an agency to function despite the absence of key personnel is critical. Informal procedures in a business, especially a smaller business, can appear to be part of a "family" atmosphere, and it's easy to get into the habit of informality. However, if illness, accident, or some other unforeseen event unexpectedly overtakes an owner or manager, these habits can become a huge liability. Every professional geriatric care manager should have a formal, written backup plan that springs into action should the owner/manager become incapacitated. This may seem an overwhelming task at first, but when you break it down into pieces, it becomes workable.

To begin to get a handle on how your agency operates, start with a job-task assessment. List all the tasks that are performed on a daily, weekly, monthly, quarterly, and annual basis. Listing the tasks is the first step; later you can evaluate their relative importance.

Exhibit 13–1   Preventing, Planning, Reacting, and Recovering

- Sole practitioners
  - Identify reciprocal sister agency
    - Follow ethical requirements such as advance client consent
    - Provide regular updated information
  - Plan evacuation procedures
- Establish emergency response team
  - Define decision-making authority
  - Identify and train members
  - Designate alternative members in case of absence, or
  - Establish rotation
  - Review all emergency plans periodically
- Establish emergency reporting methods
  - Provide every staff member and caregiver with phone numbers for police, fire department, building security
  - Provide staff and caregivers with emergency phone tree
  - Post emergency phone numbers in prominent locations
  - Train staff and caregivers to recognize and report possible dangers and emergencies
    - Assign responsibility for determination
    - Assign responsibility for communication
    - Assign responsibility for follow-up and "all-clear"
- Establish emergency response procedures
  - Distribute regularly updated lists of all phone numbers or e-mail addresses and phone tree contact list
  - Keep updated emergency files for all clients
    - Keep hard copies stored off-site and copies posted regularly to sister agency
  - Update and review status of clients
    - Clients who need immediate attention
    - Clients who need attention as soon as possible
    - Clients who are relatively independent
  - Identify outside resources for follow-up after emergencies, such as crisis counselors, hotlines, etc.
- Establish evacuation procedures/plans for geriatric care manager agency office and for clients
  - Have a record of plans set up for each client
  - Develop escape routes
  - Designate a gathering place away from the building
  - Develop safety check-in procedures
  - Hold regular emergency evacuation drills
    - Check evacuation supplies/bag to replace or update such items as prescriptions
  - Emphasize responsibility and need for compliance
- Develop communications procedures
  - Establish phone tree: who calls who, who keeps who informed
  - Determine procedure to reroute calls to sister agency
  - Establish priority of information
  - Provide staff, caregivers, clients, and clients' families with alternate communication plans
  - Establish notification priority
- Identify and train first aid providers
  - Keep list of qualified personnel as part of phone list
  - Designate a triage/treatment area
  - Ensure that first aid kits are available and regularly checked
- Establish damage assessment protocol and methods
  - Designate oversight person or persons
  - Update/review warranties

Exhibit 13–1   Preventing, Planning, Reacting, and Recovering (continued)

- ○ Evaluate damage
- ○ Report to authorities
- ○ Notify insurance carriers
- ○ Identify items to be evacuated—such as computers and files—if time permits without endangering people
- ○ Emphasize human safety
- Working from off-site
  - ○ Identify off-site work location, also have a backup location
  - ○ Identify functions and employees suitable for telecommuting
  - ○ Identify sources of noncomputer equipment rental
- Computers, files, and data
  - ○ Develop or refine a data backup plan
  - ○ Identify responsible persons and alternatives
  - ○ Identify off-site storage location
  - ○ Develop monthly tests of ability to restore your own files and those of your sister agency
  - ○ Identify sources of rental/loaner computer equipment
  - ○ Document all modifications/customizations to computer systems
    - ▪ Store hard copy of documentation off-site
  - ○ Have blank checks stored off-site
- Identify, protect, and insure
  - ○ Regularly look for hazards at the agency and at clients' residences
  - ○ Inventory office
  - ○ Obtain appraisals
  - ○ Regularly evaluate adequacy of procedures and preparations
- Implementation during an emergency
  - ○ Human safety comes first
  - ○ Evacuate if necessary, report to authorities, obtain medical attention
  - ○ Mobilize emergency response team
  - ○ Rescue property if possible
- Recovery
  - ○ Locate all personnel, assess and prioritize needs
  - ○ Implement emergency communications
  - ○ Inform communications center of client status particularly for out-of-area relatives
  - ○ Respond as planned but expect the unexpected
  - ○ Begin the notification process
  - ○ Ask for help if necessary; offer assistance where possible
  - ○ Contact local emergency operations centers
  - ○ Initiate move to secondary location if necessary
  - ○ Register with appropriate authorities for relief or insurance purposes
- Debrief
  - ○ Thank everyone, acknowledge efforts and ongoing inconveniences
  - ○ Provide as much information as possible about future plans
  - ○ Seek input from everyone about what worked well and what did not
  - ○ Obtain information about additional resources
- Normalization
  - ○ Thank everyone again
  - ○ Celebrate creativity and caring in the face of disaster
  - ○ Add, delete, modify details of the disaster plan

When you have your list, and you can always add to it, sort the tasks into four areas:

- Management/administrative
- Client/clinical
- Business development/marketing
- Professional/community

Preparing your list and sorting categories clarifies priorities. You can identify which tasks need to be performed on an ongoing basis, such as signing checks, and which can be postponed, such as speaking engagements.

Now is the time to designate a person to assume control in an emergency (an "agent") and give that person documented authority. This person should be able to sign checks and contracts, and conduct day-to-day business. Be sure to check with your attorney to anticipate any legal problems. Even if the agent has already filled in for the principal, he or she will find a blueprint essential to running the business in a way that the owner wants. The best way to ensure this is to create an advance directive for the agency operation.

Documents: Advance Directive and Office Manual

The advance directive should contain specific policies and procedures, written out and made explicit. It should include a mission statement as well as directions that the owner or principal would like followed under different circumstances. Put in statements such as, "If x happens, do y." The chain of command as well as a backup chain of command can also be found here. The advance directive should be signed and dated by both the principal and the agent. It should also be reviewed periodically and updated as policies and procedures or circumstances change.

The absence of the owner or manager is not the only absence that can affect an agency. Any member of the staff can unexpectedly fall victim to accident or illness or quit without notice. Once again, the way to get a handle on what to do when key personnel are absent is to

begin with the job-task assessment. Have each staff member make a list of all the tasks he or she performs on a daily, weekly, monthly, quarterly, and annual basis. Be sure to have them include informal responsibilities, such as taking out the trash, for example, or responsibilities they may have taken on themselves. Then, sort these tasks into priorities: (1) those that must be done, (2) those that should be done, and (3) those that could be done if there's time and energy. In addition, designating one or two people to be responsible for coordinating information in the aftermath of an emergency would be useful.

At this point, you can begin developing the office manual, a document and tool to pull together all the agency's policies and procedures. A copy of the office manual should be provided to each member of the staff as well as posted to the private, protected company Web site. Update the policies and procedures regularly. A phone tree, the list of who calls whom in an emergency situation, should be posted on the Web site and also placed in the manual.

Cross-Training

The agency can begin working out a cross-training program at the same time that it is developing a backup chain of command. Cross-training should begin by evaluating the staff's strengths and making everyone familiar with the procedures they need to assume in an emergency. Cross-training enables various staff members to assume extra responsibilities during the absence of a colleague, or one person can take over all of another's responsibilities, such as when the agent takes over for the principal. Cross-training should be more than a backup plan on paper; certain days should be designated when emergency responsibilities can be assumed and practiced. Not only does this familiarize individuals with their new tasks, but it also enables them to have their colleagues available for pertinent questions. Planning, practice, and flexibility are the keys because, when the need arises, it will most likely occur under stressful circumstances, so it is optimal for the staff to be as familiar as possible with their new responsibilities.

Emergency Preparedness Meetings

Regular meetings need to be scheduled during which the staff members of the agency are encouraged to think the unthinkable and prepare themselves to negotiate an emergency. An emergency is not only a disaster or an illness; it can be a fire, an epidemic, a lengthy power outage, or workplace violence. In fact, the emergency preparedness meetings should be a place to brainstorm possible scenarios, and, just as fire drills teach everyone the quickest and safest way out of a building, contingency plans for responding to other emergencies can be rehearsed. This is also a good time to discuss emotional issues. Thinking about the possible absence of a colleague or any other emergency may trigger emotional issues, particularly sadness and fear. Insecurities and emotions can be addressed and acknowledged in the meetings because simply planning for such occurrences can give rise to issues around trust and relinquishing control.

Preparing for Disasters: An Overview

Recent occurrences have shown that disasters come in many forms. Hurricanes, terrorist attacks, and earthquakes may grab the headlines, but blizzards and floods can also obstruct the safe functioning of a professional geriatric care management agency. Recent disasters have made painfully clear that the elderly are dreadfully at risk in an emergency. Each disaster creates circumstances that have specific dangers and problems, and we examine these, but there are some general precautions that can be categorized and we look at these first. Professional geriatric care management agencies must foresee the worst to prevent it. Again, the keyword is *planning*. Planning, and engaging staff and caregivers and clients in the planning,

goes a long way toward forestalling injury and loss of life.

Most natural disasters are confined to particular regions. Hurricanes bedevil the southeastern and Gulf states, earthquakes are most likely to occur along the fault lines of the West Coast, and tornadoes are more frequent in the Midwest. The regional nature of potential disasters enables a level of predictability in planning for them. Evacuation routes and shelter sites, for example, can be identified long before an actual hurricane threatens. The professional geriatric care management agency should identify which types of disasters are most likely to occur in its area. Again, identifying likely types of emergencies can be used to raise awareness when such emergencies are discussed during emergency preparedness meetings. Preparations can be put into two main categories. First, prepare the agency; second, prepare clients and caregivers.

Preparing a Professional Geriatric Care Management Agency for an Emergency

The first step to protecting the agency is to preserve the files and the equipment. Vital information is stored in hard copy and computers: insurance policy numbers and insurance agent information, bank account numbers and accountant phone numbers, attorney phone numbers and legal documents, phone numbers and addresses for the relatives of clients—and this is only the tip of the iceberg. All of this information needs to be backed up regularly, with backup hard copies stored at a secure, off-site location. In this day of computerization, information can be electronically filed, but there should still be a plan for salvaging paper files and office equipment if possible. Designate a staff member to oversee continual review of emergency procedures, perhaps on a rotating basis so that everyone becomes familiar with the process.

Staff safety is uppermost, of course, but setting priorities ahead of time can result in everyone functioning more safely as well as keeping the agency working. Find an alternate location for the staff to work from for an indefinite amount of time in case of a lengthy, major disruption. An invaluable aid at this time is to have a sister agency in another region to turn to, an agency that, hopefully, would be unaffected by the disaster.

While preparing the agency for an emergency, don't forget to take basic precautions at the office. Stock emergency supplies just as you would for a residence.

Sister Agencies

Partnering with another agency enables each one to have a backup for storing files and for relaying communications in an emergency. A hurricane is unlikely to occur simultaneously with an earthquake, so sister agencies work best if located in separate regions. At least one of them can be counted on to have access to computers. Perhaps the most important role the sister agency can play in an emergency is serving as an information center. The families of professional geriatric care management clients often live far away from their elderly relatives and they will be understandably anxious; if they can call the sister agency, the families can be apprised of whatever information is available. In the likely event of power loss, computers, cell phones, BlackBerry devices, and all the electronic conveniences that we rely on may cease to function. However, landline telephones often continue to work when other means of communications fail. Thus, the sister agency becomes invaluable as a hub for relaying information in and out of the affected area.

Preparing Clients and Caregivers

Preparing individual clients, their families, and their caregivers for disasters can be broken down into three simple steps.[1]

- Basics
- Emergency supplies
- Personal plan

The client, depending on his or her level of ability to function, should be encouraged to participate as much as possible. This is not only useful for the preparations but will go a good distance toward alleviating some stress if the emergency situation does arise. And remember to include any pets in the emergency preparation. Many evacuation vehicles and shelters will not allow pets, and the need to abandon one can cause considerable distress.

All the information gathered regarding a client's decisions and needs in preparation for an emergency should be filed and reviewed regularly. Put this information in each client's file, and also in a master document covering all clients. Exhibit 13-2 is a sample of a master document that should be stored both in hard copy and on disk. Another task of the emergency preparedness meetings is to evaluate the status of a client in the event of a disaster: which clients will need immediate attention, which will be attended to as soon as possible, and which ones may be expected to function for a short time on their own.

Basics

Knowing the basics begins with learning what types of disasters are particular to a professional geriatric care management agency's area. Earthquakes happen suddenly, whereas hurricanes give at least some warning. Individual locales may have community preparedness plans that are essential for a professional geriatric care management agency to take into consideration. Federal Emergency Management Agency (FEMA) and Red Cross services should be researched to see what plans are in place as well as consulting the local police, fire department, and city planning agencies for emergency plans. Exhibit 13-3 lists several Web sites that should be researched for useful information from experts. If at all possible, the professional geriatric care management agency should add input to local agencies to make them more responsive to the special needs of the aging person.

Exhibit 13–2   Client Emergency Management Plan

ANNUAL HURRICANE PLAN
YEAR _____

Patient Name: _____   Address: _____

Priority Level: ❑ I   ❑ II   ❑ III   Evacuation Zone: ❑ Yes   ❑ No

Residence Type: ❑ House   ❑ Condo   ❑ Apt.   ❑ Mobile Home   ❑ ALF/SNF

ALF/SNF: Facility hurricane plan has been reviewed by SBF   ❑ Yes   ❑ No

Patient will evacuate home: ❑ Yes   ❑ No

EVACUATION PLAN	NON-EVACUATION PLAN

EVACUATION PLAN

❑ Red Cross Shelter
❑ Special Needs Shelter
❑ Hospital/SNF
❑ Family _____
    Name   Phone
❑ Friend _____
    Name   Phone
❑ Other _____
    Name   Phone

Transportation to Shelter:
❑ Walk
❑ Drive Car
❑ Family Driving
❑ Friend Driving
❑ Mass Transit
❑ Special County Van: ❑ registered
                       ❑ not registered
❑ Wheelchair Van/Ambulance

NON-EVACUATION PLAN

Patient will stay at home with: _____
Relationship: _____

Home will be secured by:
❑ Shutters
❑ Awnings
❑ Plywood
❑ Other: _____

Who will help secure home: _____
Person responsible for hurricane supplies:
_____

Refuses/unable to plan*

Plan for Pet: _____

List of Medications and Supplies Attached to Plan: ❑ Yes   ❑ No

❑ Shelter Address: _____

❑ Limitations of the shelter have been explained to patient and patient understands the limitations of services and conditions in the shelter, that services will not equal what they receive at home, that conditions may be stressful or inadequate for their needs and that this is an option of last resort.

Patient Signature: _____

Plan completed by: _____   Date completed: _____

*If patient refuses to cooperate with plans or does not have the capacity to plan, next of kin needs to sign form acknowledging plan.

_____   _____
Next of Kin   Date

Source: Reprinted with permission by SeniorBridge.

Exhibit 13–3   Online Resources for Disaster Preparedness

California Governor's Office of Emergency Services
http://www.oes.ca.gov Information about emergency disaster services and specific resources for preparing for earthquakes.

Centers for Disease Control and Prevention: Emergency Preparedness and Response. http://www.bt.cdc.gov Offers news and disaster preparedness information.

Department of Health and Human Services
http://www.hhs.gov/disasters/index.shtml Information about responding to health crises during and after various types of disasters, particularly about stress issues following an emergency.

FEMA: Federal Emergency Management Agency coordinates response to disasters. http://www.fema.gov/areyouready/ *Are You Ready* is a booklet developed as an in-depth guide to preparing for potential

disasters, and it can be downloaded or accessed online.

Official U.S. Government Web site
http://www.pandemicflu.gov Information specific to tracking the avian flu.

Red Cross: Contains extensive information about available services and preparation advice.
http://www.redcross.org The main site http://www.prepare.org Particularly for seniors and others with special needs

U.S. Department of Homeland Security
http://www.ready.gov Information regarding types of potential disasters and how to plan.

U.S. Small Business Administration: SBA Procedural Notices
http://www.sba.gov/library/pubs/ Information detailing what insurance your business should acquire for full disaster protection.

Another basic essential is evaluating the client's residence. If the client still resides at home, the safety of the house needs to be assessed. How much of a storm can it withstand? Does it have safe areas inside for riding out a storm? Where are the gas connections that need to be shut down after an earthquake? How is this done? Who will do it? Where are the water and electrical outlets? In addition to the residence itself, learn who the neighbors are and (with the client's permission) exchange basic information with them, such as phone numbers, family names, or other helpful contacts. The professional geriatric care management agency should encourage the client's caregivers to constantly monitor the residence and assess it for potential risk. A group home also needs to be evaluated for safety. What emergency plans does the residence have in place? What kind of shelter does it provide? How long can it function without power?

Deciding whether to evacuate in an emergency and where to go is also part of basic planning. An evacuation plan should take into account not only the prospective shelter, but what transportation will be available and what routes to take. Will family members be available or will the client be dependent primarily on the professional geriatric care management agency? Is the best place to go another home, a community shelter, a hotel, or a medical facility? Some families have given professional geriatric care management agencies open-ended plane tickets so that clients can leave the area entirely. The choice of an evacuation center must take into account special needs of the client, such as whether he or she needs dialysis or oxygen. Exhibit 13-4 shows a sample of how to assess a client for evacuation in case of a hurricane, but can easily be adapted to other disasters.

Exhibit 13–4   Annual Hurricane Plan

Client Emergency Management Log
Evacuation Status

Date: _____

Indicate beside each patient's name below in each "Level Category" the item—a, b, c, or d—that best identifies the patient's needs/preferences.

Level 3	Level 2	Level 1	Geographic Housing Risk Level	Shelter or Transportation
A. Clients able to arrange their own evacuation plan with the assistance of family or friends **B.** Clients living in an assisted living facility & will participate in the Disaster Plan in place for the facility	**A.** Clients who are limited in their ability to ambulate, and have one or more physical limitations **B.** Clients having no family/friends to care for them. They are to register with a designated shelter. **C.** Clients receiving skilled nursing. D. Clients on medications.	**A.** Clients on life sustaining/supportive devices (i.e. oxygen, respiratory support equipment, IV fluids) which cannot be maintained at home.	**A.** Clients living in low lying areas, near the intracoastal and ocean, barrier islands and mobile homes, (East of US 1 in Broward County)	**Indicate Clients who need shelter with an "S" and Clients who need transportation with a "T"**
Client Names	**Client Names**	**Client Names**	**Client Names**	**Client Names**

Source: Reprinted with permission by SeniorBridge.

Emergency Supplies

The goal of keeping emergency supplies on hand is to be able to survive until help arrives or basic utilities are restored. For clients who decide to stay in place through a disaster, a supply of food, water, and medicine for several days is essential. Drinking water for 3 to 6 days is estimated to be a gallon of water per person per day. Store a supply of food that won't spoil or require cooking because power most likely will be unavailable.

Medical preparation for the professional geriatric care management client is of utmost importance. In addition to prescription drugs, the client may need oxygen or infusion. It is possible to have an emergency supply available in areas where sudden disasters may be the highest risk. Special arrangements need to be made for clients who need dialysis. In the case of prescriptions, keep a list of medications, prescribing physicians, prescription numbers, dosages, and purchase dates with the emergency supplies. This information should also be kept with the emergency information on file at the professional geriatric care management agency office and online. Attach a copy of the prescription to the back of the list. If the doctor agrees, an emergency supply of medications can be added to the supplies. Every time a prescription is filled, put the new medications in with the emergency supplies and then use the medications that are being replaced.

In addition, the emergency supplies should contain a flashlight, a battery-powered radio, a supply of spare batteries, light sticks in case an open flame poses a risk, a hand-operated can opener along with other items that can be found on the extensive supply checklist presented in Exhibit 13–5. This list contains many items that may not be useful for everyone, but it can be edited according to individual need.

If evacuation is necessary, have an evacuation bag packed and on hand to grab going out the door. A number of things from the "stay-at-home" supplies can be kept in the emergency evacuation bag, especially copies of important papers such as medication needs, a contact list with names and phone numbers, insurance policies, and other vital documents. Other items for the evacuation bag are a change of clothing, personal hygiene necessities, comfortable shoes, an extra pair of glasses, and a blanket or sleeping bag. Be realistic because this bag should be in place and ready to easily carry or roll at a moment's notice.

Personal Planning

Every client has unique needs and the professional geriatric care management agency should establish an emergency plan for each client. This plan should be placed in a file that includes emergency checklists and up-to-date assessments, and copies should be kept online in the agency's secure Web site, at the client's residence, and at the office. Caregivers should be encouraged to periodically review the plan. If the plan includes evacuation, there should be a trial run just like a fire drill. In some areas struck by hurricanes, or in the case of earthquakes, the usual landmarks may disappear. Street signs, buildings, trees, any kind of familiar marker may be destroyed, so having already been to the designated shelter could prove to be invaluable. For clients who have disabilities, it may be possible to register with the local police or fire department so that the clients can be put on a list of people to check up on in the event of an emergency.

Evaluate the kind of shelter that is most appropriate for a particular client. Is the client relatively independent? Should he or she go to a shelter that can take people with Alzheimer's, or do they need a place equipped to provide special needs such as oxygen or dialysis? Again, involve the client and family as much as possible because this can help reduce some of the stress of an emergency. Remember, most injuries and deaths occur in the aftermath of a disaster such as a hurricane, so the more decisions made ahead of time, the safer everyone will be.

Exhibit 13–5   Inclusive Emergency Supply Checklist

Food and Water
- Water/water purifier
- Canned meat, fruit, fish, vegetables, soup
- Canned juice
- Beef/pork jerky
- Freeze-dried foods
- Canned and powdered milk
- Coffee/tea
- Bouillon
- Cereal
- Dry pasta
- Rice
- Peanut butter
- Crackers
- Trail mix
- Salt
- Sugar
- Vitamin supplements
- Pet food

Tools
- Hand-operated can opener
- Flashlight
- Battery-powered radio
- Batteries
- Light sticks and candles
- Matches
- Pliers
- Screwdriver
- Knife
- Duct tape
- Needles and thread
- Paper or plastic plates
- Cooking pan
- Camper stove with fuel
- Plastic sheeting

Hygiene
- Disinfectant/bleach
- Soap
- Sanitary napkins or tampons
- Disposable moist towelettes
- Plastic bags
- Toilet paper
- Paper towels

Clothing, etc.
- Blanket or sleeping bag
- Space blanket
- Change of clothes
- Comfortable, sturdy shoes
- Towels
- Waterproof gear
- Gloves

Medical
- First-aid kit
- Gauze
- Iodine
- Ointment for burns, antibiotic
- Disinfectant pads
- Alcohol
- Thermometer
- Scissors
- Tweezers
- Latex gloves
- Swabs
- Prescription medications
- Extra prescription glasses

Automobile Supplies
- Gasoline can [maintain at least a half tank in car]
- Bottled water
- Booster cables
- Shovel
- Space blanket
- Flashlight and extra batteries
- Maps
- Antifreeze
- Extra hat/warm gloves

Recovery

It is appropriate that, during and immediately following a disaster or other type of emergency, professional geriatric care management staff and caregivers will secure their own safety and that of their families. However, as soon as possible, these personnel should contact the agency and let the staff member who has been designated as emergency information coordinator know their status, their client's status if they are a caregiver, and their availability. Immediately following an emergency, the most important task is to locate everyone, assess their status, and respond to the most urgent needs. Information will become the most vital resource following an emergency, and this is when having a sister agency to coordinate information will prove invaluable. Locate the services that can provide you with assistance, and offer to help where possible. In a disaster, former competitors may be the most capable allies.

After securing the safety of persons, a property damage assessment is in order. Can the central office still function? Is the backup location available? Protect and preserve whatever equipment is still in operating order. Computers, files, possibly vehicles, even the building itself will need to be checked for potential hazards and operational suitability. Begin the application process for relief resources from the appropriate agencies, such as insurance or FEMA, as soon as possible.

Remember to acknowledge the services of staff and caregivers. Later, when there is time for a full debriefing and for considering the emotional aftermath of experiencing a disaster, a fuller acknowledgment can be made, but immediate consideration and encouragement will go a long way to help everyone negotiate the crisis.

Preparing a professional geriatric care management agency for an emergency is a serious responsibility. As was mentioned earlier, seniors are very much at risk in any kind of disaster. In an emergency, something unexpected will always occur, but a little foresight will pay off in huge dividends. Planning, vigilance, and researching available resources are the keys to successful emergency preparedness.

■ NOTES

1. U.S. Department of Health and Human Services Administration on Aging. http://www.aoa.gov/eldfam/Disaster_Assistance/Disaster_Assistance.asp. Accessed September 18, 2006.

Chapter 14

Incorporating a Spiritual Perspective into Geriatric Care Management

Leonie Nowitz

In the last decade, there has been a growing interest in spirituality in U.S. society and an increasing appreciation for spirituality's valuable contribution to health and well-being.[1] In the health care literature, there is evidence that prayer and a belief in a higher power contribute to healing and a general sense of well-being. There is also growing interest in the search and creation of meaning in the second half of life as evidenced by the numerous conferences, courses, and books that address these issues under the title of "conscious aging."

The search for meaning and purpose in life often begins at times of illness, crisis, and suffering. A geriatric care manager (GCM) helps older persons and their families, friends, and paid caregivers find meaning and strength in coping with changes in function, increased caregiving, and reduced resources. A spiritual perspective offers the GCM an opportunity to broaden his or her vision of meaning and values and to be open to clients' viewpoints, struggles, and ways of finding meaning in life.

In 1975, the National Interfaith Coalition on Aging defined spiritual well-being as "the affirmation of life in a relationship with God, self, community and environment that nurtures and celebrates wholeness."[2] It is that which unites all aspects of ourselves and brings together concurrent paths of spiritual and psychological well-being. If GCMs can view more positively the frailty and finiteness of life, they can help older persons and their families find meaning and value in their situations, helping them care for each other, accept life's realities, and transmit the value of caring to future generations.

A spiritual view challenges the negative attitudes about aging in a society that celebrates youth, achievement, financial success, and power. This perspective enables GCMs to help their clients find meaning when productivity fails and they become dependent on others.

This chapter addresses the meaning of spirituality for older persons and their families and considers the purpose and spiritual tasks of life's last stages. Assessment and intervention tools for the practitioner are offered. Qualities with which GCMs need to address clients' struggles are also discussed. The final section discusses the facilitation of spiritual connections with persons who have dementia and their families.

■ THE PURPOSE OF LIFE'S LAST STAGES

According to Carl Jung, "We cannot live the afternoon of life according to the program of life's morning, for what was great in the morning will be little in the evening and what in the morning was true will in the evening have become a lie."[3] To help clients evaluate their lives, GCMs need to ask several questions. What is the purpose of life after age 65? What are clients' values, wishes, and dreams? How can clients stay true to their values and accomplish their dreams?

After age 65, there may be a transition from professional work to volunteer work and from ability to disability. Social networks may diminish as friends move away or die, which leads to an increased focus on family. Changes in family roles may ensue as a result of changes in health and dwindling resources. Everyone in the family needs to make a shift. As some members increasingly need care, others may need to assume caregiving responsibilities in addition to their current work and family roles. Though painful, transition and loss provide the opportunity to reevaluate one's life goals. Who am I without my work role, when I am disabled and need to depend on others? Why am I here? What is it I still want to do and be? These important questions were inspired by the work of Schachter-Shalomi and Miller.[4]

By reflecting on these questions and attending to clients' thoughts and values, GCMs can help clients redefine themselves. GCMs can help their clients find meaning in loss by offering a loving presence and allowing a trusting relationship to develop. This process may involve listening to clients mourn and find meaning in their losses as they reflect on their lives, struggles, and strengths, and acknowledging the gifts clients have given and continue to give to others. The GCM needs to transcend the dominant culture's status- and youth-driven values and respect each client's feelings regardless of age, function, and status. When the GCM takes this approach, it can help clients shake off the culture's focus on autonomy and independence and instead see themselves as who they are based on a lifetime of experience.

It is important that GCMs acknowledge and respect a client's values. If a GCM notices a client's kindness, wisdom, dignity, depth,

joy, integrity, wholeness, confidence, or peacefulness, the GCM should tell the client. This respect will help clients reestablish a connection within themselves, with other people, and with God, if they so choose.

Kenyon notes:

> Advanced human aging may also be a time for the possibility of a transition from having to being. Something new may now be taking place that goes beyond loss. Inner activity may increase. Silence provides an opportunity for simply being with oneself which can be peaceful or anxiety provoking through confrontation with new aspects of ourselves. The experience of inner silence and being can result in an increased ability to be present to others, involving the ability to be more open to others and less preoccupied with self.[5(pp4-5)]

To provide a broader framework, it is helpful to consider traditions that offer another perspective. The Hindu tradition embraces loss as a natural part of the life cycle and thinks of the third stage of life as one in which one frees oneself from daily roles and moves to the performing of rituals and the reciting of sacred texts with all energies directed toward union with Brahman, the divine ground of the universe. Losses are considered "modes of liberation contributing to spiritual growth."[6(pp17-21)]

The Western counterpart to the Hindu journey would look upon late life as a natural monastic period.

> The aging process often strips the person of the distracting pleasures of the world by shrinking both actual life space and even the physical ability to participate in the adventures of life. It's as if God offers a new kind of intimacy and says to the frail elderly person, "You have lived a long life enjoying the pleasures of my creation. Sometimes you have enjoyed creation more than you have ME, but I understand because creation is so won-

derful. Now that you are housebound and can no longer enjoy the physical and mental pleasures of your past, we have an opportunity to really get to know one another before we meet face to face at your death!"[7(p9)]

Accepting brokenness in a positive light is a part of many spiritual traditions. Most religious traditions view frailty and loss as meaningful, valuable parts of life. The Jewish rabbinical traditions speak of the value of brokenness. The Kotsker rabbi recognizes that nothing is as whole as a broken heart and that the brokenness and deficits create an opening up to possibilities of humility and seeking union with God.[8] Rav Kook noted that a broken heart was beloved before God, and Reb Nachman said that in the brokenness itself is the yearning for God.[8] Similarly, Ralph Waldo Emerson said, "There is a crack in everything God has made."[9] It has been said that as we age, the cracks begin to show. Are they just about darkness and brokenness? Or are they also a place for the light of spirit to stream through?

Spirituality has many faces and takes many forms. It is important to recognize the unique essence of clients, their families, and caregivers and to be open and available to the form of spirituality favored by individual clients and the people around them. There are four ways persons commonly experience their spirituality:

- As a connection to something beyond themselves that comforts and guides them
- As a connection to all living things, earth, and the universe
- As a part of a faith tradition or having a close personal relationship with God or both
- As a process of finding answers to life's difficult questions

Some older persons tend to turn inward. Others move from the inward view toward more meaningful relationships with others.

And others experience spiritual awareness through religious traditions that sustained them in the past.[10] Moberg describes "spiritual" as referring to the very essence of each human being that relates everything consciously or unconsciously and either positively or negatively to God and that makes everyone valuable.[11]

■ SPIRITUAL TASKS IN OLD AGE

Genevay and Richards question the nature of growth in old age. Is spiritual growth separate from psychological growth, or is there one concurrent path that leads to mental, emotional, and spiritual growth in the last stage of life?[12]

Many believe that there are spiritual tasks to be accomplished in late life. The following tasks were suggested by Father Richard Sweeney at the 1991 American Society on Aging Forum and church and mental health workers at the 1997 American Society on Aging annual meeting:

1. Making a conscious effort to know oneself and clarify one's personal values
2. Establishing a sense of self-worth apart from life's externals
3. Letting go of dimensions of life where there is no longer ability
4. Seeking and sharing wisdom and love
5. Mentoring others
6. Viewing life as imperfect and facing issues of death and the afterlife

Many writers have shared their viewpoints on making meaning. Victor Frankl, a concentration camp survivor, writes about the search for meaning and how one's attitude toward one's experience creates meaning.[13] His works focus on how to turn suffering into human triumph and the importance of self-discovery, responsibility, and self-transcendence. Zalman Schachter-Shalomi and R. S. Miller, in the book *From Age-ing to Sage-ing*, talk about the concept of generativity, harvesting gifts of a lifetime and giving them back to family, friends, and society: "The archetype of the Inner Elder is a divine image representing the wisdom of the ages. This image of the Inner Elder calls forth the wisdom of older people at a time when our culture desperately needs it."[4(p139)] Allan Chinen's work offers much richness in noting the tasks of the elder: "learning to heed the dictates of the soul, being generative in inspiring the younger generations with practical counsel and noble inspiration, seeking self-confrontation and transformation through painful insight and authentic reformation."[14]

Carter Catlett Williams talks about the wonderful opportunity for self-discovery in later years. Paying attention to one's inner life, a person can make later life a time for growth, self-reflection, rediscovery, and self-exploration.[15] Finding meaning through suffering is the focus of Polly Young-Eisendrath, a Jungian psychotherapist who shares stories of people who have sustained major losses to their health and of family members.[16] She describes how they transcended these losses to develop, through their pain, compassion for and understanding of others. Through this process, they learned to accept the impermanence of life and allowed the formation of a new identity.

If GCMs view frailty and brokenness as valuable, meaningful parts of life, they can witness and be present to the suffering of clients. Often GCMs will witness great wisdom, understanding, and courage of their clients and families.

■ WAYS TO FACILITATE THE SPIRITUAL PROCESS IN GERIATRIC CARE MANAGEMENT

Psychological and spiritual growth can be nurtured by introspection and a search for meaning in life. Some ways the GCM can foster spiritual connection and growth in clients are discussed in this section.

Life Review

In reviewing their lives with an empathetic listener, clients can find meaning. Clients can review the struggles and the wisdom gained, the values lived and acquired, the mistakes made, and the opportunities missed. Healing can come from the process of facing hurtful experiences and letting go. Telling one's story in the presence of an empathetic listener allows a reworking of it.

Chinen notes that "in remembering the past, older adults transform it. The reflective individual comes to terms with mistakes and opportunities missed, learning to forgive himself and others. The elder embraces the past, not to regress, but to illuminate all of life."[14]

This process can be facilitated by the GCM (who may be a social worker or a nurse), paid caregivers, and family members (to whom the shared stories can transmit history and legacy). GCMs can help get their clients involved in senior center and day care programs. Participating in storytelling and the creative arts can enrich older people's lives and cultivate a sense of community. "When elders hear others reveal dimensions of their lives, they notice similarities and differences with their own experiences. They can be empowered to claim and reclaim the wisdom of their own lives."[17]

The GCM needs to be sensitive to each client's willingness to engage in this process and should engage with clients at their own pace.

Ethical Wills

The tradition of bequeathing a spiritual legacy in a conventional will, a codicil, or a separate document has its roots in the Bible. The desire was to pass on an instructive account of ideas and values close to the older person's heart—an ethical will.[18]

An ethical will can be used to pass values and a sense of what is important in life to future generations. If clients have no family members, the GCM can listen to clients' account of their values, a process that will strengthen the connection between the GCM and the clients. If clients are unable to articulate their values, GCMs can tell clients what they know of them based on stories the GCMs have heard that reflect the clients' values and character. This process will help clients feel that they are being understood and valued. Additionally, it helps clients recall old memories and gives them an opportunity to receive positive feedback and be seen for their deeper values.

For instance, Mr. K, a 96-year-old widower with a moderate degree of dementia, was working with a GCM. The GCM acknowledged Mr. K's generosity to his family and political causes as well as the extensive care he gave to his wife before she died. Although he did not initially remember some of these actions, he began to remember his wife, how he loved her, and how important it was for him to make her life comfortable when she was ill. As this example illustrates, when the GCM shares his or her view of the older person's values as exemplified by his or her life story, the older person is validated. This can stimulate memories in an environment of trust.

Prayer and Meditation

Prayer and meditation are common in all religious and spiritual traditions. Eighty-one percent of caregivers for people with Alzheimer's disease say they use prayer in coping with the demands of caregiving.[19] GCMs might consider praying with their clients. They might want to check with family members whether the older person has prayed in the past. GCMs would ask family members whether opportunities for prayer should be provided to the older person. If a GCM is uncomfortable praying with a client or comes from a tradition different from the client's, the GCM could find another professional on the care team (e.g., a nurse, a social worker) who is familiar with the client's religious tradition.

Many home care workers are comfortable with prayer and are willing to read from the scriptures and pray with clients, which can give clients a sense of peace and well-being.

Sacred and Secular Rituals

Performing sacred and secular rituals can help clients experience familiar memories and reconnect them with their faith and communal traditions. The GCM can find out what traditions and practices are familiar to clients and help re-create them. For instance, a traditional Christmas or Passover meal could be made. The GCM can ask clients and caregivers to help with planning (e.g., what foods they would like, what readings they would like to have) and can be present at a Passover Seder or Christmas meal. In addition, the GCM can help clients attend services by contacting places of worship to find out about wheelchair accessibility. The GCM can arrange for a friend to accompany the client and/or a caregiver to create more of a feeling of family and community.

Grief Counseling

Grief counseling to resolve the current and multiple losses of a lifetime is important to help clients heal their pain in the presence of a caring and empathic listener. The GCM can provide this counseling or can refer the client to another professional.

Focusing

In focusing, a GCM helps a client clarify and resolve all kinds of issues (e.g., unresolved relationship issues) and make all kinds of decisions (e.g., decisions about health care).

For example, Ms. F's aunt was not able to swallow food after surgery. Her physicians felt that the insertion of a peg tube was necessary to ensure adequate nutrition and hydration. Ms. F was ambivalent about this procedure. She questioned the quality of life of her aunt, who had recently experienced the onset of dementia. Ms. F thought her aunt would not tolerate being mentally and physically dependent. The GCM helped Ms. F explore her feelings about other relatives who had lived in a seriously vegetative state for several years. The GCM encouraged Ms. F to think about her aunt's life and what interests and people had sustained her. The GCM shared with the niece the possibility that the peg tube might not always be needed if her aunt's condition improved. She encouraged Ms. F to talk with other relatives and explore what Ms. F's aunt would want for herself. Her aunt had not expressed any negative feelings about being ill and dependent. After discussion with family members and review of her aunt's life and her own reactions to others who were disabled, the niece recognized that she needed to come to terms with her aunt's changed functioning. She also realized that her aunt was not as debilitated as her other relatives. The GCM listened to Ms. F's fears about the quality of her aunt's life and helped Ms. F clarify her decision regarding surgery. Ms. F's aunt got the peg tube and after several weeks regained her capacity to swallow.

Broadening Clients' View of Themselves to Include Deeper Values

Many older persons who have suffered losses of family and friends and changes in health tend to view themselves in a negative light. It is helpful to appreciate the deeper values that have sustained and enriched the client.

For example, Mrs. D, a widow who suffered from dementia, had no friends and only a distant relative. She reminisced with the GCM about her life with her husband, a famous physician, and how she enjoyed traveling. "Those were the good days, and they are no more," she said. She described her present existence as one in which God was punishing her by squeezing the life out of her little by little. She focused on her past life, talking about how she was valued for being the beautiful

wife of a famous physician. "Then I was something; now I'm nothing," she said. The GCM said, "Mrs. D, I see how valuable your past was to you in terms of your beauty and your sense of adventure. But in addition, I see a woman who has an inner beauty, who loved her husband and took care of him. You were hospitable to his friends and later you volunteered at a hospital and brought much caring to sick people. You visited them and gave so much of yourself." Mrs. D listened but did not respond. The GCM repeated her viewpoint many times because Mrs. D continued to think negatively about herself. The GCM talked to her about the wholeness of life and that if persons defined themselves by only one time in their lives they were bound to feel unworthy at other times that were different. The GCM continued to listen compassionately to Mrs. D's pain and sadness about the losses in her life. She shared what she valued about Mrs. D: "I value your courage and ability to endure the pain of so many losses, your warmth, your kindness, and your wisdom and ability to laugh at life." By reflecting on Mrs. D's lifelong values, the GCM attempted to help Mrs. D appreciate her many positive attributes and acknowledge her inner resources. The GCM brought small problems to Mrs. D from time to time, and Mrs. D reveled in the opportunity to share her wisdom by providing practical solutions. Mrs. D continued to view herself in a diminished capacity but also showed more comfort in being valued and grew more trusting in her relationship with the GCM and her caregivers.

Hearing the Spirit Beneath the Words

GCMs working with clients, especially those with dementia, need to listen to the meaning behind the spoken words. Older persons may not always be able to say precisely what they mean, but an attentive and sensitive listener will hear what an older person is really saying.

For example, Mrs. T was frightened of "men" in her bedroom. Her caregivers would check her room each evening to assure her it was empty. She was a religious woman and the GCM asked her pastor to visit her. On his visits he prayed with Mrs. T for God to protect her and keep her safe. He dealt with her feelings without specifically talking about the "men." By praying with her, the pastor acknowledged Mrs. T's fears and offered comfort and a sense of safety.[20]

Awareness of Countertransference

"Countertransference describes the personal feelings that a professional experiences in relation to a client that can affect his or her professional interventions."[21]

In facilitating the spiritual process, GCMs need to be aware of their own values. They can ask, "How can we facilitate resolution of past issues and letting go of emotional baggage that hinders at the end of life? Can we listen to older people and allow them to come to their own recognition of what they need?"[12(pp4–5)] To be effective, the GCM needs to be in touch with his or her own concerns and how he or she resolves them. The client may have a different perspective that needs to be respected, particularly when it conflicts with the GCM's view.

The next section discusses how GCMs can go about examining their own values, spiritual beliefs, and family history.

■ GCMs LOOK AT THEIR OWN VALUES, SPIRITUAL BELIEFS, AND FAMILY HISTORY

In helping clients deal with the multiple losses in their lives, GCMs are offered the opportunity to examine their own feelings about aging and dying and consider their own values. GCMs should ask themselves these questions: How do I view my own aging? What models of care do I embrace for myself? What makes me anxious and reactive to clients? With what family systems am I most comfortable and uncomfort-

able? GCMs need to consider values that are acquired from three sources:

- Their family
- Their culture
- Their professional training

GCMs need to be aware of the values they transmit to their clients and the impact of their values on their clients. The following exercise can help GCMs consider their own values at different stages of the life cycle and understand their clients' evolving values and beliefs. By answering the questions for themselves and considering how their clients might answer them, GCMs will broaden their perspective and learn to not impose their values on their clients. The questions were inspired by the work of Schachter-Shalomi and Miller.[4]

- How have you valued yourself at different times of your life?
- What were your beliefs about aging, interdependence, and family connections as a child, as an adolescent, as an adult, and as a person with an illness or a disability?
- Have your values been similar at different stages, or have they changed as you have aged?
- How has your belief system served you throughout your life?
- How does it serve you at a time of loss and diminishment?
- What is the meaning of your life now, despite losses that have taken place?

■ ASSESSMENT OF CLIENTS' VALUES AND SOURCES OF MEANING

In *Assessing Spiritual Needs: A Guide for Caregivers*, George Fitchett includes a spiritual assessment tool that can help GCMs evaluate their clients' spiritual life and struggles (Exhibit 14–1).[22] The tool contains a number of categories that GCMs need to consider.

Exhibit 14–1
Spiritual Assessment Tool

1. Beliefs of the client that give meaning and purpose to the client's life
2. Vocation and obligation: beliefs that create a sense of duty or moral obligation.
3. Experience and emotion that may be related to the sacred, the divine, or the demonic
4. Courage and growth
5. Ritual and practice
6. Community
7. Authority and guidance

Source: Copyright © George Frichett.

This spiritual assessment is part of a holistic assessment that includes the medical, psychological, family systems, psychosocial, ethnic, racial, cultural, and social dimensions that affect older persons. This tool provides a comprehensive picture of a client. The following text considers each of the seven dimensions listed in Exhibit 14–1 in turn, with illustrative cases discussed for each dimension.

Beliefs That Give Meaning and Purpose

GCMs should ask what beliefs a person has that give meaning and purpose to his or her life. These can be religious beliefs and practices of the past. There are also other sources from which persons derive meaning and purpose.

CASE STUDY

Mrs. N
Mrs. N, a 75-year-old African American woman who was divorced and living alone and was a very feisty and strong-spirited person, lost one of her daughters a few years ago. She had another daughter who lived out of town, as did several siblings. Diagnosed with Alzheimer's disease, she gradually accepted a few hours

of home care over a long period of time and sporadically visited a day care center. A woman who was very autonomous, she found it difficult to receive help. During one visit the GCM asked her what gave her the strength to deal with her memory loss and life situation. She said she had been raised as a Catholic and went to church all her life. She talked about God in personal terms, "I feel God is close to me—whatever happens during the day I talk to him at night and he listens. I couldn't be this age and in the world without God. He gives me strength in difficult times." The GCM asked Mrs. N about the times things did not work out the way she had hoped. She said, "I accept God's will. My mother died; she might have suffered more if she had lived. God does what is best." Mrs. N's faith and personal relationship with God gave her courage and strength to face her deteriorating health and the losses in her life. The GCM's interest in what gave Mrs. N strength encouraged Mrs. N to talk about her strong belief in and relationship with God.

CASE STUDY

Mrs. B
Mrs. B, who had a moderate dementia, talked about her very strong connection to nature by reflecting on the woods outside her apartment and how comforting it was to have the trees there. "I have always loved nature; my family found it a source of nourishment and strength," she said. Some of Mrs. B's frightening dreams found resolution in the woods. Mrs. B's source of healing and support was her lifetime connection with nature. Nature was a nurturing and

reassuring presence in times of difficulty. The GCM acknowledged and helped Mrs. B remember her connection with and comfort in nature.

CASE STUDY

Mr. J
Mr. J was a 95-year-old widower with severe sensory losses who walked minimally and suffered from moderate to severe dementia. Prior to his illness, he was an engineer who traveled extensively with his wife. Although his interests were wide-ranging prior to his illness, once he was ill Mr. J was confined to his apartment, where he watched ballgames and nature shows and enjoyed going to the nearby park to feed the squirrels and watch the boats sail by. These activities were the central focus of his day. Mr. J drew pleasure and a sense of connection from the park (he always loved nature) and from ballgames; these were activities he enjoyed in the past and could continue to enjoy. The GCM shared Mr. J's enthusiasm for ballgames. She also discussed with him the pleasure he got from feeding the squirrels and watching activities in the park.

Vocation and Obligation

It is important to consider the client's or their caregivers' beliefs and whether they create a sense of duty or moral obligation. Are clients or their caregivers able to fulfill these obligations, or are clients and caregivers frustrated and guilty about not being able to fulfill them? Both the older client's and the family member's sense of obligation may provide stress, but there may be positive experiences such as a strengthened relationship.

CASE STUDY

Mrs. C
Mrs. C's health was deteriorating rapidly due to her congestive heart failure and multiple health problems. Her daughter hired a GCM to assess her mother's situation and to provide counseling to her mother as her health declined. She also had the GCM arrange home care and access other resources. The daughter was very stressed but continued to coordinate her mother's medical care and call her daily. The GCM noted the stress the daughter experienced because of the time associated with Mrs. C's care and the emotional drain of her mother's illness and decline. The GCM listened to her concerns about her mother and the emotional drain of caregiving. The GCM offered to help her with some tasks, but the daughter refused, feeling obliged to continue her role as primary caregiver. In ongoing discussions, she talked about the stress and drain of caregiving. After several months of the daughter refusing to accept any help, the GCM asked the daughter why she continued to do as much as she did. She said it helped her feel connected to her mother. This helped the GCM understand the meaning of her sense of obligation and to continue to be respectful of her wishes. In time the daughter was able to let go of the daily coordination of care and continued her daily calls to her mother, which gave her that continued sense of connection.

It is important for a GCM to understand the meaning of the caregiver's caregiving experiences and to be respectful of the caregiver while acknowledging the stress of caregiving. The GCM needs to respect the caregiver's timetable and wait until he or she is willing to relinquish tasks to the GCM or to others in the system.

Experience and Emotion

The GCM needs to ask what direct contact with the sacred, divine, or demonic the older person has had. What emotions or moods are associated with these contacts and with the person's beliefs and sense of meaning in life? What past illnesses or crises in life were connected with spiritual experiences? How does spirituality affect the current situation? What sources or rituals provide comfort?

CASE STUDY

Mrs. G

Mrs. G was a 91-year-old widow, a musician who lived with her caregivers and who was visited by her two sons regularly. Her sons hired the GCM to oversee Mrs. G's care, because they were frequently out of town. Mrs. G had strong mood swings, which may have been caused by a long-standing personality disorder or dementia. A strong-willed women who was not able to walk, she viewed herself as capable and was often frustrated in her efforts to care for herself. Her sense of self fluctuated depending on her mood. During visits, the GCM listened to her fears and frustration and encouraged her to tell stories about herself and her accomplishments and to reminisce about things that came to mind. Although Mrs. G's family was Jewish, they observed no rituals. Mrs. G told the GCM many times that she did not believe in God and did not like her caregivers reading the Bible or praying. In one of the conversations, she talked about preparing for death. "I keep wondering at night how I continue to survive. Perhaps with the help of the Lord."

"Do you believe in God?" the GCM asked.

Mrs. G answered, "I talk a lot to God when anything goes wrong. I blame God with great pleasure and affection, but then I think what a hell of a job he has." She went on to say that she felt God was somewhere around but that she had told him to go away. The GCM asked if Mrs. G was concerned about seeing God. She said she was. "If he comes close, I will die." The GCM asked if Mrs. G believed God comes for persons when they die. Mrs. G said yes.

"So you're not ready to die now?" the GCM asked.

"Not at all; there is time." The GCM asked Mrs. G about whether she believed in connecting with God after death, as the soul rises to take its place with God—which is part of the Jewish tradition. Mrs. G thought that would be a great thing but thought God was too busy for her. After reflection, she said, "There is a mysterious thing that guides us. If I try to go too far I get lost. Something in us guides us; it's not a person, it's a mystery. We just have to follow it." The GCM asked her if she was talking about her soul or God. She said, "I would rather not put a finger on it." Mrs. G is not involved in any rituals or practice, but she has strong spiritual connections.

It is important for the GCM to be aware of spiritual resources that give clients meaning and strength and to be open to the conversation about such resources even if clients deny them. The GCM's interest and openness give the client the opportunity to share his or her beliefs and fears. The GCM should be guided by the client's expression and support the beliefs of the client. If the client's beliefs create fear, the GCM can listen to these fears and offer additional opportunities to resolve these fears by encouraging familiar clergy or family members to comfort the client.

Courage and Growth

Must new experiences, including problems, always be explained by a person's preexisting beliefs, or can a person let go of existing beliefs to allow new ones to emerge? When do persons' new life experiences challenge their existing beliefs in God? Do crises of faith or self-doubt result? It requires courage to enter the dark night of the soul, come to terms with a new set of circumstances, and accept changes in oneself. How can GCMs help their clients accept changes?

<hr>

CASE STUDY

Ms. H

Ms. H was a 77-year-old single woman who had had a stroke, was able to walk with assistance, and had a moderate degree of dementia, which affected her memory and made it difficult for her to articulate her thoughts. Ms. H's sister, who lived several thousand miles away, was her only living relative. The sister hired a GCM to oversee Ms. H's care and be accountable to the sister.

Ms. H was initially an opera singer and later worked in an administrative capacity for a major corporation. She was very knowledgeable about music and art and went to many concerts and museums. Her sense of self was diminished by her strong negative attitude toward being old and a societally induced emphasis on youth and beauty. It was difficult for her to say anything positive about herself.

The GCM tried to expand Ms. H's sense of self, encouraging her to modify her lifelong beliefs about youth and beauty. She tried to help Ms. H value her experience, wisdom, and knowledge and the fact that she was witty, caring, and loving. At times Ms. H was able to take this in. The GCM encouraged the caregivers to acknowledge Ms. H's strengths, points of view, and kindness, and Ms. H was receptive at times. At other times she stuck to her old negative beliefs about herself. The challenge of the GCM's work with Ms. H and her caregivers was to acknowledge her losses and traumas and help her view herself in a positive framework by mirroring positive views of her, to stretch her beyond her old beliefs.

Many clients have negative beliefs about aging and disability. To help clients accept their situations, GCMs can help clients explore their feelings toward God, if they express any feelings toward God at all. If clients do not have a religious connection, helping clients like Ms. H view themselves in more affirming ways can help them let go of entrenched beliefs that cause them to suffer.

<hr>

Ritual and Practice

It is important for the GCM to know what the client's rituals and practices are and what they were in the past. This would include traditional religious practices, services, prayers, and holiday celebrations. It would also include nonreligious rituals such as family gatherings for celebrations or birthdays. If the GCM's clients do not have family or do not participate in any rituals, the GCM needs to find out what events were celebrated in clients' lives that had meaning to them. The GCM might ask what the clients would like to do (e.g., go to church or synagogue, receive communion at home, or have their priest or rabbi visit). Would clients like to say prayers with caregivers or have scriptures or other spiritual material read aloud? What holidays would they like to celebrate and how? The GCM can work with caregivers to provide holiday foods and organize or participate in holiday celebrations. Providing a service for older persons in their homes generates a sense of community for clients and caregivers. When clients have forgotten rituals of their past, the GCM can find out about these rituals by trial and error, by saying a familiar prayer, lighting candles, or singing familiar songs or hymns from the person's religious tradition. These rituals can engender a sense of deep connection to clients' past and tradition. The GCM needs to respect clients' wishes and move in a sensitive manner.

CASE STUDY

Mr. G

Mr. G was Jewish but did not remember the rituals of his childhood in an orthodox home. During Chanukah, the GCM asked him if she could say a prayer when he lit the menorah candle. At first he declined and said he was agnostic. The GCM accepted his wishes, but he was curious and encouraged her to do so. She read the prayer slowly in Hebrew and English while Mr. G watched attentively. He later told her he appreciated her saying the prayer. Mr. G insisted on lighting the candles on all future Jewish holidays, including lighting the menorah on Passover.

Clients can be responsive to music from their tradition. Responses to the singing of melodies can range from joyful participation to the more subtle response of a smile or tapping finger. It is important to follow the older person's lead in this. It is helpful to involve pastoral connections and staff familiar with the rituals to say prayers and sing religious songs. In these ways, the GCM will help clients build a sense of connection to the past and create a sense of well-being.

Community

Is the person part of one or more formal or informal communities of shared beliefs, ritu-als, or practices? What is the person's participation in these communities? The GCM may ask what it means to the client to be part of the community and how active the client is in the community. The GCM should consider both spiritual and other communities of family, friends, organizations, neighbors, and caregivers. The GCM may have to educate the clergy or lay volunteer if the client has dementia or is aphasic as to how to respond appropriately to the client. It is important to stress to the spiritual leader how valuable his or her visit would be to the client, as would other types of connection with the community of faith.

Past versus Current Communities

Frail, homebound clients tend to have small communities. Families may live far away, and the clients may have lost touch with friends who have moved or are too ill to visit. Other friends and family members may have died. Because of illness, clients may not currently be connected to religious organizations. If a client is not part of any faith community, the GCM should assess past involvement in and current willingness to be part of a faith community. Would clients want to participate in services outside their home, or would they like the members of their former community to visit? It is important to talk with clients about their current community as well as their emotional connections to organizations or communities that had meaning to them in the past. The GCM can help access important people from the client's past by asking the client and his or her family for names. The GCM can encourage clients to contact whoever they were close to or offer to make the calls on behalf of clients. In addition, the GCM can arrange for new opportunities to widen clients' circles, such as attending day care programs or respite programs, having friendly visitor volunteers, and participating in activities the client likes.

CASE STUDY

Mr. R

Mr. R was a 95-year-old client who was a successful artist and was cognitively impaired. The GCM encouraged Mr. R's caregivers to take him to art shows where his work was represented. He was significantly affected by his dementia, but he loved to see familiar faces at these shows and receive acknowledgment for his work. The connection to the art community affirmed his self-worth. It is important for a GCM to involve a client with those who have had meaning in the client's life (e.g., former associates, neighbors, friends).

Home Care Community

The community of home care providers often becomes the surrogate family, providing great meaning for and connection with the client. It is important to support the home care staff so that they maintain good relationships with clients and care for clients' well-being. Many home care workers are spiritual people and view their work as the work of God, so they take naturally to caring for and loving their clients.

CASE STUDY

Mr. H

Mr. H suffered from dementia and physical incapacity. He was often agitated. His care workers were religious and had a daily ritual of saying prayers at the morning shift. At times he told them to stop. At other times, he joined the workers in their prayers. GCMs need to be vigilant that the caregivers are not imposing their viewpoints on clients, making clients uncomfortable.

Authority and Guidance

The GCM should consider where clients look for guidance when faced with doubt, confusion, tragedy, or conflict. To what extent do clients look within or outside themselves for guidance?

CASE STUDY

Mrs. L

Mrs. L's family lived out of town and hired a GCM to oversee her care. Mrs. L was visually impaired and at home in bed after a fall in which her arm and leg were injured. She could hardly move. She talked to the GCM about the difficult hospital experience. She hated not being in control and was glad to be at home in her bed. "I'm just lying here wondering what purpose I have. I don't know, but I know I've been through a lot of difficult struggles. I'm a tough egg. I've gone through difficult times but met people who had substance—that's what made the difference."

"So you valued the connections with people?" the GCM asked.

"Yes, that is right—I really liked them a lot."

"Do you wonder about the meaning of your life now?" continued the GCM.

"Yes, I don't know what I'm needed for, but that's all right, I am here and observing."

"So instead of thinking of what to do, you're just living in the present moment."

"Yes, that is what I am doing," said Mrs. L. She was quiet for a few moments. "I love listening to the music and to the voice that is coming from you."

"I appreciate that," the GCM responded. "I know you have meaning to your family."

"For a time I didn't think so, but they seem interested in me now."

"How do you feel about that?" the GCM asked.

"Oh, I love them visiting and talking with them; I really enjoy that." The GCM asked Mrs. L about her grandson. "That's right, I am a grandmother," said Mrs. L. "I remember Steve's visits a long time ago." The GCM reassured her that the caregivers and the GCM cared and loved her and that she meant a lot to them. Mrs. L said she was glad to hear that. The GCM's goal was to follow up on Mrs. L's statement about the purpose of her life and encourage her to reflect on the meaning of her life. GCMs need to listen to the thoughts and feelings that guide clients and to follow the clients' lead as they reflect on their lives.

CASE STUDY

Mrs. N

A GCM worked with an adult daughter who had difficulty caring for her autocratic, independent mother, Mrs. N, who had a significant dementia, was visually impaired, smoked incessantly, and lived alone in a tiny apartment. Mrs. N, a refugee who worked and brought her family to the United States, where she fought for the rights of workers in a union, was a proud woman who was writing about her martyred father who was killed in Eastern Europe.

For 2 years, the GCM provided consultation to her daughter concerning providing care to her mother, who often refused it, and helped the daughter in her efforts to balance caring for her mother with caring for her own family. In the process the daughter discussed her unresolved relationship issues with her mother. She admired her mother but was saddened by her mother's limited emotional nurturing. The daughter found students to read to her mother and introduced home care in a sensitive manner, using the GCM's services intermittently when problems arose.

The daughter brought her mother to her home for holidays, despite the difficulty in providing care. Mrs. N had another stroke, and the daughter honored her wishes in not taking her to the hospital. Mrs. N's daughter moved into her mother's apartment and took care of her. The GCM talked with the daughter about her mother's condition. A hospice program began to provide care to her mother; the hospice program did not provide workers on a few shifts, but the daughter stoically filled in the gaps in physical and emotional care.

A week after the stroke took place, the daughter called to tell the GCM that her mother had died the previous night. The daughter said the experience had been perfect; it was beautiful to be alone with her mother. She had gone out with friends for dinner and came home relaxed. She sat on the floor and spoke to her mother.

> I told her gently that she was dying—that she had been sick since Monday and now it was Friday. I talked about all her accomplishments, how everyone admired her, including her home care workers. I told her I loved her and that I knew how much she loved me. It was an exquisite moment. I went on to say that I knew that she didn't believe in heaven but suggested that if it were possible that there is a heaven, then perhaps mother could meet and continue her discussions with Roger [a family friend] in heaven.

Mrs. N was very deaf, very ill, and cognitively impaired and her daughter was not sure she had heard her. But Mrs. N smiled, took a few breaths, and then stopped breathing. The GCM said it was wonderful that the daughter could be so present to her mother. The daughter said that she did not feel guilty but perfectly at peace.

Initially, Mrs. N's daughter had great difficulty providing care for her mother because her mother resisted it. Over time, with the support and encouragement of the GCM, she was able to help her mother come to accept the help she needed, while the daughter did what she found possible. Despite her sadness at her mother's earlier emotional unavailability, the daughter was able to care for her mother consistently or use the GCM when she was not able to do so. She was able to help her mother die by being present to her both physically and emotionally, acknowledging her life's gifts and enabling her mother to leave her life with good feelings about herself and her daughter, and with hope for the future. The GCM's support, acknowledgment of the daughter's feelings throughout the difficult caretaking period, and help in providing the daughter with home care assistance and the GCM's presence when needed were all important to the daughter. The daughter was able to rise above her ambivalent feelings and provide care and nurturing to her mother in a loving manner. The GCM witnessed the daughter's inner resources and strength as her mother died and supported all the daughter did for her mother. By being present to their clients' struggles and providing emotional support and concrete assistance, GCMs can help people solidify their own authority to care for their parents.

Ways to Affirm Clients' Spiritual Needs

There are seven ways that GCMs can affirm clients' spiritual needs.

- GCMs can develop a trusting relationship with clients and help them feel safe to express their suffering. Being present to their pain helps clients feel cared for, valued, and respected.
- GCMs can be open to the meaning of illness and loss and to their clients' view of the world.
- GCMs can help clients view themselves beyond just their roles (e.g., father, wife).
- GCMs can talk with clients about clients' beliefs and what has brought meaning to their lives.
- GCMs can appreciate clients' life stories and acknowledge their strengths, struggles, triumphs, and losses.
- GCMs can respect clients' agenda, words, and ways of doing things.[23]
- GCMs can be open to learning from clients and interactions with them, being open-minded and nonjudgmental.[23]

■ FACILITATING SPIRITUAL CONNECTIONS WITH PEOPLE WHO HAVE DEMENTIA AND THEIR FAMILIES

How do GCMs overcome society's negative attitudes toward people with dementia and treat impaired clients with dignity and value, maintaining a person-centered approach? One way is to empathize with the frustrations of clients, whose symptoms will vary over the course of the illness. They will experience changes in their ability to do everyday tasks and will have to abandon work and familiar activities. They may have difficulty communicating and expressing their wishes clearly, have changes in personality and mood, and lack initiative. All these changes can lead to feelings of anger, frustration, fearfulness, anxiety, and sadness. "Living with Alzheimers means living in a world of fragments. There is a lack of connection. How did I get here? What am I supposed to do next?"[24]

To preserve the humanity of persons who have lost what this culture considers the defining quality of human beings—the ability to think and reason—GCMs need to move to an ethos of care based upon the emotional and relational qualities of human life.[25] GCMs are able to experience the person with dementia without having the emotions of the family, who have witnessed the changes in functioning of the person. In addition to listening to caregivers discuss their difficulties, the GCM should find out what the person's past interests, activities, and roles were and what has changed. What are the person's remaining cognitive abilities, and what does he or she like to do now? Listen to music? Take walks? The caregivers and friends can provide information on the client's values, such as working hard or caring for family members, as well as his or her life story. This helps the GCM better understand the person and be sensitive to the client's values and traditions.

It is important to understand each client's needs and to help the client feel respected, appreciated, loved, known, and understood. Persons with dementia need a sense of belonging—to feel part of a community, to share and give love, and to be productive, helpful, and useful. Because those with dementia lose their ability to fulfill these needs, they may feel frustrated, confused, isolated, and embarrassed.[26]

GCMs need to help clients experience positive connections with caregivers and the GCM. It is important for the GCM to be patient, sensitive, responsive, caring, encouraging, enabling, and empowering in his or her work and to serve as a model for both family and professional caregivers.

Being loved, responded to empathetically, and cared for can help the person with dementia feel more whole and provide a sense of security and peace. Bell and Troxel elucidate a positive and interpersonal approach in working with people with dementia and their families.[26]

Improving Spiritual Connections

In helping persons with dementia experience spiritual connections, it is important to have an idea about their traditions and bring familiar rituals to them to broaden their connections and sense of well-being. For persons with Alzheimer's, familiar symbols of faith connect with the heart rather than the intellect. The emotional or sensory aspects of spirituality take on a greater significance. "Music, hymns, prayers, familiar bible passages and rituals learned early in childhood can reach people with dementia and become a way to express themselves and receive comfort."[27(p2)] GCMs should ask clients and families what these familiar aspects of spirituality might be. "Touch, pictures, poetry, music and faith symbols can be used to communicate in individual contacts and in communal worship."[27(p2)] Clients may respond by joining in or showing nonverbal responses such as nodding, tapping a finger, or moving their body. Rituals of faith are usually learned early in life and can be part of a lifetime of religious practice. "Because they do not completely depend on the intellect they reach emotional levels and tap earlier memory which can connect the client to his past."[27(p2)]

If the client is religious, going to a church or synagogue or otherwise participating in a religious community can help the client feel God's presence as a reassuring haven of stability. It can also provide spiritual assurance that the client is worth more than just his or her cognitive capacity and offer hope to overcome fears about diminished capacity and the uncontrollable. For those without a specific faith tradition or belief system, spiritual needs may be addressed in other ways, such as sharing a sunset, listening to music, holding hands, praying together, or watching services on television.

Improving Family Connections

There are practical, emotional, and spiritual components to working with families whose relatives have dementia. In the following example, a GCM helps some adult children through the various stages of their father's illness and an adult daughter is able to experience her father in a holistic frame, beyond just his illness.

CASE STUDY

Mr. K

A GCM was contacted by the daughter of a 93-year-old man who had dementia, Mr. K. She lived out of town and needed assistance in providing care for her father. Her stepsister lived near her father. The GCM's relationship with the K family spanned 5 years. During this period, the GCM met regularly with the daughters on a schedule that fit into their visits with the father. She focused on understanding how the experience of dementia affected them and helped them listen to each other's perspectives. The GCM encouraged discussion about Mr. K's changed functioning, his forgetfulness, and his intermittent confusion. She encouraged them to reflect on the changes in his behavior, to share their feelings, to empathize with each other, and to work together. The GCM shared information about dementia with the daughters, acknowledging the changes they experienced and recommending books, tapes, and educational meetings to them. She encouraged the daughters to seek support from their partners and friends.

The GCM helped the daughters grieve over losses in their father's functioning while remaining receptive to Mr. K's remaining ability to share his love, his point of view, and his sense of humor. His daughters shared their good experiences in taking him to the ballet, watching him enjoy art shows, and helping with his care. They continued to share a warm and loving relationship with him.

The GCM engaged the daughters in discussions along the continuum of care from 8 hours a day to two 12-hour shifts of care. The daughters thought a day care program would be helpful for their father. The GCM helped Mr. K get accepted into a day care program that he enjoyed and that provided stimulation for him and oversight of his home attendants. The GCM helped the daughters plan in small steps care for the future, arranging visits to facilities and helping them decide to have the father remain in his home unless it was medically necessary to transfer him to a nursing home. The GCM visited Mr. K and his caregivers and oversaw his care. She provided feedback to his daughters on a regular basis.

Mr. K died peacefully in his home at the age of 98. The tribute that his daughter wrote to him after his death speaks of her love, care, and spiritual growth and the importance of her connection to her father. In this poem she recognizes the contribution her father made as an artist and as a communist: his struggle to make art accessible to the people and for a living wage for artists.

Were you kidding around with me or was
*   this for real?*
I found this both disturbing and amusing
I struggled to make sense of what was
*   happening*
You didn't know who I was?

I began to feel like I was your memory
you were 93 years old, the main man in
*   my life*

*we were kindred spirits, though we were
      separated by 59 years
and you were always there when I got home
      from school*

*Your loss of memory coincided with the
      collapse of the Soviet Union.
I was careful to protect you from knowing that
      your cherished system was crumbling*

*I wondered if you lost your cognitive
      memory to spare yourself the
pain of watching the capitalist class
      toot its triumphant horn
I remind myself that you were 23 when the
      Russian revolution shook
the world up, and you with it.*

*Your loss of memory coming as it does in
      the middle of these celebrations
makes me feel like the context of my youth
      is slipping away
I rush to remember the historic moments
      that became family mantras
the Spanish civil war, the state murder of
      Ethel and Julius Rosenberg
the FBI's witchhunt against communists,
      gay people and labor unions*

*Have I now become a messenger of this
      history that you no longer remember?*

*As you aged, body connection became our
      major communicator.
It was difficult to watch you lose your memory
one of my mirrors was gone
but like you I am learning to be in the moment
not lacking history but assuming it
At some point I stopped reminding you that
      I was your daughter
Our relationship had been transformed by
      your loss of memory
we just were
Because of you I now understand that
      memory is most importantly
about our bodies and our hearts.
without these we cannot do justice to
      our histories*

*Your memory of the struggle was
      embedded in your body and in
      your heart
but the details were gone*

*You had a physical and emotional memory
      of justice and fundamental truth
You had an emotional essence
You were an essence in your stillness
You are the essence of Harry. That's what
      I get:
little fleeting moments of the essence of Harry.
It is a different way of seeing the world and
      I take it as a gift.[28]*

This daughter's experience of her father throughout her life as a wonderful caregiver helped her value the positive connections between them that continued despite his dementia.

GCMs' work with families whose relatives have dementia challenges GCMs to help families go beyond grief to find the positive in the situation. The GCM can help the family shift their expectations of their relative, see their relative beyond the dementia, accept the situation, and live in the present. The family member can try to appreciate the relative's deeper values and the values of mutuality and caring throughout the life cycle. GCMs can encourage family members to draw on their inner strength and spiritual resources. Family members can think about how their parent cared for them or how they wish they were cared for. In being fully present to family members, GCMs can help them shift to being present to their relative, as they resolve their grief. Dementia offers persons the opportunity to treasure the moments they share together and live more fully in the present.

■ CONCLUSION

By incorporating a spiritual perspective, GCMs can be a resource in building compassionate communities of care. This perspective broadens the GCM's scope in working with chronically ill and elderly clients and their families in an attempt to help them find meaning and value in their lives.

By viewing the client's frailty as a potentially meaningful part of life, the GCM can share with the client the contributions he or she has made and continues to make. In reviewing his or her own values and spiritual beliefs, the GCM can discern the differences between personal values and client values and be open to and interested in the diverse ways clients find meaning in their lives.

As delineated in this chapter, the spiritual process can be facilitated in many different ways. It is important to enable family members and caregivers to experience the client's spirit beyond his or her illness, and encourage the client to share personal spiritual resources by valuing him or her, carrying out rituals, and being present to the client. In this way, the client's sense of connection to himself or herself, the community, and God can be enhanced.

■ NOTES

1. Atchley B. Atchley on aging and spiritual growth. In: Seeber J, ed. *American Society on Aging, Forum on Religion and Spirituality.* 1998;10:6.

2. National Interfaith Coalition on Aging. Spiritual well being: a definition. Presented at: National Interfaith Coalition on Aging; 1975; Athens, GA.

3. Jung C. *Modern Man in Search of Soul.* New York: Harcourt Brace; 1933.

4. Schachter-Shalomi Z, Miller R, eds. *From Ageing to Sage-ing: A Profound New Vision of Growing Older.* New York: Time Warner; 1995.

5. Kenyon GM. Aging and possibilities for being. *Aging and the Human Spirit.* 1992;2:4–5.

6. Leder D. *Spiritual Passages: Embracing Life's Sacred Journey.* New York: Tarcher/Putnam; 1997.

7. Thibault JM. Review of spiritual passages: embracing life's sacred journey. *Aging and the Human Spirit.* 1997;7:9.

8. Magid S. Wrestling with despair: a Jewish response to worry and depression. Presented by the Drisha Institute and the National Center for Jewish Healing; June 14, 1998; New York.

9. Emerson RW. *Essays: First Series.* 1841 New York: Thomas Y Crowell Company; 1926.

10. Atchley RC. The continuity of the spiritual self. In: Kimble MA, McFadden SH, Ellor JW, Seeber J, eds. *Aging, Spirituality and Religion.* Minneapolis, MN: Fortress Press; 1995:68–73.

11. Moberg DO. Spiritual well-being defined. In: Ellor JW, ed. *American Society on Aging, Forum on Religion and Spirituality.*1997:2–3.

12. Genevay B, Richards M. Spiritual growth and psychological development: a concurrent path as we age. *Aging and Spirituality.* 1997;9:4–5.

13. Frankl VD. *Man's Search for Meaning.* Boston, MA: Beacon Press; 1959.

14. Chinen AB. *In the Ever After: Fairy Tales and the Second Half of Life.* Wilmette, IL: Chiron Publications; 1989.

15. Williams CC. Explorers without a map: charting a course to value and meaning. Presented at: American Society on Aging Annual Conference; 1998; San Francisco, CA.

16. Young-Eisendrath P. *The Resilient Spirit: Transforming Suffering into Insight and Renewal.* Reading, MA: Addison Wesley; 1996.

17. Snorton TE. From struggles, dilemmas, and events in ages past. *Aging and Spirituality.* 1995;7:3.

18. Riemer J. *So That Your Values Live On: Ethical Wills and How to Prepare Them.* Woodstock, VT: Jewish Lights Publishing; 1991.

19. Alzheimer's Association, National Alliance for Caregiving. *Who Cares? Families Caring for Persons with Alzheimer's Disease.* Washington, DC: Alzheimer's Association, National Alliance for Caregiving; 1999.

20. Personal communication with Marty Richards, 1999.

21. Genevay B, Katz RS. *Countertransference and Older Clients.* Newburg Park, CA: Sage Publications; 1990.

22. Fitchett G. *Assessing Spiritual Needs. A Guide for Caregivers.* MN: Augsburg Fortress; 1992.

23. Simon D. Healing and the spirit: tapping spiritual resources to facilitate a more positive experience of life's final stage. Presented at: American Society on Aging, Summer Series; July 1998; New York.

24. Gwyther L. Helping congregations maintain a connection to spirit in the Alzheimer's disease experience. Presented at: Annual Meeting of the American Society on Aging; March 1999; Orlando, FL.

25. Post SG. *The Moral Challenge of Alzheimer Disease.* Baltimore, MD: Johns Hopkins University Press; 1995.

26. Bell V, Troxel D. *The Best Friends Approach to Alzheimer's Care.* Baltimore, MD: Health Professionals Press; 1997.

27. Richards M. Meeting the spiritual needs of the cognitively impaired. *Aging and Spirituality.* 1994;7:2.

28. Gottlieb A. In Living Memory [videotape]. Toronto, Ontario: VTape; 1997

Chapter 15

The Geriatric Care Manager and Family Caregivers of Frail Elders

Miriam K. Aronson

■ BACKGROUND

Family caregiving is the backbone of the American system of long-term care for the elderly and disabled. Today, it is estimated that approximately 44 million adults provide unpaid assistance and support for their relatives and friends, with an attributed economic value of $257 billion annually, a staggering figure that exceeds the combined costs of nursing home care ($92 billion) and home health care ($32 billion).[1] Those who provide this unpaid assistance are generally referred to as "informal" caregivers, in contrast to paid agency or private caregivers, who are the "formal" caregivers.

More elders are alive today than at any other time in history, and the numbers are growing. Advances in public health and medical management of acute and chronic diseases have contributed to increased longevity and the "graying" of the population. With the fastest-growing population segment being those who are over 85 years, a vulnerable group with greater needs for health care, the pressures on the acute and long-term care systems are escalating both logistically and fiscally and generating societal concerns. The nature and scope of caregiving has been changing. On average, chronically ill and disabled recipients of informal care were older and more disabled in 1999 than 1989.[2]

The development and expansion of the Medicare and Medicaid programs over the last 40 years have provided greater access to health care for the elderly and the disabled and support for nursing homes and other long-term care services. However, over the past two decades, there has been a shift from institutional care to more community-based and home health care. Medical advances and the greater availability of home care technology have dramatically shortened hospital stays and thus shifted the responsibility and many of the costs for posthospital management from paid institutional health care workers to family members in the home. Although at-home care is the preference of many people, there is little infrastructure to support it and most of this care is provided by family members.

Given the dramatic increase in the numbers of frail elders, their needs for care, and the budgetary constraints of public and private insurance programs and other funding sources, the role of the family in providing long-term care will inevitably increase. With this increase in needs for care, there will come increasing needs of caregivers for information, education, guidance, and emotional support and more public and private providers to deliver these services. Geriatric care managers (GCMs) have an important role in providing these services for caregivers.

Family structures today are more diverse than ever before: in addition to the traditional nuclear family, there are single-parent families, homosexual families, blended families, and grandparents raising grandchildren. Most women are in the work force, seeking a better life for their families and themselves. This is a sharp departure from prior generations when women were at home and available to provide child care and, when necessary, parent care. In blended families, which result from remarriage after divorce or widowhood, there are often increased numbers of parents and grandparents.

Family caregiving is fraught with dilemmas. New roles and responsibilities are acquired—often unexpectedly—with no job descriptions, little preparation, and few, if any, role models. The caregiving duties are heaped upon already full plates of work, family, and personal responsibilities. For many individuals, caregiving is a long-term commitment, often lasting years—so long, in fact, that gerontologists speak of the "caregiving career." The average woman today will spend more years providing parent care than she did child care.

This caregiving is not without substantial costs. There are adverse physical, emotional, and social effects.[3] In fact, research has revealed that caregivers experience excess morbidity and mortality. They develop stress-related illnesses. Depression is prevalent among them. They also suffer shrinking social networks. And there are consequences in the workplace—time lost, opportunities missed for advancement, and economic losses in terms of earnings, benefits, and pensions. These economic impacts will also have repercussions for the caregiver's own later years.

Untrained, undersupported, and emotionally stressed, family caregivers may, paradoxically, also negatively affect their frail elder's well-being. Whether intentionally or inadvertently, the care they provide may be inadequate. Overburdened or burned out caregivers may become neglectful or even abusive to their care recipient.

■ WHO IS THE FAMILY CAREGIVER?

Generally, the family caregiver is a spouse, partner, child, or other relative who provides a range of assistance for an elderly or disabled person. Typically, the family caregiver is a "dutiful daughter or daughter-in-law," but men are becoming increasingly involved. For some individuals (about 20%), friends and neighbors fulfill this role. These "informal caregivers" may provide care in conjunction with others, paid or unpaid, and may live with or apart from the individual receiving care, that is, the care recipient. The caregiver is often self-defined or identified by the care recipient, but, in fact, even this is not so clear-cut. Factors such as differing family structures, estrangement, conflict, burnout, illness, disability, competition for being "the best child," differing values, and unrealistic notions of the care recipient or caregiver are factors that may affect the actual caregiving situation.

■ THE GCM AND THE FAMILY

First, the care recipient should be assessed to identify needs and wants. In assessing the caregiving situation, the GCM must get an accurate assessment of the care recipient regarding his or her strengths and challenges, ascertain diagnoses and prognosis and projected time frames for changes, identify prominent personality traits, screen for cognitive impairment, screen for depression, observe her or him in the home as regards lifestyle and functioning, and discuss expectations, wishes, values, and beliefs. Ask about what assistance or services the client thinks he or she needs (see Exhibit 15–1).

The GCM must also query the financial status, including income, assets, benefits currently being received, health and long-term care insurance coverage, and eligibility or potential eligibility for entitlement programs. Ask about family and the support network, present and potential caregivers, and cultural variables. The typology of caregiving situa-

Exhibit 15-1   Types of Assistance the Care Recipient Wants/Needs

	Indicate Yes or No	
	Elder	Caregiver
Shopping		
Socialization/Companionship		
Errands		
Transportation		
Household Maintenance/Chores		
Assistance with Money Management		
Housekeeping (cleaning, laundry, meal preparation)		
Supervision for Safety		
Assistance with Medications		
Assistance with Personal Care		
Advocacy		
Other		

tions varies and includes the frail elder living alone in his or her own home or with a paid caregiver, living with a helpful spouse or partner, living with a difficult spouse, having cooperative and supportive children, having fighting children, having alienated children, having fighting children and stepchildren, having several children but only one child who "does it all," living in a facility with positive family involvement, or living in a facility with little or no family participation. And, within every context, different families may have varying levels of functionality.

It would be beneficial to have a reliable informant present at the initial assessment to corroborate the information. Getting a comprehensive picture is often a multistep process. The individual with cognitive impairment may not be an accurate historian. The frail individual may have relinquished certain responsibilities to family or friends and may not have an accurate grasp of the current situation. Or, the individual may be wary of the GCM. It may take time to develop rapport. In most cases, the information may have to be pieced together from a number of sources: the elder, family members, available documents, neighbors, friends, and physicians, and this may be a multistep process. Although the family caregiver(s) may be an important part of the assessment of the care recipient, it would be desirable to assess the caregiver(s) separately, in addition.

■ FAMILY MEETINGS

A family meeting may be a desirable first step in the process; however, there are a number of logistical issues in setting this up. The objective here is not the form, but rather the substance. The goals of the family conference are to establish a dialogue with the family caregivers, share information, identify needed interventions, and begin to develop a care plan that may include care by both informal (family providers) and paid care providers. There is no single approach but rather a good deal of heterogeneity to contend with. There are a variety of care recipients and caregivers, different beliefs and values, conflicting needs and wants, differing circumstances, and myriad issues, including autonomy, control, risk taking, resistance, denial, and financial considerations and constraints. The range of personalities and capabilities must also be factored in. Further, it is desirable to include long-distance caregivers in the discussions, whenever possible. Conference calls can be very useful to get everyone on the same page.

Following are a few case illustrations.

CASE STUDY

Ms. G: I'm the Client and I'll Do It My Way

Ms. G, a cognitively intact, feisty, 80-year-old widow living alone, developed serious mobility issues and lost her ability to function without help in her two-story home. She now had to depend on her son and daughter-in-law, with whom there was a long-standing estrangement, and her neighbors and acquaintances to help her. She tried to hold it together with informal care, but found her life becoming very constricted. Despite this reality, which she verbalized easily, she refused to spend money on help when she had "so many friends." In reality, she resented her friends' help "because they kept telling her what to do." Her extended family did not live nearby and did not provide any hands-on assistance. Frustrated by her pain and diminished mobility, Ms. G began toying with the idea of moving to a nearby senior living facility.

When Ms. G mentioned this to a cousin in a telephone conversation, the cousin suggested that she consult a GCM to help find the best arrangement. The relative located and screened a GCM and Ms. G agreed to an in-home consultation. Although she did have folders of her personal and financial information on her kitchen table, she was very sparing with the information she shared. The GCM's first impression was that, aside

from the equity in her home, the client had modest means. However, as the GCM was preparing to leave, Ms. G added: "By the way, I do have long-term care insurance. . . .And I have these investments that I've left sitting in a brokerage account for years." It quickly became apparent that the first impression was not accurate. Between her pension, Social Security, interest income, and long-term care insurance, this individual had the resources to support herself in a facility of her choice for years to come.

After assessing the client and having several telephone conversations with her family and physicians, the GCM assisted with the development of a care plan. Although it was suggested that live-in home care would be a viable option for her, the client rejected this unequivocally. She wanted to enter an assisted living facility. Previously, she had gone to tour a new facility and had visited neighbors and friends who moved there. The GCM escorted the client to visit several facilities and helped her make an appropriate choice. She chose to have a trial respite admission before committing to a permanent stay. The GCM coordinated the needed medical and nursing assessments and clearances and documentation for the long-term care insurance carrier. She also helped mobilize the concrete assistance that would be needed for the move, made arrangements to maintain the house intact while Ms. G was to be gone, and accompanied Ms. G on the day of admission. All the while, the GCM and client were dealing with her anger at her son for not being there, her anxiety about the move, her disappointment about her physical limitations, and her fears for the future (see Chapter 16 on GCMs and relocation).

With the consent (and, in fact, encouragement) of the client, the GCM maintained contact with her son and daughter-in-law, who gradually became more active in helping the client with the permanent move, began visiting more often, and were trying to repair their relationship.

Although Ms. G was physically disabled, she was capable of her own decision making and wanted to be in charge of her life. Even though there was not a warm relationship with her son and daughter-in-law, they were very aware of her wishes, her capacity, and her style and were much relieved when she finally decided to move into assisted living. There was no family conflict over her decision. Rather, it was Ms. G who didn't want to relinquish the status quo, even though it no longer served her needs.

Sometimes, frail individuals struggle to maintain their lifestyle long beyond its appropriateness and resist attempts by their loved ones to help them get the assistance they require. They manage to put up barriers to intervention, and, at least in the short term, the family members often back down, as in the case of Mr. M.

CASE STUDY

Mr. M: I'll Do It Myself

Mr. M, a 92-year-old retired entrepreneur, widowed for 10 years, lives alone in a well-appointed apartment in an elevator building with a doorman, near his very involved daughter and son-in-law. Over the last few years, Mr. M's health has been failing. He has a heart arrhythmia, congestive heart failure, diabetes, and mild cognitive impairment. He voluntarily stopped driving about three years ago. His walking is slow and, at times, unsteady—he refuses to use a walker or any other assistive device. His short-term memory is "shot" and his judgment and safety awareness are compromised. On multiple medications, including blood pressure medications, heart medications, a diabetes drug, and an anticoagulant to prevent blood clots, his daughter sets them up weekly and he self-administers them. He requires frequent monitoring of the blood levels of the anticoagulant, regular physician visits, and self-measurement of his blood sugar daily. His daughter, employed full time, takes him to his medical visits, calls daily, and visits frequently. A food market, pharmacy, and diner are within easy walking distance and all have a delivery service. He has a Personal Emergency Response System with a wristband activator, but "would rather call his family than use it." He writes his own checks and uses a charge card for ordinary expenses, but his son-in-law manages his assets.

Mr. M is still saving for his old age. "You never know when you're going to need care." At this time, he refuses to acknowledge his vulnerability and will not even consider getting some part-time in-home assistance, insisting that he can do everything himself. When his daughter suggests that a little help would be a good thing, he becomes angry and hostile and threatens to "fire anybody she sends." As concerned as she is, she becomes derailed by his threats.

The GCM assessed Mr. M and concluded that, because of his multiple medical conditions and medications, his cognitive impairment, his gait instability, his diminished safety awareness, and his social isolation, he is at risk for exacerbation of his chronic health problems, medication errors, compromised nutrition and falling, and would benefit from assistance with shopping, food preparation, medication management, escorting to medical appointments, and increased socialization.

Here, there is a disparity between the needs of the elder for care and his desire for autonomy. Concerned about her father's vulnerability, the daughter says she would like to be proactive; however, she is reluctant to assert any authority: "I just can't act like his mother. I'm worried about his quality of life. I don't want to make an invalid of him or he'll give up." She has chosen to be reactive to the next crisis, rather than proactive in trying to prevent it.

In the following case, there is a disparity between the needs and wants of both elders, as well as those of their caregiving children. The situation is complex because both the care recipient and the nominal caregiver are ill.

Mr. and Mrs. K: Willing to Accept only Family Assistance

Retired professionals in their seventies, Mr. and Mrs. K reside in a single-family suburban home. Mr. K, previously the dominant member of the couple, developed dementia and became increasingly dependent on his wife for his daily activities. With this role reversal, Mrs. K became quite controlling. Recently diagnosed with breast cancer, requiring surgery, radiation, and chemotherapy, Mrs. K denied having any pain or disability and continued "business as usual"—doing everything for her husband, maintaining the home, performing her volunteer activities, and taking him everywhere with her. Resistant to bathing, grooming, and changing his clothes, he was difficult for her to manage; however, she absolutely refused to hire a health care aide or seek other assistance, insisting "he doesn't want me to. And we really don't need any help." She allows him to walk around with stained clothes and messy hair, explaining, "I was never much of a homemaker anyway." Rather, she expects—or demands—that her son, a hardworking professional with a young family of his own, come after work twice a week to do his father's personal care and that her daughter, also with full-time employment and young children, drive an hour each way twice every week to bring groceries and prepared food. These adult children choose to meet their mother's hard-to-comply-with demands. They both are disappointed with their mother's denial and are embarrassed by the inadequate care their father is receiving, but stand by. Both fear the time when either parent will become more ill and require more assistance than they themselves can provide.

They consult a GCM, who meets with them and their mother and makes a home visit to assess the parents' situation. Interim steps are suggested, including hiring a part-time home health aide and enrolling Mr. K in a couple of days of social day care, to gradually introduce outside help, provide respite for Mrs. K, and encourage some independent socialization. Mrs. K summarily rejects this and things remain status quo.

The role of the GCM here was to assess the care recipients and caregivers, evaluate the current situation, discuss their concerns, educate them about available resources, and help the family develop a care plan that incorporates introduction of some formal caregiving assistance. Mrs. K is controlling and stubbornly resistant, and the children choose to maintain peace between themselves and their mother "for as long as the situation does not get any worse." They are planning, however, to "insist" that their parents obtain paid caregiving assistance when the next crisis arises. Sometimes, the unrealistic notions of the care recipient or caregiver prevail and it takes a dramatic change in circumstances to appropriately address their needs for assistance.

■ ABUSE AND NEGLECT

The stubborn, entrenched vulnerable elder may become insulting and even abusive to the family caregiver, who is attempting to help him or her. Rather than providing positive feedback, the elder may accuse the relative of thinking the person is crazy, wanting the person's money, wanting to hurt the person, wanting to take the person's decision-making power away, wanting to put the person away, or a whole litany of other alleged injustices and adverse outcomes. Elders may call their previously dear relative all kinds of horrific names. They may threaten to call the police, get a lawyer, take the relative to court, or write them out of the Will. They may complain vociferously to neighbors or friends, thus embarrassing and humiliating the willing caregiver. They may be so steadfast in their resistance to care that the family caregiver chooses to retreat, often with guilt, shame, and worry. And with this self-imposed lack of attention, the elder can become neglected.

Neglect is a form of abuse. And self-neglect, an elder who refuses to access needed services or care to remediate problems, is the most common reason for referral to a state protective services agency.[4]

Another scenario is abuse between caregiver and care recipient. This can flow both ways—the care recipient verbally abusing the caregiver or being physically combative; or the caregiver's losing patience with the difficult elder and abusing him or her. This can occur with informal and formal caregivers. The important message here is that abuse is abuse and elder abuse is against the law and reportable to the authorities, so it is best to try to intervene before abuse occurs.

Abuse and neglect are more likely when there is a history of mental illness or substance abuse in caregiver or care recipient, when the caregiver is financially dependent on the care recipient, when there is a prior history of abuse, or when the elder is of an advanced age or cognitively impaired.[5]

■ DOCUMENTS AND EMPOWERMENT OF CAREGIVERS

There may or may not be empowering documents such as a power of attorney or a health care proxy. Where these documents do exist, it is a good idea for the GCM to ask the client to bring them to the consultation. These documents can help to clarify the wishes of the care recipient and help the GCM and the caregiver to craft an appropriate care plan and structure the caregiving situation.

Even when documents are available, the caregiving arrangement may be muddied for various reasons: documents may have been prepared perfunctorily by the elder, with little thought given to what kind of needs would have to be met. Or they may have been prepared years ago, when the situation of the care recipient and the designated caregiver were far different. For example, the care recipient was healthy and married and had a healthy, attentive spouse, and the appointed child caregiver lived close by. Now, that child may no longer live near the care recipient or may have become ill or undergone a change in life circumstances; the elder, given the choice, would not select the same caregiver. Or, even though the frail elder may not be managing his affairs well, he may not entirely understand the need for substituted judgment and may perceive empowering his designees as giving up control and "allowing people to do things behind my back."

It is the role of the GCM to ascertain what documents there are and provide assistance to the elder and the family in understanding and implementing them; or, when appropriate, to assist them in locating legal counsel to make desired modifications or additions. Where there are no documents and the elder is no longer able to express his or her wishes, the GCM will counsel the family on available options under these circumstances. When there are documents but there is also conflict, it is important that the GCM abides by the documentation.

CASE STUDY

The Case of Mr. F: The Man in the Middle
Shortly after his wife's death, Mr. F, a 70-year-old widower with a daughter and a son, met a woman, who quickly became his significant other. Although they weren't officially living together, they were together most of the time. They had a lot of common interests, traveled extensively, and developed an active social life. Although his children were "not crazy about her," they deferred to his wishes and included her in family activities. However, early in the relationship, fearing that the friend was "after his money," the children convinced their father to take legal steps to protect his assets and their financial interests.

After a few years of a tenuous truce among himself, the friend, and the children, things began to change: he developed dementia and began to require supervision and assistance with bill paying, decision making, and managing his medical care. Essentially, because she was geographically the most available, the friend managed his medical care—arranging for and escorting him to medical appointments, which she has been doing without any legal documentation. While she is the de facto caregiver, the children are the power of attorney and health care proxy and do the bill paying and financial management.

Now that Mr. F is no longer able to control his interpersonal situation, the level of conflict is escalating: the friend wants a better defined social and financial role and more formal control. The children are wary and want to take an increased role themselves, although they do not have much time available to pitch in. They really want to introduce some paid caregivers. The father is in the middle, becoming increasingly anxious and even paranoid at times. The children report that the friend has started to decrease the amount of time she spends with Mr. F as his needs are increasing, and he is often left home alone and unsupervised. They are concerned about his safety and quality of life. The children and Mr. F consult a GCM.

Here, the role of the GCM is to assess the situation and find out what the client's abilities and challenges and wants and needs are; determine the role, availability, capability, and willingness of each of the present and potential caregivers—the significant other and the children—examine the power of attorney, health care proxy, and other documents; and help to structure or restructure the current caregiving arrangements.

The father's dementia was moderate with deficits in prioritizing, decision making, and managing instrumental activities of daily living. He was able to do his own personal care, but was losing weight because of difficulties with meal preparation and there had been medication errors with adverse consequences. He was also socially isolated when his friend was not there to go with him to activities. He was still driving his car and emphatically wanting to continue, no matter what anyone thought.

The GCM provided information and education for the family about the dementia and also about the potential resources in the community. Given the level of conflict in this case, the GCM encouraged the client and family to seek additional consultation from the lawyers involved in the case and to make sure that the documentation is consistent with the wishes of the client and will remain so with the progressive nature of his dementia and his changing needs.

After the meeting, more information was still needed. The GCM was unable to ascertain the client's wishes, because he indicated at times that he wanted his friend to move in and take care of him, and at other times in the discussion, he seemed to contradict himself. He did clearly state that he wanted the GCM to work with him. It was also enigmatic that the friend had cut down on her amount of involvement, while allegedly professing to want more. The GCM requested a subsequent meeting with all the caregivers (the family and the friend) to try to clarify their roles and expectations before a plan could be discussed. The level of intrafamily conflict here is problematic, and Mr. F is caught in the middle. The GCM will try to help the parties involved understand the problematic dynamics and encourage them to work toward resolving them.

The elder's preparing legal documents when he or she is capable of making sound decisions for his own well-being is a good strategy for avoiding, or at least minimizing, conflict and, hopefully, avoiding court proceedings. Where no documents have been prepared and an individual's decision-making abilities become impaired, such as by dementia, stroke, head injury, or other situation, it may become necessary for conservatorship or guardianship proceedings, to enable a family member or designated other to access the elder's resources for care. Although the court orders empower the designee to make the needed transactions, they do not always ease the tension when

there is lack of insight or paranoia. Such was the case of Mr. A.

CASE STUDY

Mr. A: I Want My Money

Mr. A, an 80-year-old widower with Alzheimer's disease, had only one son, whom he professed to trust and to love, but for whom he would sign no documents granting access to any of his bank and brokerage accounts or real estate. When Mr. A was scammed by a "friend he met on the street," the son decided it was time to step in and limit his father's vulnerability. Because Mr. A would not sign anything or relinquish any financial control, the son applied for a conservatorship, which was granted by the court. However, Mr. A could not understand this change in circumstances, in spite of repeated explanations. Although his son paid his bills and provided him with cash as he needed it, Mr. A would go to the bank and demand his money. When the bank personnel refused his request, he would have a catastrophic reaction, for which police intervention was sought by the bank on several occasions.

■ ASSESSING THE CAREGIVER

Although caregivers are the backbone of the long-term care system, many are also the invisible or hidden victims, too. Assessing the caregivers, present and potential, is an important step in developing an infrastructure that will support and assist them in caring effectively for their relative and continuing to care, while preventing adverse consequences for themselves. Caregiver assessment is not a single activity—it is not an end, but a means to an end: good care. It is also a dynamic and ongoing process, because needs of both the care recipient and caregiver are subject to change over time.

The caregiver assessment may occur as part of a family conference, a consultation with the family member and care recipient, or as a separate structured interview. Ideally, it will occur in a person-to-person meeting, but if not, the telephone may be the next best thing. E-mail can be an adjunct but not a substitute. A good assessment includes assessment of attitude and verbal and nonverbal communication. Questions should be open-ended and answers should be probed further, as indicated. Of special concern are a history of mental illness or substance abuse, financial dependency on the care recipient, lack of knowledge about care recipient's condition, and values and beliefs that are divergent from those of the elder. Suggested information to query is contained in Exhibit 15-2.

■ ONGOING ASSESSMENT: CHANGING NEEDS AND SITUATIONS

There should be a caregiver assessment at the time of the initial assessment of the care recipient and probably at least semiannually thereafter; however, this is only a guideline. Additional assessment will be necessary with the change of condition of the care recipient or the caregiver. Changes in the care recipient can include worsening of physical symptoms, needs for additional care such as necessitated by a catheter or a feeding tube, changes in medication schedule, resistance to care, changes in activities of daily living (incontinence, loss of mobility, inability to feed him/herself, difficulty swallowing), development of depression, or development or escalation of behavior problems. Hospitalization or moving from one residence to another often triggers changes in condition. Alterations in the caregiver's situation and availability may include changes in health, changes in financial status, marriage, divorce, illness, depression, surgery, job promotion or demotion, unemployment, moving to another area, illness of partner, or illness of a grandchild.

Assessing the Caregiver

Except for a few states that have tools for public eldercare programs that include questions about caregivers, there are no standardized assessment tools available at this writing. Most of the questions should be qualitative as suggested earlier and in Exhibit 15-2. In addition to the interview, the GCM may choose to

Exhibit 15-2   Caregiver Assessment Components

Caregiver's place of residence
Caregiver's self-described current relationship with elder
Caregiver's past relationship with elder
Caregiver's health limitations
Caregiver's family responsibilities
Caregiver's job responsibilities
    —Locale, hours, travel requirements, predictability
Caregiver's financial constraints
    —Money for phone calls, transportation, dependency on elder?
History of mental illness?
Substance abuse?
Is caregiver empowered by care recipient?
    —Health care proxy, durable power of attorney, other
What does caregiver know about care recipient's condition/illness?
Stress level expressed
Amount of burden caregiving imposes

use screening instruments such as a Depression Scale, the Zarit Burden Scale, and the Caregiving Strain Scale also. Whatever format the GCM chooses, it is essential for the GCM to be sensitive to the fact that caregivers do not see themselves as "patients," and too much probing may be a "turn off." As with the care recipient, good rapport will contribute to good assessment. (See Chapter 17 on GCMs and Normal Aging Family, and Chapter 3, on Psychosocial Assessment.)

Connecting the Caregiver and Care Recipient Assessments

Caregiving is an interactive process and requires information about both people involved. Conditions change. Situations change. The information from the care recipient assessment must always be connected to the caregiver assessment and vice versa. And, in the course of their ongoing relationship, when discussing issues involving the care recipient, the GCM should also query the state of the caregiver. Is he or she very stressed? Does he or she feel overwhelmed and unable to meet the physical or mental challenges of caring? Is the caregiver depressed? Is he or she on the verge of burnout?

When a problem is identified and a change in condition necessitates a transition, for example, from informal caregiving to addition of formal care providers or from community to institution or vice versa, the type and amount of information and support needed by the caregiver will change as well, and here is where the connection must impel action.

■ CAREGIVER COMMUNICATION

The GCM–caregiver relationship is an ongoing one and communication is an essential component. The caregiver can provide updates and additional information; share observations, thoughts, and feelings; and ask questions. During these conversations, the GCM has the opportunity to get additional assessment, provide additional information

and education, identify unmet needs, and modify the care plan, as necessary.

■ EMOTIONAL ISSUES

Caregiving is an emotion-laden experience.[6] Both care recipient and caregiver are dealing with a host of emotions, including love, anger, loss, grief, anxiety, guilt, depression, and shame. Individuals deal with these in various ways. Sometimes they are spurred into action; other times, they are immobilized by them. Sometimes, they are stoic; sometimes, their emotions spill over. The emotions of the elder and the other family members may not be in sync with each other. The GCM must monitor the emotional temperature of each and educate and intervene, as needed.

■ CAREGIVER BURNOUT

Caregiving is an intense experience and, when too intense, can result in burnout. Symptoms of burnout include feeling overwhelmed and angry, feeling that others are taking advantage, feeling alone and resentful, and being able to do less for oneself. The GCM must be tuned into the possibility that this can happen and must try to help the caregiver prevent this. Work with the caregiver involves helping the caregiver to take care of him- or herself—encouraging sharing of responsibilities, time off, time for the self, pursuit of enjoyable interests, exercise, and use of relaxation techniques. Some situations may require introduction of paid caregivers or even transition to institutional placement for their loved one.

■ GCM ROLE

Providing information and education for both family and paid caregivers is an important starting point. Not only do caregivers need to know, they also want to know how to cope with their situation and avoid as many minefields as possible. But stereotypes and misinformation abound and different caregivers—even members of the same family—may have differing beliefs. Often, the GCM needs to help them sort these out.

Informal caregivers also need encouragement and emotional support. Caregiving is a hard job and, with some elders, can be a thankless task. These elders not only don't express appreciation, but they may also accuse the caregiver of "hurting them," or "doing things behind my back," "stealing," or "free-loading." And because not all families are harmonious, siblings may be nasty to a caregiving brother or sister. Both common sense and research tell us that targeting family interaction problems and intervening will be a positive mediator of stress and burden.[7]

Some caregivers may require mental health interventions, including counseling, support groups, individual therapy, group therapy, and psychoactive medication. The GCM must be sensitive to these needs and make appropriate referrals.

Another role for the GCM is to help overcome the fragmentation and lack of coordination among service providers. The GCM can help the caregiver and care recipient cross the great divide that often exists.

Caregiving is a big job, with the nature and scope subject to change as the care recipient's condition changes. Levels of stress and burden change at different points in the continuum of care.[8] The GCM needs to work not only with the family and paid caregivers but with all other providers as well—public and private community agencies, physicians, categorical disease organizations, housing providers, lawyers, home health care agencies, hospice, clergy, and hospital, nursing home, and assisted living personnel.

Although the GCM's knowledge is broad-based and comprehensive, the GCM needs to refer clients to experts, as needed, and to communicate with the experts and incorporate their recommendations in the care plan. For example, a clinically depressed caregiver may require a psychiatric evaluation to determine the best course of treatment. Or an elder may require a lawyer to help sort out the person's situation and prepare for later disability. A long-distance caregiver may need to evaluate comparable entitlements in two different areas, and the GCM may need to consult a colleague in the other area for needed information.

GCMs also need to be advocates for the clients. They are in the best position to identify the gaps and inconsistencies in various systems and to advocate for change. They need to speak for the often invisible and underserved frail and disabled, who cannot speak for themselves.

■ CONCLUSION

Caregiving is a major health and public policy issue, affecting elders, families, and our aging society. Although informal caregivers are the backbone of the long-term care system, they are an at-risk population, needing help and support themselves to continue in this essential role. GCMs are well suited to provide services that caregivers need.

■ NOTES

1. *Caregiver Assessment: Principles, Guidelines and Strategies for Change: Report from a National Consensus Development Conference.* San Francisco, CA: Family Caregiver Alliance; 2006.

2. Wolff JL, Kasper JD. Caregivers of frail elders: a national profile. *Gerontologist.* 2006:46(3): 344–356.

3. Feinberg LF, Wolkwitz K, and Goldstein C. Ahead of the curve: emerging trends in family caregiver support. Available at: http:// www.aarp.org/caregiver. Accessed March 2006.

4. Pavlou MP, Lachs MS. Could self-neglect in older adults be a geriatric syndrome. *J Am Geriatr Soc.* 2006:54:831–842.

5. Epplin J. Identifying elder abuse in the home care setting. *Ann Long-Term Care.* 2006:14(1):15–16.

6. Aronson MK, Weiner MB. *Aging Parents, Aging Children: How to Stay Sane and Survive.* New York: Rowman & Littlefield; 2007.

7. Mitrani VB, Lewis JE, Feaster DJ, et al. The role of family functioning in the stress process of dementia caregivers: a structural family framework. *Gerontologist.* 2006:46(1):97–105.

8. Messinger-Rapport BJ, McCallum TJ, Hujer MF. Impact of dementia caregiving on the caregiver in the continuum of care. *Ann Long-Term Care.* 2006:14(1):34.

Chapter 16

Integrating Late Life Relocation: The Role of the GCM

Cathie Ramey and Cathy Jo Cress

■ THE PSYCHOLOGY OF MOVING AN OLDER PERSON

What Dorothy exclaimed after returning from Oz is the strong feeling asserted by the majority of older people over the age of 65, "There is no place like home." Most older people do not want to move and prefer to remain in their own home.

The ability to age in place—growing older without having to move—becomes an increasingly important housing issue for older Americans. A recent survey found that 83% of people between the ages of 65 and 74 years and 86% of those age 75 years and older want to remain in their own homes as they age.[1] In 2001, 80% of the 21.8 million households headed by seniors were owner occupied, and 20% were renters.[2,3]

Most older people are more likely to be homeowners and less likely to be renters. The majority of elders have a high level of attachment to their own homes. If older people move, they tend to move locally. The census data from 2002 to 2003 shows that approximately 4% of adults age 65 and older moved during that one-year time period as compared to 14% of the population as a whole.[4] So, the decision to leave the home is akin to leaving a warm, comfortable nest. The family memories are there, the familiar paths are there, a lifetime of history lies within those walls.

■ PUSH TO MOVE

There is a "push-pull" effect in play when older people and their families are considering the possibility of a move in later life.[5] The "push" is usually a crisis surrounding the older person, forcing the elder or the family to consider relocating the elder to a more supportive living environment. Examples of push effects are loss of social support, declining health, deferred home maintenance, decreasing finances, and questionable home safety. All of these factors contribute to a lessening ability to maintain an elder's existing level of function or independence in the current environment.

An example of a health "push" is a decrease in visual acuity. Perhaps the older person's vision declines to the point that he or she can no longer see well enough to prepare meals safely. The inability to access nutritious meals is also a common push factor in relocation.

Another health push arises when the lack of fit between the older adult and his or her environment begins to limit independence. An example of this is when, as the result of a fall, the older adult breaks his or her hip and can no longer negotiate steps. The resulting inability to leave the home environment or get upstairs to a bedroom limits the elder's ability to function in the outside world as well as his or her own small world. Both declining vision and limited mobility are health exigencies that may prompt thoughts of moving.

Another circumstance that pushes toward the need to move is the loss of social supports. A spouse dying and close friends or relatives moving away are common events that result in loss of social support. The rug can be pulled out from under an older person if a friend who provided companionship or transportation to appointments dies, moves to a higher level of care, or moves away. Not only does the older person lose a friend, but he or she also loses a primary source of transportation, which may in turn limit present and future social opportunities, access to medical care, and the ability to shop for food, clothing, and other necessities.

Declining physical safety often creates an urgency to move. This safety dip can be on the part of the older adult, as observed by the effects of health decrements, or in the condition of the home. Home safety concerns and deferred home maintenance often share a symbiotic relationship. Loose stair railings, leaky roofs, old furnaces, and seeping gas appliances all result from deferred home maintenance and create an unsafe living environment. If the older adult lacks the ability to access qualified home maintenance and repair services, the push to move will surface once again and a change in living environment may be considered. When the home environment is deemed no longer able to support the needs of the older adult, relocation may ensue.

Home modification has emerged as a vital resource to enable children, adults, and older adults who have mobility problems to remain in their homes.[6] Without such modifications, these individuals face the difficult choice of moving to a facility or remaining in unsafe, unsupportive environments, which do not facilitate independence or an active and participatory lifestyle.[7]

This calls into question the availability of sufficient financial resources to pay for much-needed assistance in the face of declining health or support networks. Aside from structural changes to the home, an older person's lack of ambulation may require paid caregivers. If the older person has insufficient financial resources to afford care or modify the house, this financial crisis may push an older person to consider moving.

To summarize, social support, health and functional abilities, home environment, safety, and finances are all factors affecting the degree of push an older adult or an elder's family may experience leading to the need for late-life relocation.

■ PULL TO MOVE

There is also a "pull" to move. The pull is usually not prompted by a crisis or decline but by the anticipation of an enhanced lifestyle in retirement resulting from the availability of desired social, recreational, or health opportunities. When the move occurs early in late adulthood, coinciding with retirement, it is called the "amenity move."[5] This move occurs when relocation offers an improved lifestyle or home environment for the older adult. Whether it's the pull of the vacation-style retirement community, warm weather, or reduced house payments, the amenity move pulls the older adult out of his or her existing home and into a new environment. An example of this is a 65-year-old Wyoming native who wants nicer winter weather or year-round, warm-weather recreational opportunities in Phoenix.

Another type of relocation is called the "kinship or assistance move."[5,8] This move is precipitated by the desire to live closer to family or to services to meet present or future needs. It may be similar to the situation of the elderly Stanford University alumnus who discovers the newly built senior living community adjacent to the university on the Stanford campus. By selecting this senior housing option, this elder can access the medical expertise of a world-respected hospital, enjoy the stimulating academic environment of his alma mater, plus return to a setting with familiar, pleasant memories.

Another comparable example is the pull for an older person who anticipates gradual disability in aging and thus moves into a long-term care community that offers three levels of support. These three levels include (1) independent living in a private apartment, (2) assisted living, where help with many activities of daily living (ADLs) and instrumental ADLs (IADLs) is available, and (3) skilled nursing, where, in addition to assistance with ADLs and IADLs, the older adult receives care for any health condition that requires skilled nursing care.

Family is often a pull factor for older adults. A senior may want to move closer to family for two fundamental reasons: (1) to be near children and grandchildren, and (2) in anticipation of future disability coupled with an increased sense of vulnerability. This sense of vulnerability creates a desire to be near adult children for hands-on as well as psychological support.

■ FAMILIES MAKE THE DECISION TO MOVE THE ELDERLY PERSON

When a geriatric care manager (GCM) works with an older person, it is important for the GCM to remember that most times the client entity is twofold, consisting of both the older person and the family. The family might be fragmented, dysfunctional, long distance, or around the corner; however, families and the older person usually make the decision to move together, unless totally estranged from each other or the elder is conserved.

Family is involved in the decision to relocate because the triggering event has, to a greater degree than previously experienced, drawn them into the support system of the older adult. The trigger to begin a move might be prompted by the failure of a planned support system that has kept the older person at home. This may mean that Meals on Wheels was ordered, but the older person does not like the food and is no longer eating well. If the only other perceived choice for providing support to the older adult requires home care or the adult child bringing food by, this choice may tip the balance and prompt the family to consider placement.

If caregiving for the older person has increased to a level no longer able to be met by the formal and informal support systems, relocation may be considered. For example, consider the family member who cannot cope with the need to change his incontinent mother's diapers and the only other option available is hiring paid care to cover this caregiving task. If the paid care is too expensive, placement may be the only alternative.

Another family-related trigger for placement is the lack of consistent, stable services. When the elderly parent needs increased home care and dependable paid caregivers cannot be found, the family may be left feeling overburdened and over the edge. Finally, there is another circumstance that results in the family's decision to relocate the older person: caregiver burnout. Making care arrangements, flying long distances on a regular basis to supervise care, covering shifts if they live nearby, and receiving call after call at night are all experiences that may lead directly to caregiver burnout. Like a proverbial sandwich, the family members are situated between meeting their personal and family needs and attending to the care needs of their elderly parents. (See Chapter 15 on GCMs and caregiving, and Chapter 17 on GCMs and the normal aging family.)

■ WHEN A GCM PREVENTS A MOVE

Good geriatric care management can prevent a move, in most cases. However, it may require the availability of alternative solutions to a variety of challenges, including meal preparation, home care, and ADL deficits. For example, if Meals on Wheels is rejected by the older adult who cannot prepare his or her own meals, you as the GCM might make arrangements for the older person to go to a senior center for a nutritious hot lunch each day. Additionally, if the older person is capable, you could ask a family member or a neighbor to buy a microwave and healthy microwaveable meals so the older person could prepare meals at home.

If the senior requires home care staffing and the paid caregiver staffing is not stable, you could find a new staffing agency. If the older person is incontinent and an adult day care health center is available, the older person might be placed there during the day and additional care can be arranged for nighttime.

Accommodations like these may tip the balance toward keeping the person at home because you make new arrangements and take away the burden of sorting through the vast continuum of care from the burned-out adult child.

It is important to remember, however, that in the event an alternative plan of care is not enough, and either (1) the person is ready to move or (2) the family's needs cannot be filled by a GCM, then a move must be considered. Evaluating the physical environment in combination with an understanding of the client's ability to perform the ADLs enables you to understand the level of care the client needs. This is the basis for recommending when a client should consider a move to another setting. (See Chapter 5, Care Planning and Geriatric Assessment.)

■ THE GCM's ROLE IN MAKING A MOVE

If you as a GCM want to add moving to your product list of services, it is important to plan ahead and develop a database of moving resources in your community. The database could include the names of moving companies,

professional organizers, lists of all good antique dealers, second-hand furniture stores, estate sale and consignment companies, as well as charities that accept donated items. Remember, a successful move consists of the completion of a series of multiple steps prior to the move, and you will need resources for all of them.

An additional resource for you is the National Association of Senior Move Managers. This service provider can be of assistance with the physical task of relocation. Senior move managers offer a range of services that may include organizing, downsizing, and planning as well as packing, floor plan design, coordination of estate and consignment sales, unpacking, and setting up the new residence. For a complete list of services and senior move managers in your area, visit the association's Web site at http://www.nasmm.com/.

Your role before, during, and after the move of an older adult is multifaceted. Not only might you provide move management services as well as postmove support and advocacy, but you might also assist the family and the older person through any difficulty or crisis that occurs before the move.

You are there to assess the needs of the older person and the family, to determine to what level of care the client should move in relationship to the budget, and to develop a clear understanding of the specific needs or wants of the relocating older person. You will also provide opportunities to enhance perceived control by the client as well as ensure, as much as possible, that perceived expectations for the move match the reality of the outcome. Examples of activities that support perceived control are (1) allowing the client to select which personal items he or she will take to the new living environment, and (2) encouraging him or her to participate as much as possible in the selection of that new environment. In addition, choices in food selection, social activities, and clothing for the day enhance perceived control. You can also guide the client and family in the establishment of expectations equal to the reality of the new environment. Arranging for the client to make premove visits to the new living environment to meet staff and fellow residents, to sample the meals, and to familiarize him- or herself with the physical property can help achieve this goal. If a client is unable to visit his or her new residence beforehand, showing the person pictures of the administrative staff, the grounds, and common rooms, as well as of the apartments or rooms, would be helpful.

You can use assessment results to help the family find the level of care the older adult requires. Once the level of care is determined and a residence is selected, you can then actually assist with the many components of the physical move: packing, storing, mailing, helping the elder and the family decide what furniture and personal belongings to bring. Also, you should be prepared to help the older person, and sometimes the family, mourn the loss of the family home. Once moving day arrives, either the family can actually move the older person or you can make all the transportation arrangements for the transition. Finally, you can help the older person adjust to the move, monitor the transition for the family, and help the family and the older person adjust to the new setting and loss of their old nest.

■ ASSESSING AN ELDER TO FIND THE RIGHT LEVEL AND PLACE TO MOVE

Although the elder and family may decide to move, often they need assistance in determining to which level of care to move and finding that level of care within their budget and that meets their preferences. Your first task in transitioning an older adult is to determine the level of care and appropriate living environment the client requires.

For example, Ms. Greenberg might ask you to arrange a move for her mom, Mrs. Jacobson, who is presently in an assisted living facility in Miami. The daughter wants her mother to move to an assisted living facility or an appropriate level of care in Philadelphia. The daughter wants her mother to be nearer to her home in Philadelphia because she needs to provide increased care and is burnt out from making constant trips to Miami. The daughter is currently juggling a full-time job and the responsibility of relocating her mother She may need to outsource this process to you, a GCM, because of her limited time, her lack of comfort in selecting the level of care her mother requires, and her feeling that you, the GCM, are the expert in such matters.

The Moving Assessment Tool (Exhibit 16–1) can assist you in assessing the basic needs of the older person facing relocation and his or her family.

The Moving Assessment Tool provides the means to determine the needs and preferences of the client and the family for important factors, including time frame, geographic location, budget, and level of care. The first area addressed is the timetable: when does the family want the move to occur? The second area addressed is geographic—where do they want the older person to move? If it is within a city, how far do they want the older person away from critical contacts, such as family? For example, if Mrs. Jacobson is to move to the Philadelphia area, how far from her daughter's home does her daughter want Mrs. Jacobson's new residence to be? Is having public transportation close an issue? What about stores and medical services? The next assessment area addressed is the budget. The family or older person will usually have a range within which they can afford to rent or buy. This is critical to planning a move. You can't plan a Mercedes move on a Volkswagon budget. Additionally, if the older adult is restricted to low-income housing or skilled nursing that accepts Medicaid, you need to determine the availability of that in the city or county to which he or she is moving.

The next step prior to moving the client is to determine the required level of care. GCMs can use psychosocial assessment and functional

Exhibit 16–1 Moving Assessment Tool

Date _____

Completed by: _____

Client Name _____

Address _____

City _____ State _____ Zip _____

Time Frame: _____ Week(s) / Month(s) (circle one)

Actual Moving Date: _____

GEOGRAPHIC LOCATION:
1st Choice: City _____ County _____ State _____
2nd Choice: City _____ County _____ State _____
3rd Choice: City _____ County _____ State _____

FINANCES
Monthly Housing Budget: $_____

Revenue Sources

❏ Medicare ❏ MediCal ❏ Pension ❏ Social Security ❏ Retirement Income

Notes: _____
_____

REQUIRED LIVING ENVIRONMENT:
Independent

❏ Gated Active Adult Community ❏ Senior Independent ❏ CCRC ❏ Life Care

❏ Apartment (Senior) ❏ Apartment (Community at Large) ❏ With Family

❏ Town house / Condo / Duet ❏ Purchase ❏ Lease/Rental

❏ Detached Single Family Home ❏ Purchase ❏ Lease/Rental

Comments: _____
_____
_____
_____

Assisted Living

❏ Dementia Care

❏ Assisted Living Facility ❏ Residential Board and Care ❏ Foster Home

Comments: _____
_____

Skilled Nursing
Medical Spend-Down Accepted ❏ Yes ❏ No _____ Projected Date

❏ Rehabilitation ❏ Long Term ❏ Dementia Care ❏ Medicaid/MediCal Beds
❏ Feeding Services

Comments: _____
_____
_____

Exhibit 16–1   Moving Assessment Tool (continued)

PROXIMITY TO:
Family
- ❑ Walking   ❑ Driving   ❑ Home   ❑ Work
- ❑ 5–20 min   ❑ 30 min   ❑ 1 hour   ❑ 2 hours

Notes: _____

Grocery and Drugstore
- ❑ Walking   ❑ Driving   ❑ Home   ❑ Work
- ❑ 5–20 min   ❑ 30 min   ❑ 1 hour   ❑ 2 hours

Shopping, Restaurants, and Entertainment
- ❑ Walking   ❑ Driving   ❑ Home   ❑ Work
- ❑ 5–20 min   ❑ 30 min   ❑ 1 hour   ❑ 2 hours

Church
- ❑ Walking   ❑ Driving   ❑ Home   ❑ Work
- ❑ 5–20 min   ❑ 30 min   ❑ 1 hour   ❑ 2 hours

Senior Center
- ❑ Walking   ❑ Driving   ❑ Home   ❑ Work
- ❑ 5–20 min   ❑ 30 min   ❑ 1 hour   ❑ 2 hours

Doctors' Offices
- ❑ Walking   ❑ Driving   ❑ Home   ❑ Work
- ❑ 5–20 min   ❑ 30 min   ❑ 1 hour   ❑ 2 hours

Hospital
- ❑ Walking   ❑ Driving   ❑ Home   ❑ Work
- ❑ 5–20 min   ❑ 30 min   ❑ 1 hour   ❑ 2 hours

Alternate/Public Transportation:
- ❑ 1 block   ❑ 2 blocks   ❑ 3–6 blocks   ❑ Door to Door

SPECIFIC NEEDS
- ❑ Transportation   ❑ Religious Services   ❑ Pets   ❑ Music   ❑ Crafts
- ❑ Entertainment   ❑ Special Events   ❑ Holiday Observations
- ❑ Guest Visits (overnight)   ❑ Private Dining Room

Diet and Nutrition
- ❑ Diabetic   ❑ Low Cholesterol   ❑ Low Sodium   ❑ Vegetarian
- ❑ Kosher   ❑ Halaal   ❑ Other   ❑ Food Allergies

Notes: _____

ADDITIONAL SERVICES: PRE-MOVE
- ❑ Medical   ❑ Legal   ❑ CPA   ❑ Real Estate   ❑ Interior Design
- ❑ Professional Organizer   ❑ Estate/Consignment Sales   ❑ Move Management

Other: _____

ADDITIONAL SERVICES: POST-MOVE
- ❑ GCM   ❑ Medical   ❑ Legal   ❑ CPA   ❑ Real Estate
- ❑ Interior Design   ❑ Orientation   ❑ Move Management (unpacking and setup)

Other: _____

assessment tools to evaluate the older client's ability to perform ADLs and IADLs in relationship to the person's present physical environment (see Chapter 3, Psychosocial Assessment, and Chapter 4, Functional Assessment). This enables you to establish a baseline for the level of care. Evaluating the older person's present physical environment in combination with an understanding of the client's ability to perform the ADLs enables the care manager to understand the level of care the client needs. From this baseline, you can determine which living environment options offer the required level of care. These assessments should be done with each client, in all cases, for each move. It may be more costly to the client to pay for the geriatric care management assessments, but there is no sense in spending unnecessary time and money finding a skilled nursing facility (SNF) when all the person really needs is an assisted living facility.

Once the required level of care is determined, you can assess the specific housing needs and preferences of the older person and/or the family and correlate that to the budget constraints. Once you have completed your initial moving assessment and psychosocial and functional assessments, you should be able to identify, based on your assessment results, what level of care your client requires in a living environment. The moving assessment enables you to determine geographic preferences and budget constraints. The intersections of these assessments enable you to narrow down your housing choices for the client. If, after you have completed your assessments, you have an older person who functionally and psychosocially must (1) reside in an assisted living facility, (2) in Philadelphia, (3) within the $5,000-dollar-a-month range, and the facility must (4) be within 20 minutes of the daughter's home, (5) provide weekly transportation to temple services and physicians' offices, (6) observe holidays, (7) offer a Kosher diet, and (8) allow pets, your choices are narrowed for the search.

■ ADDITIONAL CONSIDERATIONS: HOUSING NEEDS AND PREFERENCES

If the client is moving to an apartment by himself or herself, what amenities does the person want in that apartment? How large, how small? Does the person require privacy? A view? What will the budget allow? Is the person eligible for moderate or low-cost senior housing? Is there a waiting list for these apartments? Does the community have an on-site services coordinator? If the senior is going to rent a market rate apartment or senior housing, you can contact the Area Agency on Aging (AAA) in the county or the local senior center for a list of senior housing and apartments for review.

You also need to assess transportation, terrain, and social services requirements. Does the client need to be in close proximity to accessible public transportation? What about the distance to stores and medical services? Is there a grocery store or drugstore close by? What about terrain? Is it on a hill or on flat land? What is the policy and procedure for maintenance repair? How quickly does the management respond to requests for repairs? Are smoke detectors and carbon monoxide detectors installed? If not, can the person have them installed?

What about social amenities? Should you find an apartment that allows pets because the client's dog is a treasured companion? Should the apartment be near the religious or spiritual services practiced by the older person? Religious involvement is a way to engage the older person in a new community if the person includes that practice in the lifestyle. Does the person like to play bingo, mahjong, or bridge? If so, a new assisted living or senior housing facility should have those activities. If not, could you find a senior center nearby that offers them? What amenities were you looking for when you apartment shopped or house hunted for yourself? Older people are just like you.

■ EVALUATING SENIOR HOUSING, CONGREGATE HOUSING, SHARED HOUSING, AND CONTINUING CARE RETIREMENT COMMUNITIES

When you consider alternative living environments, you will find there are many types of senior living environments and many lower levels of care, below an SNF, from which to choose. One idea to keep in mind is that not all older adults want to be among seniors, so the community-at-large housing market can also be considered. All choices in your community should be reflected in your database and be updated constantly. You can get this information from your AAA, information and referral services in your community, or through the resource called Elder Locator. You can also use a real estate agent with a Senior Real Estate Specialist designation to locate properties for the older person to rent, lease, or purchase in the community of choice.

Senior Housing

The Housing for Older Adults Act of 1995 describes senior housing as follows:

> Dwelling specifically designed for and occupied by elderly; or is occupied solely by persons who are 62 or older; or houses at least one person who is 55 or older in at least 80 percent of the occupied units, and adheres to a policy that demonstrates intent to house persons who are 55 or older. Therefore, housing that satisfies the legal definition of senior housing or housing for older persons described above can legally exclude families with children.[9]

To find a variety of descriptions for the various senior housing options from which you and your client can select, do a Web search using the keywords "types of senior housing." Helpguide, a resource created by the Rotary Club and the Center for Healthy Aging in Santa Monica, California, can be found at

http://www.helpguide.org/elder/senior_housing_residential_care_types.htm and offers consumer information as well as the following in-depth descriptions of senior housing:

- **Independent living for seniors: a retirement community of peers:** For healthy seniors who are self-sufficient and want the freedom and privacy of their own separate, easy-to-maintain apartment or house, along with the security, comfort, and social activities of a senior community.

- **Assisted living facilities for seniors:** For people who do not have severe medical problems but who need help with personal care such as bathing, dressing, grooming, and eating. There is a great deal of variety both in the types of housing and the range of services provided, and not much government regulation at this time.

- **Board and care homes for seniors:** A residence for people who need minimal help with personal care such as bathing, dressing, grooming, and eating, but who need or want communal meals and easy access to social contact with peers. Facilities are state-licensed and may specialize in care for seniors, psychiatric patients, or those with Alzheimer's disease.

- **Nursing homes (SNFs):** Facilities with 24-hour medical care available, including short-term rehabilitation (physical therapy) as well as long-term care for people with chronic ailments or disabilities that require daily attention of registered nurses in addition to help with personal care such as bathing or dressing or getting around.

- **Congregate housing for seniors:** Previously considered a unique combination of private living quarters combined with shared activities, including communal meals and other social activities, but now considered a type of assisted living.

- **Continuing-care retirement communities (CCRCs):** A complex of residences that include independent living, assisted living, and nursing home care, so seniors can stay in the same general location as their housing needs change over time, beginning when they are still healthy and active.[10]

Additional information regarding the variety of assisted living options for seniors can be found on the Assisted Living Federation of America Web site at http://www.alfa.org/files/public/ALFAchecklist.pdf.

In addition to the previously mentioned living environments, two others should be included: life care facilities and active adult communities.

- **Life care facilities:** The Episcopal Homes Foundation Web site describes life care as the following: "Life care is an arrangement by which persons pay an initial accommodation fee and monthly maintenance fees in exchange for living accommodations and services. All levels of care are provided, including acute care, physicians' and surgeons' services, skilled nursing care, and personal care on premises of the retirement community, with no change in fees based on level of care."[11] Other life care facilities may vary their services included or their financial arrangements.

- **Active adult or planned adult communities:** Planned adult, active adult, and gated golfing communities for active adults over the age of 55 offer homes for purchase as well as a variety of social and athletic activities for residents. Golf courses, tennis courts, swimming pools, theaters, special interest groups and clubs, social events, and travel opportunities create a vacation environment for the over-55 adult who selects this type of housing. Monthly homeowner fees may cover maintenance and/or housekeeping services. Meals are usually not included.[12]

When conducting evaluations of various living environments, you are making evaluations of the same factors you would rate in an SNF: overall environment, health and safety features, resident environment and comfort, food service, if applicable, staff, and programming. American Association of Retired Persons provides a checklist for evaluating an assisted living facility on its Web site at http://www.aarp.org/families/housing_choices/assisted_living/a2004-02-27-assistedlivingchecklist.html.

For additional checklists to assist you in the evaluation of all types of senior housing, you can access the resources available at http://www.helpguide.org/elder/senior_housing_residential_care_types.htm.

■ LIVING IN THE COMMUNITY AT LARGE

If the senior is buying a condo or town house, it is important he or she is connected with an appropriate real estate services provider. There are now real estate agents called Senior Real Estate Specialists (SRESs)(see http://www.seniorrealestate.com).

Real estate agents are able to acquire an SRES designation by enrolling in a course provided by the Senior Advantage Real Estate Council (SAREC). To view the requirements for the SRES designation, view the SAREC Web site at http://www.seniorsrealestate.com/sarec/servlet/perspective/requirements.

Make sure you interview the real estate agent in depth before referring the client or the client's family to this person. The real estate agent used by a GCM should be someone who has experience with seniors, is a good listener, has a genuine concern for the senior's welfare, is patient with the needs of the GCM and the senior, and is available to see a senior through the stressful process of selling or buying a home.

Additionally, the real estate agent should have a history of executing contracts diligently and completing all paperwork in a timely and orderly fashion. His or her license should be in good standing and free of any disciplinary action by the state department of real estate or local board of real estate agents. The SRES designation is a good place to start in the process of finding a real estate agent for a client; it is one of several criteria that should be used when selecting a real estate agent to work with the client or client's family. Because relocation is a process, not an event, the people involved determine how smoothly the process takes place.

If the senior is downsizing and renting a home, town house, or condo in the new community, many real estate agents manage and lease properties for homeowners and could act as a resource for finding available housing. However, a home or apartment that is leased requires a signed contract. A contract required by any housing facility, whether in the community at large or in a senior living community such as a CCRC, life care community, senior independent facility, assisted living, board and care, or SNF, should be reviewed by a family member and an attorney before it is signed. Housing available in the community at large on a month-to-month rental basis is another option to explore.

■ RELOCATING TO A SKILLED NURSING FACILITY

When relocating an older person to an SNF, you must evaluate many of the same living requirements you looked at for independent apartment living and assisted living. In terms of finances and budget, it is important to anticipate the need for Medicaid assistance. A critical budget question is: Is Medicaid a factor now or in the future if a spend-down is anticipated? If Medicaid is not a factor now but could be in the future, it is important to know if the SNF has Medicaid beds for Medicaid-eligible residents. Verifying eligible Medicaid beds today could prevent an involuntary move of the client tomorrow.

As in other living environments, services and amenities play an important role. If the client is at an SNF level, do religious services need to be on site? Does the person need special services for feeding, bathing, toileting? Does the person desire animal therapy services? Does the facility need to be within driving distance or public transportation reach of family? Is bingo a must for this particular client? All these needs and preferences must be determined through your assessment before the move is planned.

■ CREATING AN IDEAL MODEL

After you have done the psychosocial assessment and the moving assessment, develop for the client an ideal model of the ideal residence where the senior will move. This model should include the following information:

1. Level of care
2. Budget
3. Geographic area
4. Specific services or amenities that must be available (e.g., a Catholic mass, pets allowed, near enough for the wife to visit, and a great view)

Following are a few examples of ideal plans.

CASE STUDY

Example 1: Mr. Remer

Mr. Remer ideally will be moved to an SNF in St. Joseph, Missouri, within a mile of his daughter Katherine, within a budget range of $3,000–$4,000 a month, where the facility allows spend-down to Medicaid eligibility. The facility will ideally allow pets (he would like to bring his 15-year-old dog), will have Lutheran services or general religious programs, and will have a recreation program that offers art therapy because he was a commercial artist when he worked.

The preceding describes Mr. Remer's ideal model, and your job is to find the living environment that approximates this ideal to as great a degree as possible.

CASE STUDY

Example 2: Mrs. Murphy's Father

Mrs. Murphy has a father in Kansas City and wants you, a GCM in Los Angeles, California, to find a placement for her dad in the Redondo Beach, California, area, where Mrs. Murphy lives. You contact a GCM in Kansas City and arrange for him to do the psychosocial and functional assessments and the moving assessment. You then, through phone conversations and e-mail, determine with the family members (1) the budget, (2) kind of space that would work best (Mrs. Murphy requests a view of the ocean and a single room), and (3) the kinds of services that must be in place. Next, you develop a model from that information and then find an appropriate facility using the model as your guide.

■ NARROWING DOWN SENIOR HOUSING TO PREVIEW

The selection of the type of senior housing the older person will move to should be made by the family and the older person based on (1) the results of your psychosocial and functional assessment, (2) your premove assessment, (3) their preferences, (4) budget, and (5) housing availability in the community. Other factors to include when selecting a living environment that offers services below the level of skilled nursing are (1) the size of the facility that would work best for the older person, (2) apartment size (small and cozy, or large and spacious), (3) privacy, (4) physical floor plan, and (5) amenities (does the person want to cook and have a kitchen?).

After the client and family have selected the level of care and type of senior housing, you should review the client profile and narrow down the choices to 10 possibilities or fewer. If the community offers few choices, you might not need to narrow down the list and might need to call all facilities that fit the profile on paper. For example, finding an assisted living facility with an ocean view in the Redondo Beach, California, area may be difficult. Therefore, it is imperative that the facility be evaluated by more than an "on-paper profile" to ensure the best environment with the finest fit for the client is selected.

Once you have made evaluation phone calls to each potential housing option and have confirmed the specific features that match the ideal profile, the family and older adult are brought into the process once again. They may be given the list of properties to visit on their own, or they may prefer that you visit and evaluate the choices with them or by yourself and report back to them. Because you are working for the client, on their dime, so to speak, remember to visit only properties that match your client's profile. If further research of other properties is required, you must secure permission to do research beforehand.

■ RESOURCES FOR RESEARCHING SENIOR LIVING: ASSISTED LIVING AND SKILLED NURSING FACILITIES

If the client and family have hired you to search for that ideal living environment for the elder person, numerous state and local governing bodies and resources can help you in your search.

If you are searching for an SNF, contact the local AAA for a listing of all senior housing, a list of licensed facilities in the appropriate city, and licensing regulations in the corresponding state. Your state's licensing body is also a valuable resource. You should be able to get a list of facilities and information on specific facilities such as any citations, the number of beds, as well as information on the availability of special units such as an Alzheimer's unit from this government body. To find the appropriate agency in your state, access the Web site of your state's Department on Aging.

For California, the California Advocates for Nursing Home Reform (CANHR) can provide valuable information. Otherwise, ask the local AAA if a group such as CAHNR exists in the geographic area in which you are searching.

You can contact the Long Term Care Ombudsman for help in choosing facilities as well. What you want to find is not just a list of facilities and whether they accept Medicaid, but also the number of citations each facility has received, which is a critical piece of information. You must recommend a facility with the fewest, preferably zero, citations; this is critical to giving weight to the best and safest SNF or SNFs.

Once you have assembled this information in your database, it is essential that you update it regularly because the information is constantly changing. As the expert, you must know the continuum of care in your community to help you stay abreast of this information. Some facilities go out of business or change their acceptance criteria; citations can happen at any time.

Once you have contacted all the housing resources and created your skilled nursing or assisted living list, narrow down the list of potentially ideal facilities to only facilities with minimal, preferably zero, citations. It is important to remember that quality of care and safety in an SNF or assisted living facility are the highest priority factors you are evaluating for. If the ideal model is not available with zero or minimal citations, consult the ombudsman for other suggestions. You may have to alter your mo   del rather than recommend an unsafe facility.

If you are searching for senior apartment complexes or homes to buy, narrow down your list to only the complexes or the homes that match the ideal model (say, the ones with an ocean view, tennis courts, and bingo). You should also add to your database of relocation information the contact information for 202 Housing (i.e., government-subsided housing for the elderly in your community). If the older person's budget requires a housing subsidy, and the person's level of care is appropriate for an apartment in your ideal model, you should readily be able to identify the appropriate site.

After you have established your pared-down priority list, you can, with the client's approval, accompany the client to preview these properties or preview them on the client's behalf.

■ VISITING AND EVALUATING YOUR LIST OF SKILLED NURSING FACILITIES

The next step is to physically evaluate the facilities on your list by making a site visit. This, of course, must be done with the client's or family's permission. The family may want to do this themselves to cut costs. But if they wish you to do the job, then you can use the Facility Evaluation form shown in Exhibit 16–2.

Because there are so many factors to weigh when selecting an SNF, it is recommended that you review and incorporate where appropriate these additional supplementary facility evaluations, which can be found online at the following Web sites:

http://www.medicare.gov/Nursing/
    Checklist.pdf
http://www.carepathways.com/
    checklist-nh.cfm
http://nursinghomeguide.org/pub/
    eval_checklist.pdf

You should have already determined the basic fees of each SNF and are visiting only those in the client's budget range.

Exhibit 16–2   Facility Evaluation

Evaluator: _____   Date: _____

General Information:

Name of Facility: _____

Address: _____

Phone #:   _____

FAX: _____

E-mail: _____

Facility type: ❑ Profit ❑ Nonprofit ❑ Private ❑ Government
                              ❑ Religious Affiliate ❑ Other: _____

Contact Information (Include Position, Phone #, Fax, E-mail):

Name: _____   Administrator / License # _____

Name: _____   Director of Nursing _____

Name: _____   Social Worker _____

_____

_____

Fees:

Basic Fees:

    Single Room   _____

    Double   _____

    Triple   _____

Deposit: _____

Included in Fees:

    Medications: ❑ Yes ❑ No

    Telephone: ❑ Yes ❑ No   If no, how much? _____

    Cable TV: ❑ Yes ❑ No   If no, how much? _____

    Laundry: ❑ Yes ❑ No   If no, how much? _____

Other Amenities: _____

Immediate Availability: ❑ Yes ❑ No

Payment:

Medicare: ❑ Yes ❑ No

Medi-Cal: ❑ Yes ❑ No

Long-term Care Insurance: ❑ Yes ❑ No   If yes, will facility bill LTC insurance
                              company directly? ❑ Yes ❑ No

Other: _____

Recreational and Social Activities:

Daily Recreational Activities: _____

Weekly Recreational Activities: _____

Seasonal / Holiday
  Recreational Activities: _____

Exhibit 16–2   Facility Evaluation (continued)

Religious Services and
    Chaplain Visits: ❑ Yes ❑ No
                       If yes, denomination: _____
                          Describe services: _____
                       If no, is transportation available to and from
                          religious services? ❑ Yes ❑ No

Other social support:

Addressing Grievances:

Resident Council: ❑ Yes ❑ No
Family Council: ❑ Yes ❑ No

Other formal / informal avenues
    to address complaints: _____

Number of citations: _____

Type of citations: _____

Medical and Other Health-Related Services:
Availability of:
    Dementia Care: ❑ Yes ❑ No If yes, describe service(s): _____
    Dental Services: ❑ Yes ❑ No If yes, describe service(s): _____
    Optometry / Ophthalmology ❑ Yes ❑ No If yes, describe service(s): _____
    Podiatry: ❑ Yes ❑ No If yes, describe service(s): _____
    Respiratory Therapy: ❑ Yes ❑ No If yes, describe service(s): _____
    Physical Therapy: ❑ Yes ❑ No If yes, describe service(s): _____
    Occupational Therapy: ❑ Yes ❑ No If yes, describe service(s): _____
    Speech Therapy: ❑ Yes ❑ No If yes, describe service(s): _____

Closest Hospital: _____

Other Hospitals: _____

Specialty Clinics: _____

Transportation:

Medical appointments: ❑ Yes ❑ No Describe service(s): _____
Social and recreational activities: ❑ Yes ❑ No Describe service(s): _____

Capacity:

Total # of beds: _____
# of private beds: _____
# of semiprivate beds: _____
# of triple beds: _____
# of current residents: _____

Staffing Ratios:

Shift 1   Shift structure: _____   Ratio: _____
Shift 2   Shift structure: _____   Ratio: _____
Shift 3   Shift structure: _____   Ratio: _____

Private care allowed?   ❑ Yes ❑ No

Private care encouraged?   ❑ Yes ❑ No

continues

Exhibit 16–2   Facility Evaluation (continued)

Type of Staff:
   In-house: ❑ Yes   ❑ No
   Registry: ❑ Yes   ❑ No

Staff interaction with
   residents (describe):   _____

Is there enough staff to
   feed the residents?   ❑ Yes   ❑ No

General Environment:

Presentation: _____

Common Areas: _____

Odors: _____

Hallways: _____

Doors: _____

Bathrooms: _____

Window(s) / Doors
   to the outside: _____

Access to outside: _____

Dining Rooms: _____

   Feeding tables?   ❑ Yes   ❑ No

Other Considerations:

Types of residents accepted: _____

Types of residents
   not considered: _____

Alternative diets: ❑ Yes   ❑ No

Visitation Policy: _____

Evaluator's signature: _____

Next, make an on-site visit to the facilities that fit the client's profile. Make an appointment on a busy day at the facility; ask to go to lunch and for a meeting with the activity director. Request to meet with the facility director, not a subordinate staff member.

Prior to entering the facility, survey the surrounding neighborhood, the condition of the street and surrounding buildings, and note whether the building is in good repair.

When entering the front door, your initial screening tools are sensory: how the facility feels, smells, and tastes are things you cannot evaluate on the phone or from a list. When you walk into the facility, how does it feel? Does it feel welcoming, like a pleasant new home for your client? Use your intuition here—the same intuition you would use for yourself if you were picking a new apartment or buying a home. On all facility evaluation checklists there is a general environment question; this is where you put your answer to the question "how does it feel?"

Next, use your sense of smell. Most graphically, do you smell urine? What do you smell in the facility—urine, strong disinfectant, lack of cleanliness (any GCM who has worked with disadvantaged clients knows this smell)? Again, use your intuition and use the same guide that would assist you in choosing your own new home.

Is the temperature comfortable? What's the noise level? Peek in the corners. Go down hallways—are they free of clutter and is the lighting good? Look up and see if there are smoke detectors and sprinklers. Enter bathrooms—are they clean and uncluttered? Check out the toilet seats. Is the bathroom safety-adapted? Walk through the dining room and check out the kitchen. Note what the general condition of all these areas is and evaluate what the facility feels like, smells like, and looks like. Try thinking "would my mother like this?"

Next, use your sense of taste. Have lunch in the dining room. Does the food smell and look palatable? Does it taste good? Is the environment in the dining room relaxing and does it encourage residents to relax and enjoy their food? Are residents rushed through their meal? Are residents given some dietary control by being offered a choice of foods on the menu? If residents need help with eating, how is this help offered? Can the facility provide special health-compliant diets?

Go into a resident's room similar to the one the elder you represent will use. Look at the condition of the doorknobs and the phone. Does the resident's room have personal furniture? Are the doors marked with memory boxes or do they display the resident's name and picture? Are there water glasses and pitchers in the rooms?

Visit the recreational areas and talk to the activity director. What are the activity choices, by day, week, and season? Does the facility observe rituals such as birthdays, holidays, and culturally appropriate events? Is art or music therapy available? How often? Does the facility offer religious services or chaplain visits?

Go to the public areas. Is the furniture comfortable and nice looking? Look at the residents. Are they clean and well dressed? Try to talk to three residents or visiting family members. Ask how residents like living here. Ask important questions such as: Do staff members respond when you need help? What is the best thing about living here?

Observe the staff interaction with the residents. Do they seem to enjoy their exchanges with residents? Are they attentive to residents' needs? Are they friendly?

Finally, meet with the facility director. Ask these questions: What is the waiting period for admission? Is the administrator licensed? Is there a deposit, and what is included in the fee (medications, telephone, cable, laundry)? Does the facility do background checks on staff? What is the ratio of staff to patients? Remember, the lower the staff to resident ratio, the better. What is staff turnover? What is staff training? Are snacks available during the day and evening? What is the facility's emergency plan? Can you see it? Remember the horrible events in SNFs in New Orleans, post Katrina in 2006. (See Chapter 13, Preparing for Emergencies.)

Are citations posted? Try to bring the last inspection results with you. Has the SNF corrected these? Ask for a copy of the resident agreement or contract and marketing literature about the facility.

■ NARROW DOWN TO THREE CHOICES

Finally, the time has come to make the final decision. The family and the older person should make this decision. If you can, create an electronic spreadsheet that lists all factors in your patient profile and any others you might add and ranks each category for each facility. If the client and/or family have previewed the locations, then you can do this task with them. You or your client can double-check your evaluations by making one more unannounced visit to three facilities and asking any unanswered questions you or the client might have. If you are doing the evaluations alone, be sure to obtain permission from the client and family prior to these additional visits because they must pay for the hours you spend. Once you or you and the client/family complete the spreadsheet, send the spreadsheet or a general facility description along with marketing literature that you received from the facility to the family. It is now the family's and older person's time to make the final selection of where to move.

■ GETTING THE OLDER PERSON AND FAMILY PSYCHOSOCIALLY READY FOR THE MOVE

Usually, older persons experience the emotions of very traumatic loss when they move. They lose their familiar surroundings, familiar faces, and sometimes their independence. They lose personal items that orient them to their past and present, such as pictures of family, furniture that may link them to their life experiences, the garden where familiar plants came up every year giving them joy and a sense of sameness every spring. If a long-time pet cannot be taken with them, they may also lose one of their trusted companions. Coping with this momentous lost is often like coping with death because, in a real way, this move can trigger a grief response.[13,14] Such a response was noted in one older women, Mrs. Butler, who looked around when first placed in a nursing home and said, shaking her head, "I guess I'm at the end of the road."

Your role in muting this potentially devastating loss can be to offer emotional support and counseling. As a GCM, you can arrange help to lessen the pain of this loss by listening to the older person's grief and accepting it as real. You can make sure that familiar and treasured items move with the senior to make a bridge from the past to the present, orient the moved elder, and create a familiar living environment.[14]

Included in the familiar and treasured is the older adult's pet. If there is a pet involved, your search should be for a facility that accepts pets. The beloved pet companion provides an even more important bridge to the present than furniture can.

If someone is being moved to a different city and has not seen the facility or met the staff, ask the GCM or family in the area to send pictures of the facility and staff members and create an album for your client. Place all pictures in an album and identify by name or site, especially the client's new room or apartment. Another option is to consider making a video of the facility, showing the client's new living environment and surrounding areas such as the dining room, the grounds, the lobby, or recreation room. Additionally, if possible, have staff members introduce themselves to the client individually by name and identify their role in the new living environment. With the use of a laptop computer, the client can view this video in advance of the move and have a better idea of what to expect. Hopefully, some personal belongings can be sent ahead so that the room or apartment looks and feels familiar when the senior arrives.

Meeting the Psychosocial Needs of the Adult Child Before the Move

Adult children have their own trials and tribulations before a parent's move. Often, they have a very difficult time coping with the slow pace with which the older person accepts the traumatic loss of moving. This is something you can warn adult children about as the process begins. Also, offer encouragement by reassuring the adult child that the move will take place and that you are there to help. That knowledge can often slow down their demands for a speedy process.

Adult children are harried at times because they are taking care of younger family members while arranging the move of their elderly parent. You can take the burden off the adult child by finding others in the continuum of care to complete the move or by providing agreed-upon services for a fee.

If the adult child has to find time to tour facilities, make the process easier by offering several time choices so that the task can be squeezed into an already busy schedule.

Counseling the adult child about this life transition is often as important as counseling the elder making the move and is a good fit for a GCM's skills. Adult children are often coping with their parent's mortality, a specter that hovers over the parent and the child, "Is this the end of the line?"

Once the place to move has been determined by the older person and the family, you can fill many roles in a move.

Packing and organizing are areas you can cover, or you can find a moving specialist to do this. If you choose to offer this service, managing the move can include premoving preparations and activities. A major theme in premoving is to keep the older person involved constantly and have the person take part in all decisions. That way, the person will feel more in control and it may minimize relocation stress syndrome.

■ WORKING WITH THE PHYSICAL PART OF THE MOVE

Once you have chosen a place and level of care to move to, make arrangements with another GCM or family member or someone very reliable to carry out the receiving end of the move, especially if this is in another geographic location. This should be done well in advance of the move.

Premove activities should include helping the client decide what to take to the new home, completing a checklist of what needs to be done before the move, assisting the older person in going through possessions, and arranging the donation, sale, or family distributions of the older person's belongings. More of your job is creating an inventory of all items to be moved, organizing items before the move, arranging for the mover, ordering boxes, and then packing. Packing responsibilities may be outsourced to a reliable senior moving company in your area. You can add disconnecting all utilities and stopping all present support services (cleaning, caregiving, Meals on Wheels, etc.) currently in place.

Assisting the older person to sort through possessions is an excellent GCM task. If the move location is far away from the area you serve, connect with a family member living nearby or another GCM to have them take the measurements of the final move site. This will enable you to select furniture and belongings that will fit in the space available in the new home.

There is potential for experiencing great loss through the disposition of personal belongings, furniture, pictures, even clothes, because they represent the older person's whole past, present safety, and family history. Although you might want an aide to do an inventory here, the crux of the sorting is not just what will be moved and what will be discarded but helping the older person through the trauma of leaving his or her past. Understand that the person is also discarding the present safe space by determining what items go and what items stay.

A general rule of thumb: when in doubt, take the comfortable old friend. Help the client choose the chair he or she sits in every day, perhaps the recliner that is slightly tattered but like a cozy home to sink into. If there is a huge collection of an item, take a few and store, sell, or distribute the rest. If the client has a collection of craft items or sewing materials, for instance, suggest donating them to the local senior center craft group. (This is also good advice for those who have to sort and donate the hobby items of a spouse who has passed away. This group likes to know that a "perfectly good" item is being used, not wasted.) Even if the person will not cook, if there is a small dining or kitchen area, take a place setting for two or four in case the person has guests over. Unless your older client is moving to a single-family home or private home in a senior community, label all furniture and personal belongings with the older person's name. This is a good task to delegate.

After you know how much stuff the senior would like to move, you can execute two sorting events. The first sorting is to determine what will actually fit into the new space. The second sorting is for those items that mean the most to the senior and will provide a basis for feeling safe and surrounded by familiar things in a new home. With these two filters you can begin to pare down the inventory of what goes with the older person and what must be given away or sold.

If your client is moving to a facility and space is limited, consider buying juvenile furniture for any pieces that are needed. It is sized smaller and fits more easily in smaller living quarters. You also may be able to get juvenile furniture at second-hand stores. Most assisted living facilities have a move-in coordinator. Check if one is available and work with that staff member to make the move.

■ DISBURSEMENT AND DISPOSITION OF PERSONAL BELONGINGS

The family meeting to discuss the disbursement of family belongings is another opportunity for you to smooth the way. You can participate in a minimal way by suggesting family members visit the Web site Who Gets Grandma's Yellow Pie Plate? (http://www. yellowpieplate.umn.edu) and by suggesting the adult children have a family meeting with their parent or parents to discuss what family items go to whom after the move. Have a list of all items in the home ready for the family meeting. If this will be a contentious meeting, consider a licensed Marriage and Family Therapist, or Licensed Clinical Social Worker who specializes in mediation. In the presence of strong words such as, "You got the Lenox dishes because Mom loved you best," you can facilitate this highly charged meeting. Sometimes the family prefers to do this in private. The elder who is moving must have a strong voice because, through the disposition of their belongings, he or she is passing history on.

Sometimes just knowing that a treasured item is passed on as a legacy helps the older person turn the loss into a gain and helps the adult children feel both nurtured and better prepared for the next stage of their parent's life. The family meeting can be a time whereby an agreement is made delineating which personal and household items go to which child. Keep this list handy for the actual physical moving stage. Once again, late-life relocation is a time that may include a role reversal or dependence by the parent on the adult child (see Chapter 17, Geriatric Care Management Working with Nearly Normal Aging Families).

■ PERSONAL BELONGINGS: MOVING TO A SKILLED NURSING FACILITY OR ASSISTED LIVING FACILITY

If the older person is moving to an SNF or congregate facility, put the person's name on all furniture and bedding, consider laser printing all old family photos that cannot be replaced, and give the originals to family. Take familiar bedding, buy a bright inviting new comforter, and take the person's pillow. Ask whether the client wants flannel sheets, which are comforting. Bring along items that bring contentment. Take a radio, glasses, a watch, and a calendar. Make sure you take chocolate, knitting or hobby items, the person's TV, beloved books, and pen and paper. If the person is religious, bring religious objects.

If the person is moving to an SNF, bring bedclothes that are easy to get on and off and warm socks. If you have a local source of easy-to-get-on-and-off clothing for people with disabilities, order from there. All clothing, furniture, and personal belongings should have the new resident's name written on them (for clothing, use washable laundry markers). Check whether the facility will allow you to put a picture of the older person and, if allowed in the facility, the person's pet, on the door of the residence. Also ask family members to write a short biography of the older person and post this on the door so aides see your client not just as another older resident but someone with a history who made a difference in life. With client and/or family approval, you may be asked to write this personal biography. Use the Moving to a Skilled Nursing Facility Checklist (Exhibit 16–3) to help you assemble everything the client will need for the move.

■ MOVING DAY

Being on hand on moving day is a good idea if the family or client agrees to this arrangement. You can supervise where items are placed, offer support to the older person, and act as a traffic director. It is your job to make the move happen. Your role is to see that everything transpires as planned and everything arrives as expected. Remember, life offers the unexpected and there is no perfect move. It will not always be smooth sailing. If the antique dresser is left behind, make new arrangements. If the antique dresser arrives but is in the wrong place or won't fit, find a solution. Just like a care plan, what you plan often falls apart and requires reevaluation. Use the creative skills in your GCM repertoire and find new solutions.

To make moving day as simple as possible for your client, do as much as possible to prepare for the physical relocation that day. Pack a special bag just for moving day that contains any medications and instructions, special belongings, a change of clothes, toiletries, and special personal items the client might need (should there be a delay) or simply want to keep close. Preferably, the new living environment can be set up and readied for occupancy before the client arrives. If not, check whether you can arrange for a temporary "guest" room for the client to use until everything is set up.

■ AFTER THE MOVE: POSTMOVE SUPPORT

Family is an integral part of the successful relocation outcome for the older family member. Arrange in advance a visit from the adult child after the move. If appropriate, you or a family member can stay with the client on the first day to assist him or her with learning the physical layout of the new environment. If you are retained to do so, provide support, especially if the client is anxious or not looking forward to the move. After learning about and then mastering the new environment, the client is freer to work on social activities and tasks of adjusting to the transition.[15]

If family members cannot provide postmove support, and if the move is local, arrange to visit or to have church members, friends, or former social or interest group members such as those from a book club or craft group to visit. If the move is to a new city with a church or synagogue of your client's denomination, arrange for the institution's representative to visit your client as soon as possible. If the client was in a book club in the former city or town, check whether a similar group exists in the new town and investigate the possibility of a member visit for your client. Familiar people and activities can offer sameness even when the physical environment changes.

Exhibit 16–3   Moving to a Skilled Nursing Facility Checklist

Date _____

Completed by: _____

Client Name _____

Address _____ Phone ( ) _____

City _____ State _____ Zip _____

Facility Name _____ Room Number ____

Address _____ Phone ( ) _____

City _____ State _____ Zip _____

Medical Supplies
Prescription Medications

1. _____ 2. _____ 3. _____ 4. _____

5. _____ 6. _____ 7. _____ 8. _____

9. _____ 10. _____ 11. _____ 12. _____

Other _____

Over-the-Counter Medications

1. _____ 2. _____ 3. _____ 4. _____

Medical Equipment

❑ Wheelchair ❑ Walker ❑ Cane ❑ Transfer Board ❑ Other

1. _____

2. _____

3. _____

4. _____

Personal Grooming Supplies

❑ Electric razor   ❑ Toothpaste

❑ Toothbrush   ❑ Soap

❑ Deodorant   ❑ Perfume

❑ Hand lotion   ❑ Incontinence supplies

❑ Hair brush   ❑ Other _____

❑ Hair spray   _____

❑ Preferred shampoos   _____

Clothing

❑ Sleepwear (button up the front)   ❑ Sweat / fleece jackets (front closing)

❑ Warm socks   ❑ Sturdy shoes and socks

❑ Sweats / warm-up sets (several)   ❑ Underwear

Bedding

❑ Pillow   ❑ Sheets (hospital beds require single sheets)

❑ Blanket   ❑ Bright, colorful bedspread

Exhibit 16–3   Moving to a Skilled Nursing Facility Checklist (continued)

Furniture

❑ Favorite chair or recliner
❑ Favorite afghan or quilt

❑ Armoire (for TV/DVD/CD player or personal belongings)

Electronics

❑ Radio (the person can see without glasses)
❑ DVD player
❑ Remote controls

❑ CD player and favorite music CDs
❑ TV

Stationery

❑ Pencil
❑ Pen and paper
❑ Monthly calendar

❑ Greeting cards (variety)
❑ Stamps

Religious objects

❑ Bible

❑ Other significant religious items

Jewelry

❑ A watch

❑ Inexpensive costume jewelry

Miscellaneous

❑ Books
❑ Snacks (chocolate, etc.)
❑ Pictures (home and family)
❑ Knitting/crocheting
❑ Cards
❑ All items are labeled

❑ Pet Supplies
  ❑ Food
  ❑ Food and water dishes
  ❑ Leash
  ❑ Grooming supplies
  ❑ Bed or kennel

Your role does not always end after the move. If the client lives in your town, monitoring the effects of the move include making sure what you said would get there, got there and what the facility said it would provide is provided. If the client is moved to a different town, if the family wishes, make arrangements for another GCM to do the important follow-up process.

Older people who move can experience difficulty in coping with the relocation. They may resist being in the facility or new domicile. An older person will usually accept a move if the transition is smooth. You as the GCM are there to ensure a smooth move.

The facility itself can present problems such as not offering activities, staff, or the type of meals it said it would. If you move a pet, there can be pet problems.

As the older person adjusts to the move, you can add more activities from the continuum of care. For instance, if family members are not visiting or friends can't find the time to stop by, try to arrange for a friendly visitor, paid care provider, or new book club member to visit your client. If the meals are not satisfactory, talk to the facility director to have the food adjusted until the resident is satisfied. If the older person is not going to meals or sits at a table where he or she is not accepted, work with the facility to make adjustments.

You will wear many hats throughout the relocation process for each client. At certain points in the process, you will be a logistical coordinator, at other times, an information specialist. Additionally, and possibly most important, you will be the advocate for, supportive advisor of, and confidant of the older adult client in search of a new place to call home.

■ MOVING A PERSON WITH MEMORY LOSS

The process of relocation for a senior experiencing memory loss has a unique set of challenges that older adults and their families often encounter. It is imperative, therefore, that the GCM take great care when assisting families and clients with this transition.

As the GCM works with families through this often difficult and emotional process, you will need to be aware of family dynamics, the medical, cognitive, and emotional needs of your client, and available community resources when creating a transition plan. Your role may also include locating appropriate living environments for the family to choose from, facilitating the actual move, and providing post-relocation support to the older adult and his or her family members.

To assist you with this challenge are the client's family and doctors, the staff of the new living facility, and community agencies such as your Area Agency on Aging (AAA). These are all valuable resources that you can consult with when creating a transition plan for a senior with memory loss.[16]

Relocation is not a one-size-fits-all experience for seniors with memory loss or their families. Your role is to transition your client (as well as his or her family) with the least amount of trauma possible through the use of a relocation plan custom tailored to his or her unique circumstances.

■ CONCLUSION

Relocation of an older adult is a multifaceted process involving the older adult, the family, numerous professionals, and select service providers. Relocation is accomplished over a variable amount of time and is unique to each individual. This transition requires the GCM to focus on the relocation of the social and psychological facets of the individual a well as their physical relocation, and the physical relocation of their personal belongings. The GCM supports the older adult through the process of relocation by providing insight, assistance, and support through each stage of the journey. Initially, this is done by offering the senior opportunities to participate in the decision-to-move process and by providing information to facilitate the selection of the new living environment. The GCM provides coordination and assistance with management of personal belongings and their physical relocation to the new home. And finally, the GCM is the trusted professional who provides follow-up assistance to the senior and the family, once the move has been completed. Friend, advisor, confidant, coordinator, facilitator, educator, resource expert; the role the GCM plays in relocation is invaluable and sets the stage for the older adult to achieve an optimal relocation outcome.

■ NOTES

1. Gaddy K. Special care environments: an overview of state laws for care of persons with Alzheimer's disease. *Bifocal: Newsletter of the ABA Commission on Legal Problems of the Elderly* (Washington, DC), 2000;21(2).

2. U.S. Census Bureau. Housing vacancies and homeownership (CPS/HVS). Available at: http://www.census.gov/hhes/www/housing/hvs/movingtoamerica2002/tab6.html Accessed September 28, 2006.

3. U.S. Health Department Administration on Aging. American housing survey for the United States in 2001, current housing reports (H150/01). Available at: http://www.aoa.gov/prof/Statistics/profile/2003/11.asp. Accessed August 7, 2005.

4. U.S. Census Bureau. Geographic mobility: 2002 to 2003. March 2004. Available at: http://www.census.gov/prod/2004pubs/p20-549.pdf. Accessed July 3, 2006.

5. Wiseman RF. Why older people move. *Res Aging*. 1980;2(2):141–154.

6. Pynoos J, Overton J, De Meire M. *Home Modification Resource Guide*. Los Angeles, CA: University of Southern California; 1996.

7. Peterson K. *Home Modification*. Los Angeles: Andrus Gerontology Center, University of Southern California; 2005.

8. Wiseman RF, Roseman CC. A typology of elderly migration based on the decision making process. *Economic Geography*. 1979;55(4):324–337.

9. U.S. Department of Housing and Urban Development. Senior housing—what you should know. Homes and Communities. January 31, 2006. Available at: http://www.hud.gov/offices/fheo/seniors/index.cfm. Accessed September 20, 2006.

10. Rotary Club and the Center for Healthy Aging of Santa Monica. Choosing senior housing and residential care. Helpguide. June 23, 2006. Available at: http://www.helpguide.org/elder/senior_housing_residential_care_types.htm. Accessed September 20, 2006.

11. Episcopal Homes Foundation. Retirement communities with life care. 2006. Available at: http://www.ehf.org/cw/cwlifecare.html. Accessed September 20, 2006.

12. New Lifestyles. Types of senior housing. 2004. Available at: http://www.newlifestyles.com/resources/articles/Types_of_Senior_Housing.aspx. Accessed September 20, 2006.

13. Dimond M, McCance K, King K. Forced residential relocation: its impact on the well-being of older adults. *West J Nurs Res*. 1987;9(4):445–465.

14. Young H. Moving to congregate housing: the last chosen home. *J Aging Stud*. 1998;12(2). Available at: http://0-web20epnet.com.opac.sfsu.edu/citation.asp?tb=1&_ug=sid+75B9572D%2DD37. Accessed December 28, 2004.

15. Lawton MP. Three functions of the residential environment. *J Housing Elderly*. 1983;5(1): 35–50.

16. Spencer B, White L. *Moving a Relative with Memory Loss: A Family Caregiver's Guide*. Santa Rosa, CA: Whisp Publications; 2000.

Chapter 17

Geriatric Care Management: Working with Nearly Normal Aging Families

Anne Rosenthal and Cathy Jo Cress

■ INTRODUCTION

Eugene O'Neill's play *Long Day's Journey into Night* tells us the wrenching tale of a dysfunctional family, marked by strained relationships and unresolved conflicts. Most aging families are healthy, not dysfunctional, but are knocked off balance by losses sustained when older family members decline or die, caregiving takes up huge blocks of family members' time, or significant family relationships and continuity disappear. These losses can disrupt even a healthy family. A "nearly normal" aging family can be righted if they have historically been compatible, cohesive, productive, and stable.

This chapter discusses the work geriatric care managers (GCMs) do with healthy aging families who at times are "nearly normal," caught in the vice grip of an elder's deterioration. It covers many hurdles healthy aging families face in supporting a progressively disabled older relative. This chapter gives the GCM maps to guide "nearly normal" families through the exhausting overload of long-distance caregiving, to identify and relieve caregiver overload, to work as part of a team to help the older person, and to navigate through family meetings among baby boomer siblings who, 50 years later, may be still chafing over who "Mom loved best."

■ DIFFERENTIATING BETWEEN THE HEALTHY AGING FAMILY AND THE CHALLENGED FAMILY

Although in the spectrum of aging families, there will always be a blur between healthy families and difficult families, GCMs can differentiate between the two. You can refer to two sections in Chapter 18, Difficult Families: Conflict, Dependence, and Mutuality, to help distinguish between the truly difficult family and the healthy, nearly normal family. You can evaluate family interaction to distinguish between a difficult family and healthy family. Then, you can use the guide "How Difficult Families Present" to assess whether the aging family served by the GCM is dysfunctional or nearly normal.

■ GERIATRIC CARE MANAGEMENT WITH FAMILIES

A recent survey by the National Alliance for Caregiving and the American Association of Retired Persons found that 22.4 million U.S. households, nearly 1 in 4, are providing care to a relative or friend aged 50 years or older or have provided care during the previous 12 months.[1]

GCMs often find themselves assisting family caregivers. What are these caregivers providing? Typically, they spend 18 hours a week taking the person they care for to physicians, managing the older person's finances, helping with grocery shopping, and providing hands-on personal care. Two-thirds of the caregivers also are employed. Of these, slightly more than half have had to make workplace accommodations, such as arriving late, leaving early, dropping back to part-time work, or even passing up promotions, to provide elder care. How can GCMs assist families in dealing with the conflicting demands of jobs, families, and caregiving?

There is much GCMs can do to offer families direct and indirect assistance. It behooves GCMs not only to be experts on community resources but also to be adept at understanding and communicating effectively with many different types of families, especially families that are in crisis.

In other words, GCMs are experts in knowing how to save families' time and money and prevent situations from taking an emotional toll on family members. Some of the areas where these resources can be conserved are home care services, community-based programs, and facilities. GCMs can also help families keep their finances in good shape through options such as long-term care insurance and publicly funded programs.

From GCMs, families also learn more about the illnesses with which their family members cope. GCMs are familiar with the symptoms and course of chronic diseases such as Alzheimer's and vascular dementia as well as stroke, Parkinson's disease, and arthritis. Families will benefit from GCMs' suggestions about what adaptive equipment can make the older person safer; the most effective ways to communicate with a distressed, demented individual; and other matters.

Frequently, families contact a GCM during a point of crisis. For instance, Mrs. L came with her adult son and daughter to the office of a GCM to discuss a possible placement for Mr. L. Mr. L had been recently hospitalized

for a debilitating stroke and was ready to be discharged from the hospital.

The daughter and son wanted to see their father cared for at a skilled nursing facility, but their mother wanted to care for her husband of nearly 50 years at home. The adult children expressed an objection to the home arrangement primarily because their mother had always been extremely dependent on her husband.

Mr. L had been a successful businessman, active in the community and civic affairs. His wife, coming from an earlier generation of women, knew little of managing anything outside the home, let alone managing the team of home health staff—nurses, a physical therapist, an occupational therapist, and a speech therapist—that would be caring for her husband. Mrs. L could not arrange for the durable medical equipment (e.g., a hospital bed, a wheelchair, and a commode) that he would need to remain at home. In fact, Mrs. L had never even written out a check!

The GCM met with the family together to discuss each member's concerns. The GCM assessed Mr. L's aptitude for making judgments, his reasoning ability, his memory, his orientation, his cognition, and his motor skills. The GCM also assessed whether the home was safe for someone with limited mobility who was using a wheelchair.

The GCM was able to assure the family that it was feasible to have Mr. L remain at home. Although he had some recent memory deficits, he seemed to be able to make sound judgments on his own behalf. He clearly expressed his desire to remain in his own home. Because the house had stairs, the GCM recommended that a ramp and strategically placed grab bars be put in and some area rugs be removed.

Together, the GCM and family were able to agree on a plan of care. The home care agency best equipped to care for Mr. L was contacted. It was Medicare certified, and Mr. L qualified for services at home that would not have to be paid for out of pocket.

The family members were grateful for the savings in time and cost. A coordinated schedule of care that supported Mr. L at home was established. His wife was pleased with the experienced help.

The adult children were able to return home to their jobs and families, knowing that the GCM would be monitoring the home care, following up with any additional matters that arose, contacting them regarding any change in their parent's status, and keeping them current on the situation at home.

The physician was able to obtain details from the home health staff, which helped him in treating Mr. L.

Although Mr. L eventually died peacefully at home in his sleep, the story does not end there. His wife continued to live in the same home. The GCM counseled the wife regarding her grief over the loss of her husband. After a period of mourning, she became interested in becoming more independent. She was supported and assisted in learning how to write out checks and take more control of her daily life. She has taken three cruises and regularly travels to see her family.

Recently, Mrs. L was hospitalized. The adult children, all of whom have busy professional schedules, contacted the GCM to assist with their mother's care. The GCM visited Mrs. L in the hospital. The GCM offered assurances that she would take care of whatever was necessary to settle Mrs. L back in at home. In addition, the care manager met with the hospital nurses and discharge planner to understand more fully Mrs. L's recovery care. The GCM remained in close contact with Mrs. L's family members to ensure that they agreed to the recommendations made for the assistance Mrs. L would need once she returned home.

The family saved time and money. The GCM was able to identify services for which Mrs. L would qualify under her insurance program. Mrs. L, who always prided herself on her cooking skills, reluctantly agreed to receive home-delivered meals. Later she admitted to being grateful for the nutritious meal and for the friendly volunteer who brightened her day. An attendant would come during the week to do light housekeeping, to stand by while Mrs. L took a bath, and to run errands until Mrs. L's strength returned. Mrs. L would be able to resume her visits to her family, enjoying new grandchildren. The family members know that when Mrs. L returns home, the GCM will be only a phone call away.

Adult children commonly face many problems. Three examples follow. In each case, a GCM steps in to help the adult children solve the problems:

CASE STUDY

Problem Situation 1

An older woman fell and broke her hip. She was hospitalized for hip replacement surgery, and the hospital says she is now ready to return home. The woman's daughter is panicking because she is scheduled to leave for a trip to Europe in 2 days and she doesn't know how her mother can manage without her. She calls a GCM to ask for help.

The GCM asks the following questions:

- Does the mother want to return to her home or go to a care facility to recuperate?
- Can the mother complete activities of daily living (e.g., dressing, eating, toileting, bathing) on her own?
- How are the mother's cognitive functions? Is she oriented to time, place, and person?
- How is the mother's judgment and reasoning ability?
- What is the mother's living environment like? Are there obstacles (e.g., stairs, bathroom adaptive equipment, rugs) that should be dealt with?

The GCM talks to the hospital discharge planner regarding the following matters:

- What will Medicare cover if the mother is at home? What will Medicare cover if the mother is at a care facility?
- What will the GCM do if the mother returns home? Determine the amount of home care required and recruit the home care worker?
- What will the GCM do if the mother transfers to a care facility? Locate the facility and arrange for admission?
- How will the GCM help the mother to deal with her questions, anxiety, and planning during her daughter's absence?
- What support system can be put in place during the daughter's absence? Is there a local family who can offer support? What will the GCM do if the daughter would like to retain ongoing care management services?
- What will the GCM do to communicate with the daughter, monitor the mother, and communicate with the mother's hired caregivers during the daughter's absence?

CASE STUDY

Problem Situation 2
A working professor has concerns about his mother, who lives out of state. The mother is in an assisted living facility, appears quite depressed, and is now displaying some paranoid ideations. He is the only relative and is 3,000 miles away. He thinks he should relocate his mother to live with him, but he is not sure. He asks for the advice of a GCM.

The GCM explores with the son the quality of his mother's living situation. Is she happy where she is? What is the quality of the care she is receiving? Are there other levels of care available in the facility should she require a higher or lower level of care?

The care manager visits the mother in her facility and has more discussions with the son to determine answers to the following questions:

- Who visits the mother now?
- What is the son's home situation like? What kind of social stimulation is available for the mother there?
- What has been the quality of her visits to his home in the past?
- If the mother moves to his home, what modifications would be necessary for her safety?
- What are the financial aspects of the two options being considered (i.e., relocation to the son's home, remaining in the care facility)?
- Are there facilities to be considered in the son's area should the home arrangement not be feasible?
- What about the mother's paranoid ideations? Does she have a history of emotional disturbance? What is the nature of the psychiatric intervention she has received at the care facility? Could that intervention be improved? If the mother relocates to the son's residence, can the mother's emotional problems be adequately addressed?
- How does the mother feel about her son's wish to relocate her to his home? Is she comfortable with the idea?
- What are the son's motivations for wanting to initiate the move? Are there other family members to consider?
- If the mother remains where she is, what could be done to improve the quality of her life?

Problem Situation 3

An older divorced woman with a history of dementia secondary to alcoholism is addicted to buying items from a home-shopping channel. The older woman is indiscriminately ordering hundreds of dollars of items each week. She has a live-in attendant who helps with personal care. The older woman's sister calls a GCM because she is concerned there will be no money left to use for the older woman's long-term care.

The GCM asks the following questions:

- What is the attendant's role with regard to the impulsive shopping? Can she be enlisted to intervene?
- What seems to trigger the older woman's impulse to make phone purchases?
- Can the older woman be diverted?
- Is the older woman cooperative?
- Does the older woman lack the capacity to consider the consequences of her actions? If she does lack this capacity, should a conservatorship or a guardianship be considered?

Exhibit 17–1   Alarm Bells List for Visiting Long-Distance Relative

- Unpaid bills
- Missed appointments
- Clutter in a home that was once always neat
- Weight loss
- Memory loss, change in short-term memory
- Poor grooming by a person who was once meticulous
- Getting lost
- Wandering
- Refusing to go with friends on outings or to religious services
- Refusing any suggestion or conversely agreeing to everything without consideration
- Mood swings, getting angry quickly
- Refusing to go to medical providers
- Can't take care of activities of daily living: cooking, bathing, dressing, housekeeping, etc.
- Entering contests, credit card maxed out on shopping channels

■ WORKING WITH LONG-DISTANCE CAREGIVERS

Families continue caring for older family members even if they live long distances apart. Nearly 7 million Americans are responsible for the care of an older family member who lives an average of 300 miles away.

Why are there so many long-distance care providers in the United States today? Baby boomers move frequently with their jobs. We are a mobile society and many of us have moved away from our birthplace, where our parents still live. Many parents of baby boomers retire to warmer climates (Arizona, Florida) while their adult children live far away with their job and family.

What Can a GCM Do for a Long-Distance Family?

Long-distance family members spend an overwhelming amount of time caregiving. They

What do these three problem situations have in common? In all three, families are facing problems and GCMs provide assistance using their problem-solving skills and understanding of short- and long-term planning. All three families benefit from a GCM's assistance. In all three cases, the GCMs assess the situation, learn what the family's preferences are, make appropriate recommendations based on what is feasible, implement the recommendations once the family members approve them, follow up and monitor the situation, and adjust services and GCM involvement as the family's needs change.

spend time caregiving over the phone and more time flying and driving to give care for older family members. The GCM can save the long-distance family member both time and money by taking over many of the caregiving tasks for the family. The GCM can also save the long-distance caregiver more money by assuming some of the adult child's duties. Many times, long-distance family caregivers are employed. They are leaving early, getting to work late, and dropping back to part-time hours to deal with the burdens of long-distance caregiving; thus they are losing money. Oftentimes, they exhaust their vacation or family leave time to care for long-distance family members.

The GCM's involvement with long-distance family members and their aging relatives can save caregivers from being overcome by their daunting task. Long-distance caregivers, like all caregivers, are sandwiched between the needs of their aging parents, their teenagers, their own adult children, work, and caregiving. This is an explosive combination that can result in mental and physical problems for the long-distance caregiver. Depression and anxiety can result from the stress of long-distance caregiving; these dedicated adult children can end up with depression, anxiety, and weakened immune systems that may lead to physical illness.

The stress of long-distance caregiving can also result in spousal and child abuse, troubled marriages, and divorce. The intervention of a GCM in a long-distance caregiving situation can be an incredible win-win opportunity for the long-distance caregiver, older family members, and the whole extended family.

Adult children living at a distance from their older relatives face complex emotional and logistical issues. How do they know what to look for if they suspect their parents are having problems? Exhibit 17–1 describes some alarm bells that should go off in the long-distance caregiver's head when he or she visits an older relative.

You as a GCM can alert long-distance family members to these warning signs. If they observe these red flags on a long-distance visit with their older family member and then ask you to begin services, you have many excellent options to offer the family. Your first step is to complete a psychosocial and functional assessment (see Chapters 3 and 4 on psychosocial assessment and functional assessment). Administering a mental status questionnaire is also suggested to assess cognitive functioning. Your next step is to report these findings to the long-distance family member and request that you be able to make an appointment with the older person's primary physician and take the older person to the appointment. It is a good idea to call ahead to the registered nurse in the office and explain your geriatric care management role plus fax in a summary of your assessment findings so the physician and/or nurse can read them before the appointment.

Next Steps for the GCM Assisting Long-Distance Family Members

The next step is to find out, after the initial assessment, if the long-distance caregiver wishes you to monitor the older family member weekly, monthly, or at all. Ask if the family members want you to be on call for emergencies. Both are a good idea. If they agree and they want to hire you, help them understand there are many tasks you could offer assistance with.

Work with the long-distance family members and older client to map out a plan in the event the older family member is hospitalized. This is sometimes best done in a family meeting with the GCM present or with just family members present. This plan starts with deciding which hospital the older person wants to use. This appears basic, but sometimes a person can favor one hospital over another, or one hospital is better equipped than another is. The discussion should include where the older person might go after hospitalization. Does the older person want to go home with care providers if needed? If care or rehab is required after hospitalization, does the older family member want to go to a skilled nursing facility for recovery or to home using Medicare-covered physical therapy, occupational therapy, and paid home care? Would the adult children prefer to have the older person come to their home to recover? If the older person needs to move permanently because of disability, where does the person want to move? Does the person want to downsize to a smaller home? Would the person move to a nursing home? Would he or she move to an adult child's home? (See Chapter 16 on moving.) Having a plan like this in place cuts down on crisis management and replaces it with preventative maintenance for the client and family.

Find a neighbor, old friend, or nearby family member who is willing to check on the older person on a regular basis, report regularly to you, plus notify you of any crisis. This sets up a monitoring network and safety net through the elder's continuum of care. You can also locate an emergency response system and put it in place, if there are no caregivers nearby. You should be the emergency contact in addition to the long-distance family members. Your value as a GCM is that you are there and the long-distance family members are far away.

Create a care plan for the older person (see Chapter 5 on geriatric assessment and writing a care plan). You can also help the family hire ongoing care providers if needed, monitor household maintenance problems, and generally manage the older family member for the long-distance family.

Additional ways you can help long-distance family members and give them peace of mind are shown in Exhibit 17-2.

Exhibit 17–2   Assisting Long-Distance Family Members

- Arrange regular visits from religious groups if appropriate.
- Telephone or e-mail or send monthly report to long-distance family on a regular basis.
- Arrange services from the community such as Meals On Wheels.
- Accompany older person to all medical appointments.
- Monitor neighbors or friends or anyone who might take advantage of the older person, carry out any sweetheart scams, or exert an undue influence.

Creating a Caregiver Binder

If the long-distance family members want to manage the care and monitoring of the older person, suggest they make a binder containing information about the older family member, much like the client data book that you may have on each client in your GCM office.

Suggest including the following sections:

- Emergency contacts: Make a list of all the person's emergency contacts—telephone numbers, e-mail addresses, addresses—such as for neighbors, friends, and family members.
- Physician information: Complete information including name, address, telephone number, e-mail address, and specialty of older person's physicians.
- Pharmacy information: List the name of pharmacy, address, telephone number, exact meds, dosage, over-the-counter medications, vitamins.
- Religious information: List the person's clergy contacts if he or she has religious/spiritual connections.
- Local support agency information: List local agencies involved in the person's care, including names and contact info. Examples: Meals On Wheels, home care agency.
- Neighbor information: List the neighbor's name, address, phone number, e-mail address.
- Friend information: List information on any old family friends in the area, including name, address, phone number, and e-mail address.
- Emergency plan for household: _____

The National Association of Professional Geriatric Care Managers has an excellent binder available in the GCM Store on a Web site called *Caregiver Planner—A Notebook to Organize Vital Information*, by Betsy Carey Evatt. It has most of the tabs mentioned in Exhibit 17–2, and the family member can add more.

You can also coach family members by having a conference call or a family meeting to decide how to share tasks. Delegate responsibilities so that one family member is not doing it all. You can also task long-distance family members with doable responsibilities

they can achieve without increased stress. See Exhibit 17–3 for some examples.

You can encourage the long-distance care providers to make good use of their time when they visit their parent. They should make an appointment with the physician during their visit and establish a relationship with the doctor, if they do not have one already. On a visit to the older family member, they should also meet with an elder-law attorney and discuss estate planning and ensure there is a durable power of attorney, living will, and all appropriate legal documents in place.

Exhibit 17–3   Long-Distance Care Provider Tasks

- Take home a copy of the yellow pages from the area where the parent lives for reference.
- Find all legal documents, take them home, and put them in a binder. (If these include original signed documents, make copies and put originals in a safe deposit box or safe place.) Key legal and financial documents might include the following:

    ○ Legal documents
    ○ Birth certificate
    ○ Social security card
    ○ Divorce decree
    ○ Will

- Set up a filing system at the long-distance caregiver's home for the older person and include all pertinent documents involving the older person.
- Have all mail forwarded to one of the long-distance caregiver's addresses and manage mail for the older person.
- Set up online chat room in which family members can discuss the older person's issues.
- Manage round-robin letter if family members choose that form of communication.
- Be a relief care provider—stay with the older person on a regular basis (1 time per month, once every 6 months)—to give the primary caregiver respite.
- Invite care receiver to your home for visit/respite.
- Gather all insurance information and take it to a financial planner to make sure policies are current and appropriate:

    ○ Auto
    ○ Homeowners
    ○ Medicare
    ○ Medicaid
    ○ Medigap
    ○ Long-term care
    ○ Disability

CASE STUDY

A working daughter became concerned because her mother, who lives across the country, began phoning her frequently through the day and night, sometimes up to 15 times per day. The daughter suggested that her mother come live with her or have a companion, but the mother refused to discuss the subject. The worried daughter contacted the employee assistance division of her company and was given the name of a GCM in her city as well as the names of several GCMs in her mother's town.

The daughter first contacted the GCM in her own city. That GCM gave the daughter information about the nature, depth, and scope of geriatric care management services. The GCM also provided the daughter with a guideline statement called "How to Find a Qualified Geriatric Care Manager" (see Appendix 17–A).

Shortly thereafter, the daughter flew out to see her mother. She had made appointments to interview four GCMs using the guidelines she had been given. She met with each GCM at her mother's residence, introducing the GCM to her mother as someone who specialized in helping older people live as independently as possible.

The daughter hired the GCM who responded to the guideline questions most thoughtfully and competently and to whom her mother responded most favorably. This GCM was also the most proactive. For instance, the hired GCM was the only one who asked the mother what she thought she needed to make her life better. The mother was able to state that she would like to have someone live in a spare bedroom. The GCM assessed the mother and her home and made recommendations for household adaptations such as a railing, improved lighting, and an address that was clearly marked outside the house. Additionally, the GCM recruited an attendant, who was sensitive to the mother's habit of calling her daughter.

The incessant calls to the daughter gradually ceased as the mother became comfortable with her new companion. The GCM visited the mother on a regular basis, offering activity suggestions to the companion. For instance, the mother was very fond of dogs. Upon the GCM's suggestion, the mother and her companion visited the local dog park, borrowed books from the library on dogs, and subscribed to a dog magazine. The GCM was even able to arrange visits on a regular basis from a GCM assistant with a calm and responsive dog.

Other tasks provided by the GCM to this long-distance family on a direct and indirect basis included the following:

- Phoning the daughter regularly to provide status reports and to respond to the daughter's ongoing concerns about her mother
- Arranging for weekend relief help and relief help when the regular attendant needed time off
- Making appointments to meet with medical specialists, dentists, optometrists, and psychiatrists as needed
- Replacing a broken washing machine and torn window dressing
- Locating a bill-paying service
- Locating an audiologist and reputable hearing aid specialist
- Arranging for plumbing and gardening services
- Arranging for volunteers to call regularly and arrange for intervention should the situation warrant follow-up

- Arranging for the installation of devices that help older persons better manage in their homes
- Arranging for an emergency response system to allow an older person who falls and is injured to push a button, leading an automatic dialer to contact a central system that can then contact the person or responsible parties

Some public utilities and the U.S. Postal Service offer gatekeeper/home observation programs in which service people who visit the home regularly are trained to notice anything unusual or any indication of need and report it so that someone may investigate and take action.

It is not uncommon for a GCM to contact a GCM in another town (where either the out-of-town relative or the older person lives) to coordinate efforts or to provide background information (with the permission of all parties) so that the other GCM can provide services.

■ HELPING ADULT CHILDREN AND FAMILIES MANAGE THE OVERWHELMING DEMANDS OF CAREGIVING

Middle-aged people, usually women, who are balancing family, work, and caregiving responsibilities are likely to report feeling stressed, frustrated, and sometimes even angry. Because they often care for children and parents simultaneously, these adult children have sometimes been referred to as the "sandwich generation." They feel squeezed between the needs of so many people that they are vulnerable to anxiety, depression, and weakened immune responses. Caregiving can stress even the happiest of marriages.

GCMs are able to help with practical suggestions regarding placement, referrals, and medical needs as well as some very specific recommendations that can assist caregivers in reducing their stress. For instance, GCMs may recommend that caregivers join support groups or otherwise alleviate caregiver overload.

Support Groups

Support groups can be of help if the participants are focused on a particular problem. The following is one family's experience with a support group.

CASE STUDY

Mrs. R's husband was away on business when he suffered a debilitating stroke. Until this time, the Rs were actively enjoying their "golden years." Mr. R's stroke rendered him unable to speak. He could still manage most of his daily living activities and attended speech therapy three times per week at a local rehabilitation center. However, his inability to communicate placed a tremendous burden on Mrs. R, who continued to work outside the home.

Mr. R continued to be as good-natured as ever, but Mrs. R was exhausted from worry and on the verge of mental collapse. The hospital social worker recognized the wife's fragile mental state and referred her to a private GCM. The GCM met with the wife in the hospital and, after recognizing her overwhelming situation, recommended that she join a support group for spouses of stroke victims. Mrs. R reluctantly joined the group and was immediately relieved to know that there were others who shared her experience. Through the support group, she made new friends and learned about new resources to help her.

Exhibit 17–4   Checklist of Brain Impairment Problems

Please check one box for each problem, indicating how often these problems have occurred *in the past week.*

Problem	Very Often	Somewhat Often	Never	Comments
1. Asking the same question over and over	❑	❑	❑	_____
2. Having trouble remembering recent events (e.g., items in the newspaper or on TV)	❑	❑	❑	_____
3. Having trouble remembering significant past events	❑	❑	❑	_____
4. Losing or misplacing things	❑	❑	❑	_____
5. Forgetting what day it is	❑	❑	❑	_____
6. Starting but not finishing things	❑	❑	❑	_____
7. Having difficulty concentrating on a task	❑	❑	❑	_____
8. Destroying property	❑	❑	❑	_____
9. Doing embarrassing things	❑	❑	❑	_____
10. Waking up others at night	❑	❑	❑	_____
11. Talking loudly and rapidly	❑	❑	❑	_____
12. Appearing anxious or worried	❑	❑	❑	_____
13. Engaging in behavior that is potentially dangerous to him- or herself or others	❑	❑	❑	_____
14. Threatening to hurt him or herself	❑	❑	❑	_____
15. Threatening to hurt others	❑	❑	❑	_____
16. Being verbally aggressive toward others	❑	❑	❑	_____
17. Appearing sad or depressed	❑	❑	❑	_____
18. Expressing feelings of hopelessness or sadness about the future (e.g., "Nothing worthwhile ever happens," "I never do anything right")	❑	❑	❑	_____
19. Crying and being tearful	❑	❑	❑	_____
20. Commenting about the death of him- or herself or others (e.g., "Life isn't worth living," "I'd be better off dead")	❑	❑	❑	_____
21. Talking about being lonely	❑	❑	❑	_____
22. Commenting about feeling worthless or being a burden to others	❑	❑	❑	_____
23. Commenting about feeling like a failure or about nor having worthwhile accomplishments in life	❑	❑	❑	_____
24. Arguing, being irritable, and complaining	❑	❑	❑	_____
25. Being unable to communicate	❑	❑	❑	_____

Source: Reprinted with permission from L. Teri et al., Assessment of Behavioral Problems in Dementia: The Revised Memory and Behavior Problems Checklist, *Psychology and Aging,* Vol. 7, pp. 622–631, © 1992, Linda Teri, Ph.D.

In addition to the sense of camaraderie found in support groups, there is a cathartic effect that frequently takes place because it is only in a milieu of peers that some people can share their feelings. Support groups have been developed for various kinds of geriatric problems. There are support groups for spouses, adult children, those who have family members with an Alzheimer's diagnosis, those who have a diagnosis of early Alzheimer's, dementia, stroke, diabetes, Parkinson's, and the like. Support groups are frequently organized through nonprofit entities such as family service agencies (Jewish Family Services, Catholic Family Services) and religious affiliations such as synagogues and churches. Hospitals and long-term care facilities also frequently offer support groups to the community at large. The local Area Agency on Aging, county department on aging, and senior centers offer support groups directly or can recommend support groups. Academic institutions, especially universities with medical and gerontological programs, offer support services. The Alzheimer's Association and Family Caregiver Alliance are also excellent sources for group support. You should develop a list of these support groups for use in practice.

Alleviating Caregiver Overload

Because many adult children take the "I can do it all" approach, they frequently become overwhelmed with unrealistic caregiving expectations. GCMs are in a position to point out the need to make compromises and assist adult caregivers with adjusting their expectations when they are distressed over the burden of caregiving. One helpful approach is to assist caregiving family members in setting limits on their time and energy—to assist them in knowing to what extent they are able to be directly involved and when they can rely on hired help or services to ease the burden of caregiving.

Even after family members set limits on their time, they may tend to push these limits. If this occurs, family members need to be encouraged to look at why they are uncomfortable with the limits they have established. Family members may be advised to be alert for signals that they have overextended themselves. Exhibit 17–5 lists signs of caregiver overload. Exhibit 17–6 suggests some strategies that a GCM can suggest to family caregivers experiencing caregiver overload.

Exhibit 17–5
Signs of Caregiver Overload

- **Sleep disorder.** Depression, overexertion, and nighttime caregiving may prevent caregivers from getting adequate sleep.
- **Marital problems.** Marriages can be strained because of caregiving responsibilities.
- **Reduced employment.** Caregiving demands may force family members to curtail their hours or quit a job, adding financial stress.
- **Social withdrawal.** Family caregivers may become lonely, lamenting diminished contacts with friends and fewer social activities.
- **Depression.** Caring for a physically or cognitively impaired individual may leave the caregiver feeling helpless and hopeless.
- **Guilt.** Caregivers may begin to wish the care recipient was the way he or she used to be or that someone else would take some of the responsibility. They may feel guilty about having these thoughts.
- **Anxiety.** Family caregivers may begin to feel edgy or nervous. Regardless of their efforts, they may have a sense of falling behind.
- **Physical problems.** Increased physical and emotional stress may decrease the caregiver's resistance to sickness. Family caregivers may complain about frequent colds, headaches, or backaches.
- **Fatigue.** Caregiving is physically and emotionally hard work and may lead to exhaustion.

Exhibit 17–6   Strategies for Solving Caregiver Overload

Following are some strategies that a GCM can suggest to family caregivers experiencing caregiver overload:

- The GCM can help family members to begin setting realistic expectations of themselves as caregivers.

- The GCM can encourage family members to explain to employers that flexible scheduling at certain times may be needed to help parents keep physicians' appointments. The GCM can also offer suggestions for making up the work. If comprehensive caregiving is required, the GCM can suggest that the Family Leave Act may be used.

- The GCM can encourage caregivers to talk with other family members about feelings and ask family members for their suggestions. Caregivers can ask children what they need (e.g., help with homework, a special shopping trip) and ask for their help in making it happen. Caregivers can also try to include children in caregiving responsibilities by asking them to run errands, fix a meal, or simply sit and visit with the older person.

- The GCM can encourage caregivers to plan some time for spouses, explaining personal stressors and asking the spouse to share personal stressors as well. Spouses can work together to make some changes in the partnership that will help accommodate the caregiving responsibilities.

- The GCM can encourage caregivers to seek out and use community resources. Most people are surprised at the wealth of community resources that are available at no cost. Public libraries, Area Agencies on Aging, and local senior centers have information about community resources.

- Most important, the GCM can encourage family caregivers to make time for themselves. Unless caregivers stay physically and mentally healthy, they will not be any good to themselves or others.

Frequently, family members will express a sense of relief that they have found a GCM, someone on whom they can call to help with problem solving and to listen to frustrations. GCMs can also use an assessment tool to measure caregiver burnout. (See Chapter 3 on psychosocial assessment.) Exhibit 17–7 is the Zarit Burden Interview that can be used to assess a caregiver's response to caregiving.

Family Support Assessment

It is a good idea to suggest to a family, whether long-distance or local, that they sit down with the older family member and complete a family support assessment (see Exhibit 17–8). This assessment should be completed in a relaxed family meeting at the parental home. What you are really encouraging is that the family plan for incapacity and ask the older person how he or she wishes the family to help should the person's health decline. This type of assessment and planning helps everyone have a map to follow as the parent ages. Family members will know which child will be the lead care provider and which other members of the family or community will have a role in the supportive and caregiving tasks.

Family Meetings

A family meeting is a meeting held with family members to discuss a problem, large or small, involving an older relative. These gatherings are often led by an outside party who can remain objective and keep attendees on track.

Exhibit 17-7 The Zarit Burden Interview

Do you feel:

1. That your relative asks for more help than he/she needs?*
2. That because of the time you spend with your relative you don't have enough time for yourself?
3. Stressed between caring for your relative and trying to meet other responsibilities for your family or work?
4. Embarrassed over your relative's behavior?
5. Angry when you are around your relative?
6. That your relative currently affects your relationship with other family members in a negative way?
7. Afraid of what the future holds for your relative?
8. Your relative is dependent on you?
9. Strained when you are around your relative?
10. Your health has suffered because of your involvement with your relative?
11. That you don't have as much privacy as you would like because of your relative?
12. That your social life has suffered because you are caring for your relative?
13. Uncomfortable having friends over because of your relative?
14. That your relative seems to expect you to take care of him/her as if you were the only one he/she could depend on?
15. That you don't have enough money to care for your relative in addition to the rest of your expenses?
16. That you will be unable to take care of your relative much longer?
17. You have lost control of your life since your relative's illness?
18. You wish you could just leave the care of your relative to someone else?
19. Uncertain about what to do about your relative?
20. You should be doing something more for your relative?
21. You could be doing a better job in caring for your relative?

Overall, how burdened do you feel in caring for your relative (not at all, a little, moderately, quite a bit, extremely)?

* Items 1–21 are measured as never, rarely, sometimes, quite frequently, nearly always.

Source: Reprinted with permission by Steven H. Zarit.

Exhibit 17-8 Family Support Assessment

- Which child do you want to be your main caretaker? Why?
- How can your children divide tasks so they can meet your needs?
- Will nieces and nephews be a part of care supports?
- Will friends or people in the community be a part of your web? If so, who?
- Will a rabbi, minister, or spiritual leader be part of your support system? If so, who?
- If children live a long distance away, how can they contribute to your future care needs?

Reasons to Hold a Family Meeting

There are many reasons you can suggest a family hold a family meeting. If families are having difficulty sharing tasks, a family meeting is an opportunity when you can coach family members to divide tasks and delegate responsibilities so no one person is doing it all.

Family meetings are an excellent way to help families plan for an older person's disabilities, manage incapacity, or solve a crisis with an older person including decisions such as whether a person be put on life support or move out of his or her home of many years because upkeep is a problem. They are a great way to do general problem solving with a family. It is inevitable that when you arrange a family meeting in which hard decisions must be made that adult children revert back to their childhood personas and dredge up old hurts and angers while trying to solving here-and-now problems. Many families are dysfunctional in some ways. These family systems may be the most challenging you deal with. (See Chapter 18, Difficult Families: Conflict, Dependence, and Mutuality.)

Who Should Moderate a Family Meeting?

You can moderate the meeting if you are a seasoned GCM and have skills and experience as a mediator. Five years of experience as a GCM is a good benchmark to assess whether you can mediate a family meeting. If you do not have this experience, find a licensed clinical social worker with a background in aging or a mediator with experience in aging. Family meetings can be a brutal tug-of-war.

Setting Up a Family Meeting

If the family agrees to hold a family meeting, you and the moderator can plan the family meeting. Plan an agenda for a successful meeting. Before the meeting, ask all family members, especially long-distance members, to list their concerns and the tasks they are willing to do and to mail or e-mail this list to you. Integrate these concerns and agreements into your agenda, and hold the meeting at a neutral site.

During the Family Meeting

During the meeting, be certain everyone has an opportunity to express feelings, voice preferences, and offer suggestions. Focus on the positive. Identify something each person can do. Recognize each person's limitations (for instance, medical illness, lives long distance). Create a feeling of trust and support. Keep the meeting on current concerns rather than past conflicts ("Dad paid for college for you but not for me!"). Address the needs from each family member's point of view (usually siblings). Be certain everyone has an opportunity to participate.

Although the reason for the meeting may be one major crisis or problem to solve, it is a good idea to integrate many of the items listed in Exhibit 17–9 into the meeting, if they haven't already been addressed.

After the Meeting

In a family meeting, you and/or a moderator can help the family strike a balance.

Following the family meeting, draw up the plan that was decided in the meeting of what each family member will do and when each person will do it, and send the plan to all family members for them to sign off.

Improving Family Communication

Sometimes you may need to set limits with the family. Family members may want to engage you in their arguments or may want you to share information that you are not comfortable sharing. You should model ways of showing concern without rejecting.

What should you do when you find yourself trapped in a mistake, such as getting involved in a family's argument? One approach might be to say, "You know, I realize that I have been trying to change your mind on something that you have some definite feelings about. Could you excuse me for this and explain the situation to me once more?" Another approach might be, "Although I didn't mean to, I think I've been

Exhibit 17–9   Agenda Items for a Family Meeting

- ❑ Divide up tasks if one family member is doing caregiving directly.
- ❑ Break caregiving into manageable tasks. For example:
    - ❑ Long-distance son pays for caregiving.
    - ❑ Out-of-town daughter gets all mail, pays bills; teenage son sorts it for her.
    - ❑ Local niece visits aunt on a regular basis; grandchildren send cards weekly.
- ❑ Coach adult children to ask for flexible hours at work.
- ❑ Help adult children who provide direct care to plan time alone with spouses.
- ❑ Encourage adult children caregivers to make time for themselves.
- ❑ Encourage adult children caregivers to go to support group.
- ❑ Help adult children members set realistic expectations.
- ❑ Decide who will check into all legal documents.
- ❑ Coach family members to share tasks.
- ❑ Delegate responsibilities so no one person is doing it all.
- ❑ Help adult children set realistic expectations.
- ❑ Decide who will be in charge of house repairs.
- ❑ Decide who will pay bills.
- ❑ Decide who will take parent to doctor's appointments if not the GCM.
- ❑ Arrange a schedule for all family members to call older person regularly.
- ❑ Decide who will be in charge of arranging for care.
- ❑ Decide which family member will respond to emergencies.
- ❑ Decide which family member will be main spokesperson to GCM.
- ❑ Arrange for long-distance family regularly to send cards, videotapes of family.
- ❑ Decide who will introduce new care providers to older adult.
- ❑ Decide who will contact all new possible services in continuum of care.
- ❑ Decide who will sign contracts for services.
- ❑ Decide who will have right to approve expenses and budget.
- ❑ Decide to whom all mail will be forwarded and who will manage mail.
- ❑ Decide who will set up an online chat room so all family members can communicate and share information.
- ❑ Decide who will manage round-robin letter if family chooses that form of communication.
- ❑ Arrange for family members to be relief care provider—stay with parent on some regular basis to give primary caregiver respite.
- ❑ Arrange for family members to have care receiver stay at their home for visit/respite on regular basis, if appropriate.
- ❑ Moderate and discuss problems with siblings not doing their share.
- ❑ Help siblings appreciate each other.
- ❑ Coordinate all family members writing regular notes to primary caregiver saying how much they appreciate what the person is doing and how hard it is.

arguing with you instead of listening to you. Could you help me out by explaining it to me again, while I pay better attention?"

Families who are having difficulties working as a cohesive family system may benefit from guidance from a GCM. Family caregivers can be helped to recognize and prioritize their problems so they can become empowered to develop their own solutions.

Some things for you to consider are how the family seems to be functioning. What is the family caregiver's own attitude toward aging and an older person's particular illness (e.g., Alzheimer's disease)? If the caregiver has the attitude that older people are supposed to become demented, then the older person's behavior will not be seen as a problem to be considered. What motivates the family to care? If a caregiver has a full load with a job, marriage, and children, he or she may not be looking for additional problems. How does the family work? Do the family members address problems together, or do problems split them apart? Is there domination from a single family member? Are abuse and threats, implied or real, used to control others? What is valued by the family? Will the family be receptive to suggestions?

If the family is receptive to suggestions, you can help improve how a family communicates by modeling the following communication techniques:

- You should not interrupt family members until they have finished speaking.
- You should show each member that he or she has value in the family.
- You should show each member that his or her views are valid.
- You should show each member that his or her experience of a situation is valid.
- You should help family members work together to make the load easier for all to bear.
- You should realize that family members will make mistakes and that mistakes are okay as long as the family members learn from them.
- You should remember that it is okay for a family member to state that he or she has reached his or her limit of time, emotion, or stress.
- You should encourage family members to ask each other for help.
- You should allow family members to decide whether they can be helpful.

Helping Families Develop Solutions for Their Needs

Professionals should look beyond actual medical care and understand the caregiving dynamic of an older person's family to help ensure that both the older person and the

caregivers have an adequate support system. Two older people can have exactly the same needs, but two caregivers will perceive the degree of burden very differently.

The following strategies can help you to assess the needs of family caregivers and counsel them to develop appropriate solutions for their individual needs.

Dealing with a Caregiver's Denial

Denial is a common defense mechanism that individuals use, especially when they are under stress. To deny or ignore a problem allows the individual time to temporarily adjust to the idea of the problem or may serve to permanently keep the troubled thought or problem out of conscious awareness. Caregivers wait an average of 3 years from the onset of symptoms of Alzheimer's disease or vascular dementia before bringing an older person to be evaluated, usually following a dramatic event such as setting the stove on fire. Caregivers in denial are restless and inattentive. Their ability to process information may be impaired. They are controlling but may be very tired. They may report that they do not have time to exercise, or they may overeat. The coping strategies are not to think, not to feel, not to do. Professionals need to repeat information, perhaps over a period of a year or more, until they know caregivers are assimilating it.

Dealing with a Caregiver's Emotions

Caregivers frequently attempt to control their emotions, particularly anger and anxiety, so they are not overwhelmed by them. That anger surfaces when an adult daughter looks at a mother who is falling apart physically and sees herself or when she looks at someone she has never really liked very much, such as an alcoholic and abusive father, and realizes she has to care for him or her. What motivates the caregiver may not be love but rather a sense of responsibility, ethics, and morality. Caregivers facing such predicaments struggle with a complex array of emotions. There may be a desire to be absolved from responsibility, but the family caregiver feels bound to the parent because he or she is a moral human being. You can help with this by sorting out the emotions, clarifying feelings, and finding support for those feelings, including psychotherapy.

Helping Caregivers Build a Partnership

You should encourage caregivers to talk with older relatives without controlling the older relatives. Caregivers should work with the older person to develop a list of questions before a physician's appointment, for example, rather than monopolizing the discussion with the physician during the appointment. Partnerships are difficult to achieve when individuals have not always had a caring, loving relationship. When older people do not want to go along with the program, caregivers should be accepting without attacking the person or becoming hostile. Caregivers must be helped to recognize that they cannot always be the most effective change agents. Perhaps someone else within the family system can be the catalyst.

You can work with the family physician, neighbors, or clergy as individuals who can get the older person to see the world differently. The following story illustrates how a GCM can help a family build a partnership.

CASE STUDY

Mrs. D was always, according to her four children, a controlling mother. As a result, all of her children became successful professionals in their fields; Mrs. D would not have it any other way. However, when Mrs. D turned 87, she suffered a series of strokes that would have incapacitated most individuals. Mrs. D's determination overrode her

frailty. Her adult children, with the help of her physician, who they believed was one of the few people in her life for whom she had high regard, finally convinced her to stop driving. Her life at home was quite marginal because it could not be adapted to meet all of her disabilities, including disabilities in vision, hearing, and mobility. Her children were convinced that the only solution was for her to move to a care facility, but Mrs. D refused to discuss it. The GCM helped Mrs. D's children form a partnership with her physician, who fully agreed with her children that it was not safe for her to be in her home. It took several months of medical visits; each time Mrs. D's physician brought up the subject of relocation, Mrs. D would agree to consider it, and the discussion progressed at each medical visit. When Mrs. D asked her physician where he thought she should move, he suggested her children be included in the discussion of relocation. Mrs. D finally agreed to make the move, especially because she convinced her physician to make her his only home-visit patient.

Building Partnerships with Professionals

GCMs work as part of a professional team. GCMs can offer a full-service package to their client families by developing alliances with allied professionals such as elder-law attorneys, certified public accountants, fiduciaries, trust officers, nurses, and geriatric psychiatrists and psychologists. This team approach is advantageous for several reasons: it streamlines the services offered to older clients, ensuring continuity of care; it makes for a more efficient services delivery pathway; and it avoids duplication of services.

You can be at the fulcrum of the service matrix, recommending the types of services and the extent of service required based on an initial evaluation of the client and adjusting the recommended services as the client's needs change. For example, the following case study shows how a GCM can use her professional partnerships to the advantage of her clients.

CASE STUDY

The chronically ill single son of an older client contacted a GCM to assist with concerns he had for his mother, Mrs. H. Mrs. H was living alone and seemed to the son to be losing weight, forgetting medical appointments, and was unable to keep track of bills that needed to be paid. Mrs. H had several falls but no resulting injuries. The son stated that his mother had always been a private and self-sufficient woman and that this new behavior was very much out of character. He had had a recent medical emergency and was concerned about who could look after his mother in the event he was unable. He said his mother had not yet drawn up a will.

The GCM arranged to meet with the son and his mother at the mother's residence the following week. The GCM wanted to assess Mrs. H in her home. During the course of this first meeting, the GCM was sensitive to Mrs. H's need for privacy and independence and yet was able to establish enough rapport with her that Mrs. H confessed to the GCM that she was worried about herself. She was aware that she wasn't managing as well as she once had. The GCM used this time as an opportunity to ask the mother if she was at all concerned about her memory. "Oh, yes, indeed," she replied. "I know my memory isn't what it once was because I can no longer do my *New York Times* crossword puzzles." The GCM asked Mrs. H whether she would like to know how her memory was, that perhaps it was not as poor as she thought. The GCM explained that she could administer a short memory quiz and they could determine in just a few minutes whether there should be further concern about her memory. The GCM used the Short Portable Mental Status Questionnaire. The GCM administered a 10-question mental status evaluation. Mrs. H missed 3 out of 10, scoring within normal limits. She missed the questions related to the presidents and the math calculation. The GCM also noted that the home was quite cluttered and dusty. As a result of the first meeting with Mrs. H, the GCM identified several areas where Mrs. H's quality of life could be improved. With her son's and Mrs. H's approval, she would proceed with the following suggestions:

- Although Mrs. H's memory showed only mild impairment, the GCM recommended that she see a neurologist for further testing to rule out any treatable conditions such as thyroid disorder, diabetes, dementia, or depression. The GCM offered to be available for these appointments.
- The GCM recommended a bill payer to organize Mrs. H's statements and set up a system for having bills paid on an automatic basis as much as possible.
- The GCM recommended having a home attendant to see that Mrs. H's house was cleaned up and to keep track of medical appointments. The GCM would recruit an attendant through the best home care agency. She would introduce the attendant to Mrs. H and her son, explain Mrs. H's needs to the attendant, supervise

the attendant, and follow up with any necessary adjustment in the care provided.

- For some appointments, the GCM would herself see that Mrs. H got to the appointment, accompanying her on occasion if there was important information that should be relayed to the physician. On other occasions, the son would transport his mother for routine appointments, such as dental exams, or the attendant would accompany Mrs. H using public paratransit or transportation for the disabled.
- The GCM recommended a physical therapy evaluation to determine the reason for the recent falls.
- The GCM recommended finding a bank trust officer to handle the estate in the event Mrs. H's son was not able to manage his mother's financial affairs at a later date.
- The GCM recommended having an elder-law attorney draw up a current will and help Mrs. H identify an individual who could act as a surrogate executor in the event her son was incapacitated.
- The GCM would make regular visits to Mrs. H, address any new needs that arise, and make referrals and adjustments as required.
- The GCM would be in regular contact with the son, apprising him of the results of her efforts and noting any change in his mother's condition. Likewise, the son would advise the GCM of any progression or other changes in his mother's symptoms.

As the preceding example illustrates, the GCM can be at the fulcrum of the service matrix, recommending the types of services and the extent of service required based on an initial evaluation of the client and adjusting the recommended services as the client's needs change.

Helping Caregivers Diffuse Conflict

The GCM can help caregivers manage conflict. Creative resolutions emerge out of conflict. Caregivers can be made aware of their conflict management style. They must learn to think before they talk or act. Instead of escalating conflict, they can practice deflecting the negative emotions that stir conflict. Family caregivers can be reminded that an aging person with dementia may not be aware of what he or she says to a caregiver. The following story illustrates how a GCM helped a caregiver diffuse conflict.

CASE STUDY

A demented woman with a history of psychiatric disturbance was very hostile to her daughter-in-law and criticized how she dressed, prepared meals, and kept the house. The couple came to the GCM for assistance regarding managing the mother but also disclosed during the course of the assessment that their marriage was under considerable strain because of the husband's mother's interference and criticism. The GCM was able to help the daughter-in-law deflect the criticism by framing it in the context of her mother-in-law's history of mental difficulties. The son was able to set limits with his mother. The daughter-in-law was gradually able to disregard the criticism and tolerate her mother-in-law to a greater extent.

Helping Caregivers Establish Good Communications

Some families work well together and develop a kind of partnership, where each member assumes a certain role. Other families do not want to work together at all. If two siblings were not a close part of each other's early life, it is understandable that they may not care to work together to help with the care of an aging parent. For example, a 45-year-old son relocated from Delaware to assist his mother in Oregon, who was becoming increasingly withdrawn, depressed, and confused. He contacted a GCM, who assessed the mother, found psychiatric assistance for the mother, and offered support to the son, who was a recovered alcoholic and substance abuser. The son had not abused alcohol or drugs for 10 years. The mother had another son who lived in California but expressed resentment toward his mother and chose not to become involved in her care. However, when the brother in Oregon assisted his mother with her financial and estate planning, the brother in California was outraged and asserted that his brother could not be trusted with their mother's estate matters due to his former alcohol and drug habits. The brother in California could not bring himself to become constructively engaged in his mother's care. Blaming his brother for his history seemed to be the only way he could remain involved, albeit negatively. The GCM worked with the brothers to help build trust and establish a working alliance where the division of labor was comfortably defined. For example, the brother in California managed the finances for their mother, while the brother in Oregon took care of her instrumental activities of daily living, such as transportation to medical appointments and meal shopping and preparation. The brothers did not develop a close relationship but were able to work together for the benefit of their mother.

Encouraging Families to Communicate Their Needs

You should assess the caregiving situation from the perspective of each family member. Solicit opinions from each family member, from youngest to oldest. Tasks should be identified and plans formulated. Caregivers can become overwhelmed when there is one problem after another. Breaking caregiving into manageable tasks is important. For instance, can spouses or teens in the family help with errands or phone calls? Can out-of-area siblings offer monetary support? The following story illustrates how a GCM encouraged one family's members to communicate their needs.

CASE STUDY

One son and two daughters were concerned about their widowed mother, who was becoming increasingly forgetful. The mother had remained in the home where she had raised her family. One local daughter lived close enough to check in on her mother, do grocery shopping, and stand by when the mother took a bath, but this daughter was facing surgery and had a chronically ill husband. The other two adult children lived out of town.

The adult children came to see the GCM for guidance. The local daughter was inclined to have her mother placed in a local assisted living facility. However, the other two siblings did not like the idea. The mother was willing to be placed to relieve her daughter of "the burden of my care."

The GCM helped the family organize a system that would help the mother remain at home and not overburden the local daughter. The GCM helped the family caregivers strike a balance by making several suggestions for manageable tasks the adult children could handle.

- The GCM was told that the son was financially solvent. She therefore suggested that the son finance home care so that the chore work and personal care would be done by attendants. The son agreed.
- The daughter who lived out of state arranged to have her mother's mail sent to her address and engaged her teenage son to sort the mail. Bills to be paid were forwarded to the brother. The daughter maintained close contact with her mother and attendants and ordered groceries and household items on the Internet, arranging for their delivery to her mother's home.
- The local daughter was able to visit her mother when she felt up to the task. Her visits were primarily social. The older mother was most pleased with this new arrangement and lived in her home until she died 2 years later.

Helping Caregivers Strike a Balance

Juggling the demands of an aging parent, a spouse, children, and a job is at the heart of the caregiving dilemma. Professionals are in a position to provide caregivers with models of balance. What is a well-balanced caregiver? According to Donna Cohen, PhD, director of the Institute on Aging at the University of South Florida in Tampa, and C. Eisendorfer, "It's someone who knows herself—what she can and cannot do. She's aware of the impact she has on others, can accept weakness in herself and others, and can identify strengths in others."[2(p130)] A happy caregiver can live with

imperfections in him- or herself, his or her home, and his or her loved ones.

One of the single greatest challenges of caregiving is resisting doing everything. It is preferable to be a coach and delegate responsibility; professionals and caregivers alike can benefit from this advice. GCMs can assist family caregivers in striking a balance between doing it all and feeling guilty that they are not doing enough. Most family members are receptive to suggestions that they consider other individuals and service providers who can lighten their burden. For example, a GCM who is working with a caregiver who has siblings in other states can suggest a family meeting or conference call where each adult child and possibly older grandchild is able to offer a way to lighten the load of the local family caregiver. Some family members might offer to come into town to stay with the older parent on a scheduled basis to give respite to the local family caregiver. Other family members may be in a position to send financial support to hire help at the parent's home. Older grandchildren may be able to provide visits or household help themselves. Some older people are stable enough to split their residence, living part of the year with one relative and then returning to live with another relative. This option is feasible only if the older person likes the arrangement and is well enough to do so. Caregivers might consult with a family physician if a change of residence is being considered.

Helping Families Divide Up Family Treasures

Sometimes one of the most wrenching things a family of an aging parent does is to divide up family treasures. *Nontitled property* is a term that refers to personal items that do not have a legal document (such as a title or deed) to indicate who officially owns the item. These personal possessions may have monetary worth, or they may be cherished primarily for their sentimental value. Nontitled property can include such items as follows:

Furniture
Dishes
Pets
Collections
Sporting equipment
Photographs
Books
Family documents
Linens and needlework
Musical instruments
Guns
Jewelry
Tools
Toys

Resolving who in the family gets personal belongings, the nontitled property, is often more lacerating than determining the division of titled property or financial wealth. Dividing nontitled property can cause friction between siblings that can fast-forward through their lifetime. Many times, this is brought about by old wounds from childhood ("You are the baby, and you always got what you wanted, like you are doing with Mom's good doll collection").

Aging parents have personal belongings such as Dad's 49ers shirt collection, Mom's salt and pepper shaker collection, or the old cracked plate set that sat on the ledge in the kitchen and reminded everyone of how great it was to have breakfast together. Family items contain meaning to family members beyond money. Going through all these articles and distributing them when Dad moves or Mom or Dad dies happens to everyone. This transfer of family treasures affects aging families regardless of income level or cultural background.

Possessions can be divided at many stages in an older person's life. The underlying value of Mom's or Dad's possessions in many cases is the memories they hold. Counsel families to talk about how possessions are to be divided before anything is given to anyone. It is critical to check a parent's will and see an attorney to review that will or trust before anything is divided.

Splitting up possessions when a loved one dies can lead to bitter words: "You took Dad's stamp collection and it's just like when we were kids and Dad favored you because you have his eyes." There are ways to gracefully divide family items loaded with sentiment. Every family has horror tales about how the goodies were divided when Grandma moved to a nursing home or when Dad died.

In one family, Grandma's engagement ring was passed on to her daughter, then to her granddaughter. When a grandson and his fiancée walked into a room full of his relatives, three aunts stared at the fiancée's ring finger and cackled miserably to the engaged woman, "How did *you* get Mom's engagement ring?"

In another family, five granddaughters couldn't decide who should get the grandmother's set of valuable sterling silver. Eventually, it was agreed it would be shared: each woman would have it for a year, then pass it along to another.

But there was so much stalling on passing the silver to the next sister, after 5 years they had a family meeting and decided to hold a drawing to determine permanent ownership.

Who gets personal property is frequently ignored until a crisis occurs, like the death of a parent or a parent moving. At the zero hour, when family members are grieving, selling the home they grew up in, or facing the increased dependence of an elder, adult children can have a hard time making fair or equitable decisions.

Few families have planned ahead enough to decide who should get what personal belongings. If there is no will or no separate listing identifying the wishes of the property owner, family members are sometimes left with a fractious relationship and only old hurt feelings to guide them in dividing an elder parent's personal possessions.

When they must divide family treasures, you can suggest families use a great tool called "Who Gets Grandma's Yellow Pie Plate?" (see http://www.yellowpieplate.umn.edu) developed by the University of Minnesota.* It is a format to help families divide up nontitled property and to help them take time to make the process worthwhile. It helps the families tell stories, listen to both each other and the stories, and remember. It is designed to make dividing assets a positive experience.

The University of Minnesota researchers who developed Grandma's Yellow Pie Plate have identified five factors that adult children should consider as they plan to transfer the property:

1. The adult children and aging parent if alive need to understand the sensitivity of the issue of transferring nontitled property. This means that, for example, a Menorah is not just an item but something that reminds all five children of the happy moments during Hanukah celebrations. If Mom dies, then Dad remarries, and after his death the Menorah goes to the stepmother's kids, the adult siblings may be terribly bitter not about the physical Menorah but about someone who was never at their Hanukah celebrations getting their memories.

2. The family should determine what they want to accomplish in the transfer. Does the older family member want to find family members who will lovingly care for their beloved—though not valuable—Santa collection? Do the adult children want to carry out family traditions, such as only the firstborn daughter in the family gets Grandma's engagement ring?

3. The family should decide what is "fair" in the context of the individual family and that family passing nontitled items along. Is it fair that the firstborn daughter gets the engagement ring or should the firstborn daughter pick names from a hat to see who gets it or should sons get a chance to get it also? Sometimes it is impossible for families to be fair. For example, three adult children may want the baby cereal bowl with Little Red Riding Hood on the bottom. Because there is no fair way to decide among themselves, except to break the bowl into three pieces, they may just have to work together to see who gets it or give it to the next born baby or grandchild.

4. The family and adult children should understand that belongings have different meanings for different individuals. When Mom moves, the oldest adult child may have a loving memory of a valuable silver tea set, not for its monetary value but for the tea parties Mom had with her when she was a toddler. Mom may have been too busy to have those tea parties with the other children, and they may value the set only because of its monetary value.

5. Consider distribution options and consequences. You can help the family agree to manage conflicts before they arise and avoid common obstacles before the items are divided.

GCMs and Dividing Family Items

You can be helpful to the family by researching this issue and utilizing the knowledge before an older person moves. You could guide the family by giving suggestions on how to man-

---

*For more information about "Who Gets Grandma's Yellow Pie Plate? Transferring Non-Titled Property," call the University of Minnesota Extension Service at 624-4900 or 1-800-876-8636 between 8 AM and 4:30 PM Monday through Friday. A packet of information (order number EP-6686-MST) costs $8, and a video (VH-6692-MST) is $30, plus shipping and sales tax. To arrange for someone to speak to a group about the transfer of nontitled property, call Marlene Stum at the extension service at 612-625-4270.

age conflicts over distributing family items and by offering even to be present at a family meeting about dividing treasures. If you have the skills, you could mediate or counsel at the family meeting. You can be helpful to the family by suggesting that the issue on distributing nontitled property be brought up and discussed. Oftentimes, family members think this is too sensitive an issue and never discuss this. A GCM who helps the family to plan ahead may really solve the problem.

Another thing you can do is to encourage family members to tell the stories that go along with the family items to be passed on. Before a client moves or after the death of a family member, you can facilitate a gathering of family members, especially the older family members, and have them pass on the stories that go with the items. A grandmother may believe that everyone knows that the mahogany rocker with the worn seat is where she nursed all her babies, but grandchildren who will inherit the rocker may have no idea. You can also facilitate recording these stories so that they can be passed down through generations. Having the story for posterity is a gift to the family member by itself.

You can encourage the family to take time while dividing up assets to tell family stories, listen to each others' stories, and find joy in remembering. You can help the family make dividing up assets a positive experience.

Teaching families how to hold discussions about nontitled property and options for dividing personal property such as by using family meetings and the Grandma's Yellow Pie Plate methods are good geriatric care management skills. You can also counsel older clients to express their wishes about nontitled items and, through their attorney, add them to their will or trust. For example, "I want my second son John to get my gun collection." You can counsel families dividing nontitled property on ways to divide items if there is no legal direction. For example, a 20-year-old may really need the microwave, but a 40-year-old may not need but want the battered teapot because its whistle woke him up every summer morning when he visited Grandma. You can help families by giving them guidelines that can avoid complaints of favoritism and misunderstandings. Encourage family members to put their wishes about wanting family items in writing and sending these wishes to the entire family instead of making phone calls. In this way everyone gets the request in writing at the same time.

■ ASSISTING SPOUSAL CAREGIVERS AND WORKING WITH COUPLES

When people are married long enough, one spouse is likely to have to care for the other eventually. Spouses of the chronically ill are constantly reminded of a relationship that is no longer the same. They have stated that health care providers often overlook their needs. Almost all cultures place great value on caring for the sick, and yet caregiving can continue for more decades than many marriages used to last—and without the benefit of an extended family.

A spousal caregiver may be a depressed, lonely, isolated, fatigued, anxious individual who may have physical problems, a sleep disorder, and reduced employment. Spousal caregivers experience feelings they view as negative or unacceptable: they feel anger and resentment at the partner for being sick, they feel jealousy at always being second, and they feel deprived of pleasure because they have to do too much work. GCMs can help spousal caregivers considerably. Many of the suggestions discussed in the previous sections apply to spousal caregivers, too. Spousal caregivers face many of the issues that other caregivers face, but spouses also have some special issues of their own.

Principles of Intervention with Spousal Caregivers

How can GCMs assist couples in managing the often overwhelming demands of spousal caregiving? Experts say that spousal caregivers need both the lifeboat and the oars—both the support and the skills to do the job. These experts believe that caregivers are driven by five primary forces: love, morality, equity, ethics, and greed. Other factors affecting the caregiving process include family dynamics, divided loyalties, an understanding of age-related medical and psychological problems, physical endurance, the marital relationship, and the ability to communicate.

In *The Good Marriage*, Judith Wallerstein and Sandra Blakeslee cite four basic types of marriage: romantic, rescue, companionate, and traditional.[3] Although some may argue that this paradigm oversimplifies a most complex union, for the sake of examining caregiving styles, it may be useful.

Wallerstein gives case examples of couples who develop patterns that she deems good. For example, partners in a successful romantic marriage have at their core a lasting, passionately sexual relationship. The common bond the couple in a romantic marriage share is the sense that they were destined to be together.

Partners in a successful rescue marriage had early experiences that were traumatic. The comfort and healing that take place during their life together become the central theme of their relationship. Should one partner become frail and require caregiving, it might not upset the equilibrium as much as it might in another type of marriage, such as a companionate or traditional one.

A companionate marriage, which may be the most common form of marriage among younger couples, has at its core friendship, equality, and the value system of the woman's movement, with its corollary that the male role, too, needs to change. A major factor in the companionate marriage is the attempt to balance the partners' serious emotional investment in the workplace with their emotional investment in the relationship and the children.

The fourth type is the traditional marriage, where the stronger, more dominant spouse (usually the husband) is the breadwinner. Should the breadwinner become incapacitated and aphasic as a result of a stroke, for example, the system in this type of marriage would be profoundly upset. Changing dependencies, hostility, and the unspoken wish for escape all redefine the nature of affection in this relationship.

The style of spousal caregiving is determined in large part by a person's coping style, practical abilities, and marital relationship. Consider the following examples:

- A husband devotes himself for years to caring for his wife, who has Alzheimer's. Then he murders her. What might a GCM have done to prevent this tragedy?
- A wife cares for her chronically ill husband, quits her job, and neglects herself. Her adult children want her to spend more time with her grandchildren and have a more normal life. She says it is her choice and she would not have it any other way. How would a GCM counsel the family?
- A husband who is caring for his wife with Alzheimer's states that she instructed him to call Dr. Kevorkian when she no longer recognizes him. He has told a GCM of this directive. How should the GCM react?

How can GCMs help emotionally vulnerable clients to develop the new coping styles that will be necessary to spare them further stress? How much preventive intervention can care managers offer? Is it possible to prepare spouses for the often inevitable spousal caregiving responsibilities they will face? Can advance directives or a durable power of attorney for health care play a role in this?

Mr. and Mrs. H believed so. They had been married for 50 years and were grateful for their many blessings. They had good, open communication and agreed to state in the advance directives that under no circumstance would one spouse be expected to sacrifice his or her physical or emotional health at the expense of the other. Both had experience with chronically ill parents and recognized the toll caregiving can take.

They agreed to purchase long-term care policies that included home health care as well as institutional care and to implement these policies as necessary at the discretion of the well spouse. The couple said that it was a tremendous relief to know that each of them could be cared for, not necessarily by the other, and still feel that the spousal devotion was intact.

This couple, of course, was very enlightened, and they can serve as a model for couples who may wish to communicate about this most delicate subject.

Problematic Relationships

What about a situation in which a couple has not openly discussed caregiving preferences and one spouse becomes chronically impaired both cognitively and physically? How can a care manager help the well spouse achieve a relatively satisfying life while caring for the ill spouse? A case in point occurred when a GCM was facilitating a support group for well spouses of the chronically impaired. Two of the well spouses approached the GCM for her opinion. They were interested in dating each other but were very conflicted. Both members of the support group had been caring for chronically ill spouses. Both of the ill spouses were impaired to the extent that they no longer recognized their spouses.

The GCM counseled the two group members separately and together over a period of several weeks. They both expressed an overwhelming sense of devotion and guilt. Through counseling, the care manager was able to help the couple resolve the conflict. The result was that the well couple was able to define the parameters of the relationship in a

way that would not conflict with the marriage vows and was comfortable. They shared a meaningful relationship and offered tremendous emotional support to one another.

What does the codependent caregiver look like? According to Melodie Beattie, the guru of codependency issues, that person is taking responsibility for others—too often not taking responsibility for him- or herself.[4] Codependent caregivers take inappropriate responsibility for the feelings, thoughts, behaviors, problems, choices, and life course of others. Codependent caring makes people feel used, victimized, unappreciated, and unsuccessful in their efforts. Codependent caring makes them feel controlled by the other's needs while simultaneously feeling that the caregiver's own needs are not being met.

In the context of clinical intervention for codependent spousal caregivers, GCMs might ask themselves the following questions:

- What is the caregiver's own attitude toward aging?
- What is the motivation to care?
- Is the caregiver denying the spouse's issues and his or her own?
- Can the caregiver be helped to deal with his or her emotions?
- Can the GCM help the caregiver build a partnership with the spouse and helping professionals?
- Can the GCM help the caregiver manage conflict?
- Is it possible to help the caregiver to establish good family communication?
- Can the caregiver be helped to strike a balance between the need to care and his or her own needs?

General Principles for All Types of Spousal Caregivers

True helping and healthy giving are good, and they are different from caretaking. The following guidelines are summarized from the National Council on Aging "Caregiving Tips" series.[5] They may be useful for you to suggest to stressed spousal caregivers.

- Encourage spousal caregivers to admit their feelings. Feeling tired, isolated, helpless, angry, or scared can be an indication that they are trying to handle too much without the help and information they need. Such feelings, though difficult, are natural.
- Encourage spousal caregivers to talk to their family and friends about what they feel rather than keeping everything inside.
- Encourage spousal caregivers to set reasonable expectations and not to reproach themselves for failing to be a superwoman or superman.
- Encourage spousal caregivers to admit to themselves and their friends what they want and need and what they can and cannot do for themselves. Knowing their limits is an important part of taking care of themselves.
- Encourage spousal caregivers to seek help when they need it, looking to professionals and service agencies as partners who can provide guidance and counseling. Help caregivers realize that there is nothing wrong with asking for help.
- Encourage spousal caregivers to ask questions. If they do not find the answers right away, they should continue to search for people who can answer the questions.
- Suggest that spousal caregivers take care of themselves physically; eat regular, balanced meals; exercise as part of their daily routine to maintain fitness and ease tension; use relaxation techniques such as meditation, deep breathing, and massage; and maintain a sense of humor.
- Remind spousal caregivers not to forget to take care of themselves when things are tough. This is the most important time for them to be good to themselves.
- Suggest that spousal caregivers avoid destructive ways of coping such as overeating, abusing alcohol or drugs, and neglecting or taking out their stress on others.
- Encourage spousal caregivers to maintain activities and social contacts that they enjoy and plan occasions for their own pleasure and renewal.

Sometimes the most helpful counseling is based on good listening and empathic responding. Help caregivers give themselves permission to take care of themselves, emphasizing that this is not selfish or uncaring but part of surviving. Caregiving is difficult work that involves not only doing but coping.

Expressions of Sexuality

The need for closeness and intimacy does not diminish with age. But despite the sexual revolution, our culture still views some types of sexual behavior as inappropriate.

One of the greatest fears is that older people will develop inappropriate sexual behavior. Inappropriate sexual behavior is an infrequent problem with individuals with dementia. More common than actual inappropriate behavior is the myth that confused older people will develop inappropriate sexual behavior. However, should such an unfortunate incident occur, a matter-of-fact reaction without any more fuss than is absolutely necessary is what is called for. The caregiver's reaction may have more impact on the observer or the victim than the actual incident does. For example, removing the person from the situation and explaining simply that "He forgets where he is" may be all that is needed.

Some people with dementia type illness have an increased sex drive, while others have a decreased sex drive. If the individual has an increased sex drive, remember that it is a factor of the brain injury, not a reflection on the relationship. You can assist the couple in finding a balance of sexual activity that is comfortable for both. Referral to a clinician who specializes in dementia problems might be helpful. A university-based clinic could be a good resource.

Inappropriate Behavior

Occasionally confused people will expose themselves in public or fidget in such a way that reminds others of sexual behaviors. This can be upsetting, especially to family members. Family members may benefit from knowing that the problem will probably not worsen as the dementia illness progresses.

There may be reasonable explanations for seemingly sexual behaviors such as disrobing or handling the genital area. You may suggest a family meeting to identify some of the triggers, suggest explanations, and allow family members the opportunity to vent their feelings. Solutions may arise during the process. Here is a list of behaviors with possible explanations and interventions.

- Unbuckling belt buckle: feels clothing is too tight
- Unzipping trousers: needs to urinate, forgets where bathroom is
- Fidgeting with buttons on blouse: is too warm
- Making sexual advances to attendant: confuses the attendant with a spouse
- Making frequent requests for sexual relations: forgets the sexual relations that do take place
- Handling genital area: has a urinary tract infection (should be checked by a physician)
- Pulling off pants: feels uncomfortable in clothing, needs to use bathroom
- Disrobing: is too warm, is uncomfortable in clothing

Differential Diagnosis: Sexual Acting Out versus Medical Problem

An older woman was placed in a care facility's unit for people with dementia. Her family was informed by the nurse on the unit that the older woman was wandering into the beds of other residents, disrobing, and touching her genital area. After a thorough medical examination and a family meeting, it was revealed that the woman had a urinary tract infection; she also came from a large family and was recently widowed. After her urinary tract infection was treated and she was more regularly taken to social activities, the wandering and genital handling subsided. The staff of the care facility were asked to provide more evening one-on-one attention, which seemed to address this woman's need for companionship at night.

■ CONTINUUM OF CARE RESOURCES—WORKING AS PART OF A TEAM

Just as no person is an island, no GCM stands alone. A good GCM knows a staggering array of experts who can assist clients in areas where the GCM's expertise is lacking or where there could be a conflict of interest. For example, a middle-aged son came to see a GCM because his father, with whom the son lived, was beginning to require more care than the son could provide. The father was falling on occasion and appeared to be confused at times. The son traveled regularly on business. As the consultation progressed, it became apparent that the home was held in joint tenancy by the son and his father. There was another sibling who lived out of state who had a physical disability and was receiving public assistance. The father was beginning to show signs of dementia and had not yet developed a will or a general durable power of attorney, or one for health care.

The GCM suggested that the son contact an elder-law attorney to advise him regarding estate matters. A neurologist was recommended to evaluate the nature of the father's dementia and possible interventions. In addition, the father's physician was contacted to see about an order for home health care, physical therapy, and occupational therapy that would include an evaluation of the need for adaptive equipment and equipment to make the home environment safer.

The GCM asked about the father's typical day, and the son explained that his father was alone all day, ate poorly during the day, and "waited" for his son to arrive home from work, which was sometimes not until 7 PM. The GCM suggested an adult day program that provided transportation, meals, and socialization. The father responded favorably to the social stimulation and improved diet.

While developing a will with the father, the attorney also set up a trust for the estate and a special needs trust for the son with a disability. The special needs trust would allow that son to receive an inheritance and monthly stipend without disqualifying him from receiving public assistance. The neurologist diagnosed the father with a pseudo-dementia that abated after regular participation in a social day program and an improved diet. Many of these kinds of dementia have as their underlying problem depression and nutritional deficiencies, both easily reversed conditions, if treated early. The father now resides in a local retirement facility recommended by the GCM, who assisted in his acclimation. The facility has several levels of care so that as the father's needs change, he can receive assistance without relocating. The local son visits his father regularly and knows that he can rely on the GCM to advocate for his father, especially during his frequent out-of-town business trips.

GCMs should think of the following additional professionals and service providers when assisting families with identifying resources:

- Services that may be covered by Medicare
    1. Adult day health care
    2. Assessment services
    3. Home health aide services
    4. Homemaker services
    5. Hospice services
    6. Medical social work
    7. Mental health services
    8. Occupational therapy
    9. Personal care

    10. Physical therapy
    11. Physician care
    12. Protective services
    13. Respite care
    14. Speech therapy
    15. Transportation

- Services that may be covered at no cost through a public agency
    1. Care management
    2. Chore services
    3. Health insurance counseling
    4. Information and referral
    5. Legal services
    6. Supervision
    7. Telephone reassurance

- Other services
    1. Emergency response systems
    2. Home-delivered meals
    3. Paid companions and sitters

■ HELPING A FAMILY DECIDE IF A PARENT SHOULD LIVE WITH THEM

Some family members may consider having their older relatives live with them. This can be a short- or long-term arrangement. Its success depends on several factors. There are many issues to consider in coming to this decision, and GCMs can help families consider the issues.

It is often painful for adult children to admit that they cannot ask their mother or father to live with them. They may have practical reasons (e.g., inadequate living space, poor health, no settled home) or more personal reasons (e.g., personality clashes, adolescents who require emotional attention, marital strain). But how much more difficult it is to take such an irrevocable step, inviting a parent to live in one's home, and then find out that it does not work. The ensuing aftermath and responsibility the adult child will feel for disrupting the parent's life is even more painful.

Sons and daughters who are considering inviting an older parent to live with them even though they are reluctant to do so may be comforted to know that other people share that reluctance. National surveys consistently show that the majority of young and old adults in the United States think it is a bad idea for older parents and their children to live together. One might assume that the strongest opposition to such living arrangements comes from the younger generation, but that is not true; the surveys show that the older the parents, the less likely they are to favor living with their children. Older people particularly do not want to be burdens.

Even if the older mother or father directly or indirectly suggests a common living arrangement, sentiment should not dictate the decision. Instead, the decision should be based on a careful analysis of the situation, the wishes of the other members of the immediate family, and the history of the relationship between the parent and the adult child. GCMs can aid the family in considering these questions:

- How does the spouse of the adult child feel about the common living arrangement?
- What kind of financial arrangements are being considered?
- What kind of living space will be available for everyone?
- Will the older person depend completely on the son's or daughter's family for companionship and entertainment?
- What about other friends, relatives, and contemporaries? What about recreational, cultural, and religious needs?
- Can the family honestly expect to live comfortably together? Do the personalities clash? How have previous visits been? How often did family members have a migraine headache, ulcer flare-up, or other stress-related symptom during these visits?
- When the older person visited in the past, were the family members counting the days until the older person left?
- Can the older person allow the adult child to run his or her own household?
- Would the older person—because of temperament—feel comfortable in the home and with having friends visit there?

- Will the adult children be able to make sure the older person has ongoing, accessible, competent medical care?
- Will having the older person in the house violate anyone's sense of privacy?

■ CONCLUSION

This chapter focuses on how a GCM can effectively work with adult children, spouses, and other family members to improve the quality of life for older people and ease the burden of caregiving in various situations. GCMs can help all types of families, including long-distance families, dysfunctional families, overwhelmed families, and families who are considering facility placement. GCMs can also work with couples and work as part of a professional team.

The future of geriatric care management work with families will increasingly be tied to the Internet. The Internet will allow family caregivers to identify GCMs in their community as well as GCMs in their older relative's region. The Internet will also enable family members to identify resources, services, and products that will improve the quality of their lives. However, there will never be an electronic replacement for responsive, clinically astute, and empathetic GCMs who can be instrumental in improving a challenging family circumstance.

■ NOTES

1. American Association of Retired Persons. *Tomorrow's Choices: Preparing Now for Future Legal, Financial, and Health Care Decisions.* Washington, DC: American Association of Retired Persons; 1992.

2. Eisendorfer C, Cohen D. *Care for the Elderly: Reshaping Health Policy.* Baltimore, MD: Johns Hopkins University Press; 1989.

3. Wallerstein J, Blakeslee S. *The Good Marriage: How and Why Love Lasts.* New York: Houghton Mifflin; 1995.

4. Beattie M. *Co-Dependent No More.* New York: Fine Communications; 1997.

5. Cassel C, ed. *The Practical Guide to Aging.* New York: New York University Press; 1999.

Appendix 17–A

■ HOW TO FIND A QUALIFIED GERIATRIC CARE MANAGER

Caregivers should be aware that a growing number of geriatric care managers (GCMs) are now certified and known as Care Managers Certified. They are professionals, usually social workers or nurses, who are capable of conducting assessments and providing short- and long-term care plans for clients.

It is recommended that some or all of the following questions be asked by consumers who are considering retaining a GCM:

1. What are your credentials? A GCM should have an advanced degree in social work, psychology, or gerontology or should be a registered nurse with public health experience.
2. Do you have certification as a GCM?
3. How long have you worked with the frail elderly? How long in private practice? Care managers with more years of experience are likely to be better choices than are care managers with fewer years of experience. Public agency experience working with the frail elderly helps.
4. Do you belong to the National Association of Professional Geriatric Care Managers? This association has ethics codes and standards of practice.
5. Are you available 24 hours a day, 7 days a week? If you get sick or go out of town, who backs you up?
6. How do you charge? If by the hour, do you charge for telephone calls? Travel time? What else? GCMs do much of their business by phone and legitimately charge for that time. Most ask half their usual fee for travel. Charges for other services should be spelled out in contracts or fee schedules.
7. If a service you recommended does not work out, what will you do about it? The GCM should promise in advance to correct any problem, and if that fails should arrange something new.
8. Can you provide references from clients as well as local organizations such as hospitals and senior centers?
9. Do you arrange for free, low-cost, or medically insured services when available and appropriate?
10. Do you personally provide any of the needed services?
11. Who screens the home care providers and what methods are used? Do you run a background check, and does it include criminal records?
12. Are you bonded, and do you carry professional liability insurance?
13. How often and by whom is each service monitored?
14. How frequently can I expect to hear from you? Are your reports written or phoned?

The recipients of care management service should feel comfortable with the GCM.

The National Association of Professional Geriatric Care Managers in Tucson, Arizona, publishes a list of its members. Contact information for this association appears in Appendix A.

Chapter 18

Difficult Families: Conflict, Dependence, and Mutuality

Emily B. Saltz

■ INTRODUCTION

No two families are alike. Every family is its own complex, unique, constantly changing system of important relationships. And each one, at one time or another, must deal with life's most important events and issues: birth and death, marriage and divorce, intimacy and distance, growing up and aging. Dealing with the aging process within a family is a complicated matter. It can be a struggle even for families that are close-knit, well integrated, and highly functioning, as previously described in Chapter 17, Geriatric Care Management Working with Nearly Normal Aging Families. It can be overwhelming and even destructive for the so-called difficult family, that is, the family that is marked by strained relationships and unresolved conflict.

This chapter explores the strategies and techniques a geriatric care manager (GCM) can use when dealing with families who are dysfunctional and are considered "difficult." The concepts of filial maturity and mutuality—that is, balancing the giving and accepting of care—will be explored as a way to reframe dependence in old age as a normal rather than pathological process. These concepts are addressed as a means to assist families in developing positive, reciprocal relationships during later-life transitions.

Families often seek out a GCM when they are in crisis and feel hopeless about finding solutions to their elder-care problems. Caregiving is often a demanding, full-time job for which there is no job description and no training. Many of the families GCMs meet struggle valiantly to meet the demands of this job for which they may feel totally unprepared and unappreciated.

For elders, the transition to dependence involves a role change that is frequently accompanied by feelings of loss and inadequacy. For family caregivers, this same transition evokes powerful conflicts regarding dependence and independence, which are rooted in early parent–child bonds. For many adult children, the task of meeting the emerging dependency needs of their parents triggers a reexamination of how their own needs were or were not met.[1]

The ordinary aging processes are made far more challenging when a family has a history of dysfunction. As GCMs, we face some of our greatest challenges in working with these "difficult" families. These are families who are not able to organize themselves effectively in the face of elder-care challenges and crises. Regardless of whether the family system has been healthy or dysfunctional, its members are under stress as they move from long-established roles into uncharted territory.

■ UNDERSTANDING AGING WITHIN THE FAMILY SYSTEM

The aging of a key family member presents complex familial challenges in *all* families. "Aging families must deal with the psychological and relational stress associated with loss."[2] The loss may be multifaceted, involving not just the familiar effects of physical and mental decline, but may also have significant emotional components. Loss of control, loss of continuity, loss of defined roles, loss of significant relationships, and loss of a sense of purpose: all of these effects may not have been fully anticipated.

These transitions can disrupt any family, even those that have had success in the past in sustaining family bonds, reaching consensus, and managing prior developmental crises or losses. An elder-care crisis often exaggerates unresolved family conflicts. Adult children may find themselves disagreeing over anything and everything: how much care is needed, who should provide it, who should decide, who should pay. Longstanding parent–child conflicts over such issues as control, approval, nurturing, money, and support may suddenly resurface. The geographical location of the adult children can also become highly problematic, causing conflict and resentment between those who live close to the elder and those who live at a distance. The ability of any family to manage these disagreements is almost always sorely tested.

According to family systems theory, each family is an emotional unit, and behavior within that system is reciprocal and reactive. It is a "living system" of which each member is an interdependent part. The central tenet of systems theory is that a change in behavior in one part of the system begins to change the behavior of the whole.[3] A major life cycle crisis, such as the physical and/or cognitive decline of an aging parent, simultaneously causes and requires reorganization in the system.

The problem is that reorganization is difficult. A family system is homeostatic and inherently resistant to change. Families seek equilibrium, and as long as everyone sticks to familiar roles, the system remains stable. The very nature of aging means that the prevailing patterns will inevitably be disturbed. Change or stress affecting the elder within the family system will unavoidably affect the whole.

Evaluating Family Interaction

Mindful of systems theory, GCMs can more properly evaluate the quality of interaction and the roots of conflict among family members. Dan Blazer has set forth parameters that are useful in helping GCMs to assess family interaction:

- *Compatible vs. conflictual:* Do family members easily come to an agreement over care issues, or do they argue constantly, even over relatively unimportant issues? Do old conflicts between siblings or between adult child and parent resurface during the crisis period?
- *Cohesive vs. fragmented:* Does the family present as a unit, or do they contact the GCM individually with their problems? Do family members ask the GCM to keep conversations secret from other family members?
- *Productive vs. nonproductive:* Can the family respond to the GCM's suggestions and take necessary action to create change in the elder's life? Are there individual family members who are unable to mobilize and feel powerless to act?
- *Fragile vs. stable:* Has the family been stable over time? Is there a history of emotional cut-offs or distance on the part of one or more family members? Is there a pattern of divorce, remarriage, or other disruptions in relationships that changes the balance within the family system?
- *Rigid vs. flexible:* How has the family handled previous crises? Did the members accept the need to change roles in those times? Are members able to exchange or

share important roles in managing family affairs? If one member is unavailable to provide care, can other members assume the caregiving role? Do family members respond readily to crises?[4]

It is important to remember that, at the point of intervention, the GCM is meeting the elder and the family at a single, finite point in time and that the elder has had a lifetime of experience, habits, preferences, and patterns. Indeed, the family system itself may be the product of patterns handed down from generation to generation. By acknowledging the breadth and depth of family history, the GCM has a greater likelihood of initiating or promoting necessary change within the family.

■ INTERGENERATIONAL RELATIONSHIPS

The GCM also needs to remember that, for the adult child, the act of caregiving means reengaging with the most profound and influential attachment of one's life: the parent. There are few models for negotiating the powerful parent–child bond in later life.[1] Intergenerational relationships between parents and adult children are often characterized by ambivalence. Positive feelings include love, reciprocal help, shared values, and solidarity. Negative feelings include isolation, conflict, abuse, neglect, and caregiver stress.[5]

Robert Karen stated, "We are dealing with two different sets of parents—the parent we grew up with, whom we struggle with internally, and the living parent of today. These internal parents have mythic dimensions—they may have adored us or wounded us, we may idealize them or demonize them, we may or may not have fully separated."[6] An adult child may hold on to an internal representation of the parent at an earlier stage, when the parent was more powerful or more engaged, whether for better or worse. Likewise, most parents, no matter how old they have become, have a residual wish to care for their children,

which may cause them to hold on to their own images from the past.

The task for adult children is to let go of the mythic parent so that, in the late stages of family development, we can see our mothers and fathers as actual people. Adult children need to grieve the loss of the past, the loss of the internalized early parent, so that as adults they can relate realistically to their parents in the present and provide care unencumbered by out-of-date motives and impulses.

Dependency and Loss

The task for the elder is, in some ways, even more difficult. The struggle to *accept* care within the intergenerational family can be even harder than *giving* it is. We live in a culture that emphasizes youth, independence, autonomy, and self-control and, conversely, that regards "dependence" at any stage of life as a weakness or personal deficit.[7] The transition to dependence for an older adult who has had a lifetime of self-reliance and self-determination involves a role change that is often marked by feelings of loss and inadequacy. Erlanger notes, "Loss occurs during all phases of the family life cycle, but it assumes a central role in the influences on later-life families."[8]

In the context of intergenerational family caregiving, this loss is experienced in different ways by the elder and the family members. The elder may be entering into the new paradigm of caring and giving with a disturbing sense of diminished physical and/or cognitive functioning, a feeling that is most poignant among elders who are aware of their declining capacities. In addition to personal decline, the elder often confronts the erosion of social networks, economic stability, and sense of purpose, power, and autonomy in the community and in the family itself. On the other hand, for the adult children, spouses, and other family caregivers, these definitional changes for the elder may be experienced as the loss of a central figure in their own lives.

According to Terry Hargrave, the psychological and relational stress on the family that is associated with the individual elder's role change is a primary issue that aging families must address to negotiate the later stages of family development successfully.[2] Indeed, families are frequently emotionally unprepared to deal with the raw power and significance of the intergenerational shift caused by the elder's personal and social losses. The result is often family dysfunction and crisis, emerging or deepening at the worst possible time. Furthermore, although prior stages of family life inevitably include transitions in roles and attitudes between parent and child, these earlier transitions are dissimilar to, and provide no real guidance for, the profound and difficult changes in the parent–child bond in later life. Unlike the more predictable, normative developmental process for children, the character and timing of events and patterns that occur in old age are highly variable and generally undesirable. The growing dependency of the elder is not always predictable, desired, or confined to a particular life phase.

CASE STUDY

Case Example: Nancy Narcissist

Nancy Narcissist is an 82-year-old widowed woman currently living in a traditional assisted living facility. She is widowed with one son, Devoted Dan, who is married with two children. Nancy has several health problems, including severe arthritis and hypertension. Because of her arthritis, she walks slowly and uses a walker.

Recently, Nancy has been experiencing cognitive decline, and she is having trouble managing her daily affairs. She has papers and stacks of unpaid bills piled all over her apartment, and she leaves sticky notes to "remind" herself what needs to get done. She is having a hard time walking to the dining room and frequently asks that a tray be sent to her room. The assisted living facility does provide personal care services, but Nancy has refused all offers of assistance. The facility has called Dan several times to express concern about Nancy's continued ability to stay in her apartment. They would like Dan to consider moving his mother to the memory impairment unit, but he is reluctant to broach this subject with her.

Nancy is, and has always been, very critical and demanding of her son. She calls Devoted Dan several times a day, often announcing a "crisis" and insisting that he come right away. When Dan arrives, he must endure a litany of complaints about the food, the staff, and the other residents. The rest of Nancy's complaints are about Devoted Dan himself. She tells him that, if he really cared about her, he would find her a new apartment. Despite his frequent visits, Nancy complains that she does not see Dan or her grandchildren enough. When Dan offers to help his mother pay her bills or offers to hire a companion for her, she angrily refuses.

Eventually, Nancy falls in her apartment and is hospitalized with a fractured hip. From the hospital, she is transferred to a nursing home where she remains. Dan continues to visit her on a daily basis and endures his mother's ongoing complaints and criticisms. He feels pressured, overwhelmed, and very guilty.

In the case of Nancy Narcissist, the fundamental question that Devoted Dan faces is: "How am I supposed to meet the dependency needs of my mother when my own dependency needs have not been met?" This is a good example of a son who is trying desperately to manage the increasing care needs of his mother despite his own feelings of guilt and worthlessness, as well as his mother's neediness and emotional withholding. Interestingly, despite not having received the bedrock of nurturance and warmth that one would expect to find in a good caregiver, Dan remains a thoughtful and devoted son. Why?

Myth of Role Reversal

Margaret Blenkner was well ahead of her time when, in the mid-1960s, she challenged the commonly held notion that "role reversal" is a normal development in the aging process.[9] As conventionally understood, role reversal assumes that an inevitable shift of power and control occurs within an aging family whereby the adult child becomes the "parent" to the elder and the elder becomes the "child" in need of care and protection.

Although the activities of raising a young child and caring for an older adult share some surface similarities, there are fundamental differences that the original theorists of role reversal largely ignored. Caregiving activities at the beginning and at the end of life both involve protecting, worrying, and planning for the needs of a dependent family member. They both exact a high cost physically, emotionally, and economically. And they both require the caregiver's frequent, if not constant, attention and physical presence.

The differences, however, are more profound. The relationship between a parent and a young child is asymmetrical: the parent has passed through numerous developmental stages, while the child has passed through few, if any. Ultimately, the parent's goal is to guide the child toward independence, separation, and self-identity. By contrast, no matter how diminished or impaired by time or illness, the elder brings a lifetime of experience, habit, preference, belief, attitude, wisdom, autonomy, and personality that inevitably informs and transforms the caregiving rela-

tionship. No matter how much the elder declines, he or she will always be the parent within the family system.[10]

Filial Maturity

Instead of role reversal, Blenkner introduced the concepts of filial crisis and filial maturity as normative aspects of individual and family development. According to Blenkner, *filial crisis* arises when the parent in an aging family is no longer "the rock of support" for the family and may now need to lean on others for support and comfort.[9] In a healthy family system, the adult child is able to achieve *filial maturity*, which is a state of emotional readiness to relinquish earlier roles as the needy youngster and to begin to support and provide care for the elder without infantilizing the elder. Successfully accomplishing the filial task entails a new understanding and a "different love" for the aged parent by the adult child. Lowy, among others, explores Blenkner's recognition that the adult child's resolution of the filial crisis sets the stage for the adult child to confront and eventually meet the challenges of his or her own aging process and mortality.[7]

CASE STUDY

Case Example: New Jersey Norm

New Jersey Norm is a 92-year-old widowed man who is living with his 88-year-old female companion in his own apartment in Pleasantville, New Jersey. He has one daughter, Boston Barbara, a 45-year-old married woman living in Boston, and another daughter, California Callie, a 50-year-old unmarried woman living in California. New Jersey Norm was recently diagnosed with normal pressure hydrocephalus (NPH), a condition associated with problems involving balance and gait, urinary incontinence, and dementia.

During the past year, Norm was hospitalized five times for problems related to NPH, and he recently had surgery to have a cranial shunt implanted. Despite the surgery, his condition continues to deteriorate. He is incontinent, has fallen several times, and cannot be left alone. Norm's companion feels she cannot handle his care and turns to his daughters for help.

Norm did not have a close relationship with either of his daughters. He was always an emotionally distant father who did not take a great interest in his children's lives. In fact, both daughters were aware that, for more than 30 years during his marriage, Norm was having an affair with his current female companion. Both daughters were close to their mother, and they are still angry with Norm and resentful toward his female companion. Despite these historical tensions, both daughters have accepted their new role as caregivers. Norm, however, tends to act in a passive-aggressive manner, and he is unappreciative of their efforts.

California Callie has told both Norm and her sister that she is willing to give up her career job and well-established life in California to care for Norm. She proposes that she move into an apartment upstairs from Norm and his female companion. Boston Barbara tries to dissuade her sister, but Callie insists, admitting that she never resolved her feelings of guilt and loss at not having been at her mother's bedside when she died. She sees Norm's current elder-care needs as an opportunity to "make up" for her absence in the past.

What is motivating California Callie to move back home to care for a father with whom she never felt close and has a very conflicted relationship? Is it a feeling of unconditional love despite his emotional distance and betrayal? Or is she driven by feelings of guilt over her prior absence during a critical family moment? To what extent is her unresolved guilt about her mother a legitimate motivation for moving back to New Jersey and accepting the daily burdens of her father's caregiving? Is the anger she feels at her father playing any role in her decision making? Should it?

From the perspective of filial maturity, Callie appears ready to forge a new bond that she was previously unable to have with her now-dependent father. She seems prepared to let go of her unresolved feelings about her father and what he did or did not provide in the past. She is seeking to find a way to connect with him at the end of his life, an act of selflessness that may assist her in resolving her guilt feelings about her absence from her mother's deathbed. If her father succeeds in letting his daughter care for him, it would be possible for them to achieve a new and closer relationship.

Mutuality and Generational Maturity

In a fully realized caregiving relationship, there are, of course, at least two players—aged parent and adult child—who must complete important developmental tasks. In articulating a new model of normal behavior for the adult child as caregiver, Blenkner did not address both sides of the equation. Her theories of filial crisis and maturity focused primarily on the new role of the adult child as emerging caregiver. Later writers have considered the corresponding tasks of the aging parent. They have developed new models of "mutuality in older families"[11] and "generational maturity"[12] in which the child assumes more responsibility for the elder and the elder allows this shift in responsibility to occur. In these models, the task for the elder is to enter into a reciprocal caring relationship and to learn to accept care without abandoning self-esteem, dignity, or integrity. By accepting this task, the elder enables the adult child to "enter a new phase of adulthood." The resulting mutual exchange requires both sides of the parent–child pair to redefine dependency in old age as normal behavior and to recognize that continued growth, both psychological and relational, occurs at all stages of individual and family development, including the final stages.[11] Within this framework, dependence is not seen as an indicator of decline but as a meaningful readjustment of the balance in a reciprocal care relationship between the aged parent and the adult child. By accepting the elder's dependence, both parent and child engage in a shared relationship involving new meaningful roles based on familial love and reciprocity rather than decline and incapacity.[13]

CASE STUDY

Case Example: Mr. and Mrs. Manhattan

Mr. and Mrs. Manhattan are 89 and 85 years of age, respectively, and live in an apartment in New York City. Their only son, Phil, requested care management assistance to relocate his parents to an assisted living facility in Philadelphia, where he lives. Phil has been trying to convince his parents to move closer to him for the past 15 years, but they have steadfastly refused.

During the past several years, the Manhattans have both experienced a significant decline in health. Mr. Manhattan had a stroke, leaving him partially paralyzed. He is still independent in all activities of daily living and is cognitively intact. Mrs. Manhattan's memory has been declining for several years. She needs a hip replacement, which she has refused.

Mr. and Mrs. Manhattan are socially isolated because most of their friends have died. Mrs. Manhattan is the "boss" in the relationship, while Mr. Manhattan tends to be more passive. Mr. Manhattan has secretly confided in his son that he is overwhelmed and stressed by Mrs. Manhattan's care needs, and he would like to move to an assisted living facility closer to his son. Mrs. Manhattan, however, has adamantly refused to move, and Mr. Manhattan is unwilling or unable to challenge her.

Phil feels powerless, particularly with his mother, whose dominating personality seems insurmountable. Despite her decline, he still feels like a child in the relationship. He has tried reasoning with his parents with little success. On several occasions, Phil arranged for Mr. and Mrs. Manhattan to come to Philadelphia to tour appropriate assisted living facilities, but in each instance his parents backed out at the last minute and the appointments have been canceled. He tried to hire a GCM and a homemaker in New York, both of whom his mother refused.

The GCM in Philadelphia meets with Phil and helps him to revise the unsuccessful strategies he has been using with his parents. She reaffirms the appropriateness of moving his parents to a more supportive environment and helps him to understand the dynamics of his parents' resistance, particularly his mother's. In view of his mother's cognitive impairments, the GCM suggests that Phil's continued resort to "reasoning and logic" will not work. Instead, she promotes the use of "therapeutic fiblets" as a strategy for making the transition possible.

With the GCM's encouragement, Phil begins to take a firmer, more direct approach with his mother, while continuing to provide gentle reassurance to his father. He is less intimidated by his mother's obstinate words, and he asserts a newfound sense of adult authority. With his father, he speaks more confidently that the family will be able to negotiate the necessary changes that are ahead. As a result, his parents begin to signal a shift in attitude. His father now accepts his assurances and becomes less anxious about the future, and his mother becomes less resistant.

Eventually, Mr. and Mrs. Manhattan move to an assisted living facility in the Philadelphia area. Shortly after completing the move, Phil organizes a birthday party for Mr. Manhattan at the facility. In the presence of Mr. Manhattan's new neighbors and friends, and with his wife at his side, Mr. Manhattan offers a public toast to his son, thanking him openly for enabling them to move into a new and happier phase of life. Mr. Manhattan's words—"Without my son we would not be here. We are so thankful"—resonate with Phil for a long time.

What are the power struggles occurring in this family system? What strategies does the GCM use to enable Phil to overcome his sense of powerlessness with his mother? Is Phil ultimately successful in achieving filial maturity? What is the significance of Mr. Manhattan's toast, in terms of generational maturity?

■ IDENTIFYING THE DIFFICULT FAMILY

The successful resolution in the story of Mr. and Mrs. Manhattan does not occur, of course, in all families. There are families with histories of violence, abuse, neglect, or even simple dysfunction for whom the resolution of filial crisis is not likely to occur. In these families, the adult child may be thrust unwillingly into the role of caregiver with a parent who may not have provided support or nurtured the child in the past. Achieving filial maturity in this context is vastly complicated. These difficult families are, generally, most in need of intervention, but for the GCM, they are often the most challenging to assist.

From the GCM's perspective, what exactly does it mean for a family to be "difficult"? Does it mean that the family does not listen to us or accept our recommendations? Does it mean that the family is unfairly critical of the GCM's work and complains that the GCM is failing to do the job correctly? Or is being difficult as simple as repeatedly failing to return important phone calls to the GCM? Or, conversely, calling numerous times every day?

How Difficult Families Present

GCMs will have no trouble in recognizing the common themes that quickly identify the difficult family.[14]

- *The family usually presents with certain urgency to getting their needs met:* The difficult family usually calls in crisis and expresses a sense of urgency in having their issues addressed at once. They expect the GCM to respond immediately, even if the GCM does not consider the situation to be a crisis.

- *The family spends much time in contact with potential resources in an attempt to meet their needs:* The difficult family may call several GCMs, elder care agencies, or other professionals to request help and will often spend unproductive time researching options. Even after exhaustive research, the family will not be able to reach a consensus regarding whether to even retain a GCM.

- *Relationships with agencies and individuals are often conflictive:* The difficult family will easily disagree or find fault with professionals engaged in helping them.

- *Families are unreasonably demanding with a strong sense of entitlement:* The difficult family will unreasonably perceive its own problems as entitled to or requiring special attention from the GCM. This family does not respond well to limits and may expect the GCM or other institutions to "bend the rules" to meet their needs.

- *Families are overly sensitive to criticism and disappointment:* The difficult family feels easily criticized by the GCM and may become defensive regarding the GCM's recommendations. The family also becomes easily disappointed in the GCM if his or her suggestions do not have an immediate positive impact on the situation.

- *Families may have intense emotional reactions:* Different members of the difficult family may have intense reactions to the GCM's suggestions and to other members of the family. Family members will often disagree with each other about the extent of the elder's problems.

- *Families accept little responsibility for their actions and tend to blame others when things go wrong:* Difficult families tend to blame the GCM or other institutions when the elder's situation deteriorates or when the elder resists a plan. These families easily find fault with services or staff, and they become critical or angry without trying to discuss, understand, or resolve the perceived problem.

- *Families often have unrealistic expectations of their elderly relative:* Difficult families often feel that the elder can do more than the elder is capable of, either physically or cognitively. These families may have little patience or understanding for the resistance that elders commonly show to accepting services. They may deny the existence of cognitive problems or disagree over how to handle behavioral issues.

CASE STUDY

Case Example: Unrealistic Expectations
Mr. and Mrs. Homebody are 85 and 86 years old, respectively, and living in their own home. They have one daughter, Cathy Controller, who lives 3,000 miles away and who is trying to organize her parents' care from afar.

Cathy Controller retains a GCM to assess her parents' care needs and implement a plan that would keep them safely at home. She insists that the GCM "force" her parents to accept the help that Cathy has concluded they need. She considers herself an "expert" and frequently rejects suggestions offered by the GCM. Cathy calls the GCM frequently, and it is not unusual for these conversations to last for an hour. However, she also tells the GCM that she is worried about running up the bill and that the family cannot afford to spend a lot of money on GCM services.

Some of the questions that a GCM should consider are: What is the impact on Cathy of the long-distance nature of her relationship with her parents? How would her distance affect her own anxiety about their needs? What strategies could the GCM use to diffuse the daughter's anxiety? How should the GCM handle Cathy's belief in her own "expertise" and sense of entitlement? How should the GCM handle Cathy's insistence that her parents accept help?

Individual Roles within the Difficult Family

In establishing a relationship with a difficult family in the throes of an elder crisis, the GCM will recognize familiar roles and characteristics that individual family members play. Blazer describes these roles in the context of families dealing with an elder suffering from emotional problems.[4] I have modified his descriptions to make them relevant to the GCM's work with difficult families:

- *The Preserver* is more comfortable with the status quo and resists getting help for the elder. He or she is content if the elder remains overly dependent upon the family without access to needed intervention.
- *The Victim* perceives the elder's problems as a direct threat to his or her own needs or self-interest. The victim will see his or her own emotional needs as more important than the elder's. He or she will frequently contact the elder or the GCM, but the purpose of the contact will involve seeking attention for his or her own problems.
- *The Manager* tends to be calm, organized, and analytical during a crisis, but is unable to provide emotional support to the elder or to other family members. Often, the manager lives at a distance, which can cause tension with family members who are more directly involved in daily care.
- *The Martyr* has an innate need to nurture the elder, even when this comes at the expense of the martyr or the elder himself. The martyr's seemingly endless devotion can sometimes interfere with an appropriate care plan. Most commonly, he or she will insist on carrying out the elder's wish to remain at home beyond the point that is safe or appropriate. Despite complaints of exhaustion, the martyr will avoid opportunities for respite. He or she may be motivated by guilt or an unresolved relationship with the parent.
- *The Escapee* is typically an adult child who lives far away and has withdrawn or is entirely absent during a family crisis. Involved family members will resent the escapee, particularly when there is a history of family conflict. The escapee may

withdraw from family problems in self-defense and resist being drawn back into a stressful relationship with siblings.
- *The Meddler* will interfere with an established care plan in an attempt to wrest control away from other family members, to compete with siblings, or to assert dominance within the family. The meddler needs to be involved in every decision that is made and is overly involved with details. The meddler will have frequent contact with the GCM to change or challenge recommendations.

The elder, of course, is the central figure in the drama of the "difficult family." The GCM must assess the elder's own role in the creation of family dysfunction resulting in the roles described here.

Emotional Patterns of the Difficult Family

Dysfunctional families display common psychological and behavioral patterns that quickly come to the foreground when the stress of caring for an elder becomes predominate within the family system. These patterns include the following:

- *Contentiousness:* In struggling over current elder-care issues, the dysfunctional family will often revisit disputes over events that occurred years ago. Family property and family money are commonly sources of substantial contention.
- *Denial:* Adult children are frequently reluctant to recognize or admit early signs of decline in an elderly parent, particularly when the decline involves changes in cognitive functioning. For example, rather than acknowledge behavior associated with dementia, the adult child will often attribute the elder's current behaviors to earlier personality traits that are, in fact, no longer dominant. Denial becomes dysfunctional when the adult child fails to seek

necessary treatment or assistance for the elder or allows self-destructive behaviors on the part of the elder to go unchecked.

- *Anger:* Anger occurs normally in all families, but in dysfunctional families, anger may take the form of physical or emotional abuse.

- *Distancing and cut-off:* Distancing means pulling away from the family, either emotionally or physically. Cut-off refers to an individual member's disengagement to the point of having no involvement in family life at all.

- *Fusion:* Bowen first used this term to describe a "blending" of one person into another. The assumption is that in all emotional systems, people seek closeness. The person trying to fuse will pursue a relationship, while the person trying to maintain autonomy will distance. A frequent reaction to fusion is distance.[15]

- *Triangulation:* This is a family systems term used to describe a particular pattern involving the interaction among three members of the system. When tension exists between two family members, one of them may try involving a third as an ally. Triangles often represent an attempt to avoid change or conflict. Although they do occur frequently in normal family functioning, triangles that occur over a long period of time can create rigidity within the family system and make it more difficult for families to adapt or transition to new roles.[16]

■ GCM's RESPONSE TO DIFFICULT FAMILIES

Over the course of many workshops I conducted with GCMs, I have found the following terms are the descriptors most often used to describe GCMs' experiences with difficult families: overinvolved, underinvolved, unrealistic, in conflict, angry, resistant, in denial, demanding, hostile, passive-aggressive, needy, disagreeable, noncompliant, entitled, unappreciative, threatening, and unwilling to pay.

It is obvious that, when working with difficult families, GCMs experience strong negative feelings and intense reactions, just as these families create intense reactions in the institutional systems with which they come into contact. This experience is analogous to the countertransference phenomenon in psychoanalytic theory in which the therapist develops an intense emotional reaction to the patient.

It is important for GCMs to acknowledge and understand any countertransference reactions to develop an effective strategy for intervention. Which types of emotional reactions might a GCM experience in dealing with the difficult family? Felder mentions some familiar reactions:

- Intense dislike of family members
- Condescension toward client or family
- Impatience with family decision making
- Arguing with client or family members
- Avoiding necessary contact with client or family
- Becoming paternalistic, for example, taking over decisions that should be made by family
- Becoming passive-aggressive, for example, the GCM does not follow through with own recommendations[14]

To manage and overcome these counterproductive negative feelings, we need to use the same listening and reframing techniques we use when dealing with our elderly clients. With a resistant or difficult elder, we listen carefully and show compassion regarding the source of the person's fears and resistance, we acknowledge the person's losses, we affirm the person's basic dignity as a human, and we try to motivate the person to exercise control and maintain autonomy in his or her life. We need to use the same compassionate approach in dealing with and understanding the difficult family. We need to recognize the complexity of their own family system, the causes of the dysfunction, and the magnitude of the task ahead of them. The GCM must redefine the family task as "our" problem to solve, not "their" problem for which they are at fault.

■ INTERVENING WITH DIFFICULT FAMILIES

Perhaps the most important role the GCM plays in clinical practice with difficult families is as a change agent. The GCM enables families to reconnect with each other and to transform themselves into more effective units of giving and caring. In doing so, the GCM helps the family to move toward filial maturity and to redefine dependence in old age as a normal and expected development.

To be effective, the GCM must use both clinical and practical skills in assessing families and moving them toward change despite internal barriers. We need to distinguish our clinical approach from our instinctive approach in "pushing" families who are stuck. We must examine our own feelings to safeguard against the perils of countertransference. We must always be cognizant of the parameters of our relationship: we are not literally the client's therapist, coach, or friend, but we necessarily forge personal and even intimate bonds in doing our work.

Indeed, there is often an almost magical moment that the GCM may experience in working with families when "transformation" occurs, that is, the moment when the family and the client, who at the outset appeared desperate and hopeless, become empowered to move forward, resolve the immediate eldercare crisis, and make the changes that seemed so insurmountable. Such transformation is, often, the goal of our intervention.

As GCMs, how can we make transformation possible? We must remain emotionally available for our clients and diligently exercise the listening skills that are innate to our profession. We must explore options and possibilities where options and possibilities may often seem lacking. We must project trust and confidence in our own abilities as GCMs, thus enabling families to use us as a guide and, more important, as a role model in believing that change is possible, even within their own difficult family systems.

Components of Successful Intervention

In my view, there are at least four interrelated components of successful GCM intervention:

1. *Assessment:* A comprehensive and careful assessment is the basic tool of any effective care management. Chapters 3 and 4 address the traditional components of the GCM assessment, which includes an evaluation of the cognitive, physical, and emotional status of the elder client. As discussed earlier, the GCM must also evaluate the health or dysfunction of the overall family system.

2. *Identification of intergenerational roles and conflicts:* The GCM must identify existing power dynamics within the family, redefine responsibilities to achieve generational maturity, and realign roles and tasks for each family member. The GCM encourages a new two-way nurturing relationship between the adult child and the parent that may not have previously existed. At the same time, the GCM must enable the adult child as caregiver to set limits that are appropriate to a mature relationship. The GCM emboldens the adult child to identify and remove himself or herself from triangulated, fused, or other destructive family patterns, as described previously.

3. *Caregiver support and education:* The GCM can be instrumental in helping adult children understand that ambivalence, stress, and fear are normal and common aspects of the caregiving role. Furthermore, the GCM can reassure the

caregiver that our own professional experience and expertise allow us to offer a measure of predictability where, for the caregiver, none appears. By identifying concrete options and developing a positive plan for action, the GCM enables the family to move forward.

4. *Use of self.* Perhaps the most powerful tool for the GCM is the "use of self." The GCM provides to families what the author refers to as "grounded optimism." We provide a vision of the future that is based not only on a desire for hopeful outcomes but one that is also well grounded in our own clinical knowledge, prior professional experience, and belief that change within the family system is indeed possible. By being direct, empathetic, and nonjudgmental, we become a holding environment for stressed caregivers, creating a place of safety, confidentiality, consistency, and support. Finally, we offer our clients a model of perseverance. By not giving up on the possibility of positive change and by exploring all options, the GCM enables families to feel that, regardless of the outcome, they have done all that they can to support the elder.

Role Conflicts for the GCM and Difficult Family

Every GCM–client relationship requires the GCM to consider who the client is and to examine what the GCM can realistically advocate for and accomplish on the client's behalf. With the difficult family, these questions can become very troublesome.

Who Is the Client?

GCMs are rarely retained directly by an elder; instead, families or third parties retain a GCM to directly advocate on behalf of the elder. This arrangement raises numerous questions: Is the elder the client? Or is the

concerned family member who initiated contact? What if another family member signs the fee agreement? Sometimes a GCM is hired by a lawyer or other professional acting as the elder's guardian or attorney-in-fact. Who then is the client? Regardless of the legal implications of the contractual relationship, the author contends that, in all instances, the interests of the elder should be placed ahead of other interested parties. That is not to say that we can disregard the interests or viewpoints of family members and paying parties. On the contrary, recognizing that the elder is a part of a larger family system means that we must consider the interests of all parts of that system. However, the needs of the elder and the wishes of the family may be in conflict, which causes tension in our dual role in advocating for the elder and addressing the concerns of the family.

CASE STUDY

Case Example: Mr. Homebody

Barry Burnout contacts a GCM to assist him with nursing home placement for his 87-year-old father, Mr. Homebody, who has Parkinson's disease. Pursuant to a fee agreement signed by Mr. Burnout, the GCM conducts an initial assessment and concludes that, with increased in-home care and careful monitoring, Mr. Homebody's strong preference to remain in his own home can be safely accomplished. When the GCM shares her recommendation with Mr. Burnout, he reacts angrily. He tells the GCM that, after five years of caring for his father, he is exhausted, and he thinks his father's desire is not realistic. Mr. Burnout reminds the GCM that he is the one paying for services and that he retained her specifically for assistance with nursing home placement.

This represents the classic dilemma: Is Mr. Homebody the client, or is his exhausted son Barry? This conflict can be avoided only through a careful discussion at the outset of the GCM's representation. The GCM needs to have discussed with Barry—prior to entering into a fee arrangement—exactly what her own role would be as a professional, independent evaluator of Mr. Homebody's care needs. The GCM should have also discussed the fact that her professional assessment would have to include consideration of alternatives to Barry's preference for nursing home placement. On the other hand, the GCM cannot responsibly neglect the burned-out feelings of the son. Any successful care management plan has to take into account Barry's own circumstances at this stage of family development.

Who Is Being Difficult?

GCMs often advocate for families that have already been branded as "difficult" by other institutions, such as nursing homes or assisted living facilities. These families often retain the GCM when they are in active conflict with the institution. In these circumstances, the GCM must walk a fine line between advocating for a family that has truly been wronged versus representing a family that is unrealistic and overly demanding in its expectations. The GCM's investigative and assessment skills must come into play, and the sensitivity with which the GCM reports her recommendations to the family will determine the success of any intervention.

CASE STUDY

Case Example: Mrs. Lovely

Mrs. Lovely recently moved to a memory impairment unit in an assisted living facility. She initially adjusted quickly to her new life, and her daughter, Caring Carrie, was very pleased with the facility. A month later, Carrie visits Mrs. Lovely and finds her sitting at the window, unresponsive to Carrie's questions. Her mother was not dressed or bathed. Carrie quickly notices that her mother had not taken time-sensitive medications that day.

When Carrie asks the staff about her mother's condition, no one can explain why her medications were not administered properly that day. Carrie is upset, and she requests a meeting with the facility's administrator. The administrator politely tells Carrie that, as far as he knows, his staff are doing their best. Furthermore, he tells Carrie that he thinks someone did check on Mrs. Lovely that day but that she refused to get dressed or take her medications. He suggests that Carrie consider hiring a private companion to provide Mrs. Lovely with the additional care that the facility does not provide.

Carrie feels it is the facility's responsibility to either work with her mother's resistance and to notify Carrie when there is a problem. She is angry and frustrated, and she retains a GCM to contact the facility on her behalf. When the GCM meets with the administrator, he describes the daughter as overinvolved and anxious, and he feels that she does not fully understand the limitations of what an assisted living facility can provide.

Is Carrie "overinvolved" in her mother's care? Or is she advocating responsibly for her frail mother? The GCM must do a thorough investigation of the incident from all vantages: she must look at what Mrs. Lovely's actual needs are, what Carrie's expectations are, and what the facility is able to provide. If Carrie is unrealistic about either her mother's care needs or the facility's resources, the GCM needs to reestablish appropriate expectations and facilitate improved communication. On the other hand, the administrator's somewhat dismissive response to Carrie may be a red flag. Does the facility have established protocols for dealing with resistant residents on the memory impairment unit? Did the administrator adequately investigate Carrie's concern? What is the basis for his suggestion that Carrie is overinvolved? The GCM's investigation must account for these types of questions. But no matter what recommendation she ultimately makes, the GCM needs to acknowledge the daughter's anxiety and validate her concerns in the face of her mother's decline.

Setting Limits

The familiar boundaries between professional and client are easily tested when the GCM works with the difficult family. Limit setting, both as to time and professional involvement, are essential precisely because the effectiveness of the GCM can be compromised if the GCM becomes, in effect, a part or extension of the dysfunctional family system. Signs that the GCM is losing appropriate boundaries include the following:

- *Overidentification*: Although it is professionally necessary to understand and empathize with the emotional realities of the family or the client, it is not appropriate for the GCM to routinely share details of one's own emotional "story" or personal history. Whereas some sharing may be effective, the GCM should be on guard against overidentification.
- *Overconsolation*: As helping professionals, it is in our own nature to want to take away our client's pain. The GCM should guide and strategize with the client or the family, but should not expect—or be expected—to erase the difficulties they face. The GCM can alleviate, but not eliminate, the difficult family's burdens.

- *Appeasement*: GCMs cannot always please the client. The GCM needs to be honest and direct, and sometimes the GCM may have a recommendation that the family may not be prepared to hear. The manner in which the GCM shares his or her recommendation is a matter of clinical judgment, but the GCM should not withhold information to please a difficult client or prevent discomfort.
- *Overinvestment in strategy*: It is easy to become too invested in one's own strategy. The care plan is a dynamic intervention that must evolve as family circumstances change. The GCM should always remain flexible and resist the temptation to adhere to a favored, original strategy.
- *Overinvestment of time*: GCMs often make themselves available on a 24-hour basis for responding to client crises. It is important to carve out personal time so that the GCM does not blend personal and work lives. Failure to honor the distinction can eventually lead to professional burnout.

■ CONCLUSION

It is intrinsic to geriatric care management that we intervene in family matters that are innately complex and emotionally poignant. Our intervention frequently occurs during a family crisis. Even a healthy family that is able to mobilize resources and work cooperatively faces daunting tasks in negotiating appropriate care for the elder while maintaining emotional balance. For the dysfunctional family that is less emotionally equipped for these tasks, the path to resolution is perilous.

This chapter has explored the concepts of filial maturity and generational maturity because they provide a useful framework for our active interventions with all families. By rejecting the notion of role reversal and, instead, emphasizing dependence as a normal and expected stage of late-life family development, we can help family members mature into new roles defined by filial reciprocity and mutual caring. In this way, the family supports the strengths of the elder rather than the elder's fragilities or deficits. Recognizing the elder as a complete person who can provide and accept care will reward healthy and difficult families alike.

■ NOTES

1. Sandmaier M. Oldest rifts. *Family Therapy Networker.* 1998;22:23–31.

2. Hargrave TD, Anderson WT. Finishing well: a context family therapy approach to the aging family. In: Hanna SM, Hargrave TD, eds. *The Aging Family.* New York: Brunner/Mazel; 1997:61–80.

3. Kuttner R, Trotter S. *Family Re-Union.* New York: The Free Press; 2002.

4. Blazer D. *Emotional Problems in Later Life: Intervention Strategies for Professional Caregivers.* New York: Springer; 1998.

5. Fowler L. Understanding and strengthening healthy relationships between adult children and parents. August 2004. Available at: http://ohioline.osu.edu/flm99/fs04.html. Accessed June 15, 2005.

6. Karen R. *The Forgiving Self.* New York: Doubleday; 2001.

7. Lowy L. Independence and dependence in aging: a new balance. *J Gerontol Soc Work.* 1989;13:133–146.

8. Erlanger MA. Changing roles and life-cycle transitions. In: Hanna SM, Hargrave TD, eds. *The Aging Family.* New York: Brunner/Mazel; 1997: 163–177.

9. Blenkner M. Social work and family relationships in later life with some thoughts on filial maturity. In: Shanas E, Streib G, eds. *Social Structure and the Family: Generational Relations.* Englewood Cliffs, NJ: Prentice Hall; 1965:46–59.

10. Shulman S. The changing nature of family relationships in middle and later life: parent-caring and the mid-life developmental opportunity. *Smith College Studies in Social Work.* 2005;75(2):103–120.

11. Greenberg. Mutuality in families: a framework for continued growth in late life. *J Geriatr Psychiatr Neurol.* 1994;27:79–95.

12. Silver M. Caring and being cared for in old age: the development of mutual parenting. In: Demick J, Burkik K. *Parental Development.* Hillsdale, NJ: Lawrence Erlbaum Associates; 1993.

13. Cox C. Families and the frail elderly. *The Frail Elderly: Problems, Needs, and Community Responses.* Westport, CT: Auburn House; 1993.

14. Felder R, Beauchamp D. Working with the problematic client. *Geriatric Care Manage J.* 1995;5(2):12–18.

15. Bowen M. *Family Therapy in Clinical Practice.* New York: Jason Aronson; 1978.

16. Shulman L. *The Skills of Helping Individuals, Families, and Groups.* Itasca, IL: F. E. Peacock Publishers; 1992.

Chapter 19

Supporting Clients' Quality of Life: Drawing on Community, Informal Networks, and Care Manager Creativity

Nina Pflumm Herndon and Victoria Thorpe

■ INTRODUCTION

This chapter provides concrete tools and examples to support geriatric care managers (GCMs) in focusing on developing and sustaining quality of life (QOL) for their clients that goes beyond physical comfort and includes emotional, physical, intellectual, and spiritual well-being.

■ WHAT IS "QUALITY OF LIFE?"

Providing clients with an exceptional QOL is an important goal for a GCM. Activities that encourage clients to foster their emotional, intellectual, physical, and/or spiritual QOL can help to address a client's physiological health. QOL comprises (1) social interactions and general sense of connectedness (to other people, upcoming generations, affiliations with groups, pets, or whatever brings the person a sense of meaning); (2) engagement with activities that promote a sense of purpose and feelings of physical wellness; (3) stimulation of the mind in the form of learning, creativity, or idea exchange; and (4) a sense of spirituality. Most important, QOL is a deeply personal response to one's situation and circumstances based on what brings one purpose and meaning.

Addressing a broader scope of an older adult's QOL is an important goal for geriatric care. There is a tendency within the geriatric care community to focus efforts on improving a client's QOL as it specifically relates to quality of care, whether by providing support and comfort at the end of life, attending to health care needs, drawing on community resources, or simply ensuring that the client is treated with respect and consideration by care providers. As a result, care managers have traditionally been called on by families to help ensure their clients experience all-important "quality of care." However, recent experience in geriatric care, along with new research about the aging process, suggests there is a greater opportunity to affect an older adult's QOL by expanding the notion to include how older adults can stay fulfilled and engaged in their lives, despite cognitive or physical limitations.

Similar to the focus on holistic wellness among the general population, there is a growing understanding in the geriatric care community that it is imperative to incorporate a larger sense of "health" for older adults, and to consider more of the facets that contribute to their mental and physical well-being. Indeed, the World Health Organization has defined *health* as a "state of complete physical, intellectual and social well-being and not merely the absence of disease or infirmity."[1]

Although the physical elements of QOL are of paramount importance, new evidence shows that holistic QOL, including emotional and spiritual health, can have as much, if not greater, impact on an older adult's overall well-being. In reality, this is not an either/or choice because these more holistic aspects of a client's QOL are intertwined with his or her physical QOL. For example, if a client is disconnected from friends and family and lacking emotional QOL, this can lead to a sense of isolation, which can cause negative mental and physical effects. Similarly, if a client nurtures a strong spiritual foundation, whether through a religious institution or on a more individual level, this may result in positive physical manifestations, such as an increased desire to live and a stronger resiliency against depression.

Holistic QOL is defined as incorporating four distinct, yet interrelated areas: intellectual, emotional, spiritual, and physical. Intellectual QOL includes activities that engage clients mentally, including hobbies, learning, "brain aerobics," or any form of creativity. Emotional QOL includes structured social interactions or time with family, friends, and peers who have shared similar life experiences, or other emotional connections, such as with pets or grandchildren, or even a sense of being at peace with oneself. The physical aspects of QOL in this chapter focus on activities that help clients stay physically active, increase their sense of strength despite possible limitations, and provide a sense of fun. Finally, there is spiritual QOL, which delves into how clients can maintain or build spiritual connections, whether through a relationship with church or temple or through other avenues, such as volunteering or spending time in nature.

■ WHY HOLISTIC QUALITY OF LIFE MATTERS FOR GCMs

Care managers who focus on improving holistic QOL for their clients can make a measurable, sustainable impact on overall health and well-being. Activities that encourage clients to foster their emotional, intellectual, physical, and/or spiritual QOL can help to address a client's physiological health concerns. For example, one GCM worked with a client who was depressed and withdrawn, and had little interest in social activities or even visiting with family. The GCM decided to delve into the client's spiritual well-being and began talking to him about the things in his prior life that had brought him joy and meaning. When the GCM learned that nature was especially important for the client, she arranged for him to visit a local bird sanctuary with wheelchair access, where he could view birds through a specially designed set of binoculars. This experience gave the client new interest in life; his appetite subsequently improved and he started asking to see friends and neighbors again.

GCMs are uniquely qualified to assess and address a client's needs in terms of holistic QOL. A GCM has a bird's-eye view of a client's needs without the obstacles (real or perceived) that might cloud the perspective of an adult child or family member (e.g., "Dad never liked puzzles; don't bother even trying"). A GCM can also tap into community resources to address holistic QOL that a care provider may not be aware exists, such as finding an art class for elders at a local community college (e.g., "Mrs. K says she likes to paint but I don't know how to do that"). And GCMs have a third, more practical reason to address their clients' holistic QOL—if their clients are more fulfilled and engaged, they will have better health and a more positive affect, which will result in positive feedback from all parties, more referrals, and a continued flow of new business. Plus, holistic QOL activities are an opportunity for GCMs to be creative and to bring a sense of playfulness to their client interactions.

Research Supports the Focus on Holistic QOL

Although there is a great deal of anecdotal evidence that holistic QOL, including emotional, intellectual, physical, and spiritual elements, has a strong effect on the functional QOL for older adults, these stories are also supported by a growing body of empirical, scientific research.

Benefits of Activities That Promote Emotional QOL

Much research supports the benefits of promoting emotional QOL for older adults, particularly in terms of social connections.

A study of 3,112 elders in Missouri indicated that when older adults had visits with friends or relatives, had close friends for emotional support, or had the perception that help would be available if they became sick or disabled, they had better emotional health.[2] Because of these results, the Centers for Disease Control and Prevention (CDC) recommends implementing effective prevention programs for older adults to help improve emotional health among older adults who have little social support.[2] In particular, the CDC notes that "social support can promote health by providing persons with positive experiences, socially rewarding roles, or improved ability to cope with stressful events. Social support is critical for older adults who are at increased risk for disability associated with chronic disease or social isolation after the loss of a partner."[2]

Social support can come in the form of connections with other people—friends, family, peers, and so forth, but it can also come through relationships with animals, particularly with household pets. Studies have demonstrated that pet therapy can help to improve social interaction, psychosocial function, life satisfaction, social competence, and psychological well-being, while reducing depression in elder residents of care homes. It is also thought that interaction with these animals can help break the cycle of loneliness, hopelessness, and social withdrawal that is often seen in older adults.[3]

Benefits of Activities That Promote Intellectual QOL

Although for many years scientists believed that the human brain inevitably deteriorates over time, there has been new research in recent years that refutes this assumption and shows that intellectual stimulation may help preserve key cognitive functionality for older adults.

In 2002, the *Journal of the American Medical Association* published a study by Rush Alzheimer's Disease Center and Rush-Presbyterian-St. Luke's Medical Center in Chicago, Illinois, which found a connection between frequent participation in cognitively stimulating activities and a reduced risk of Alzheimer's disease. The study, which followed more than 700 dementia-free participants age 65 years and older for an average of 4.5 years, measured participants' levels of cognitive activity and correlated these levels with the amount of time the participants spent on activities that stimulate the brain, such as reading the newspaper or books, or doing crossword puzzles and playing card games. The study found that although all of the participants experienced modest, age-related declines on memory and information processing tests, the rates of decline were lower for those who had engaged in more frequent activities that stimulated cognitive development.[4]

This research not only generated a lot of press, but it has also caused some people to confuse repetitive "brain activities" that are designed to help older adults preserve singular mental skills with activities that promote intellectual QOL. Activities that promote intellectual QOL involve more than just "training" clients to better remember a set of tasks; they encourage mental stimulation and deeper engagement. In fact, new research questions the recent effectiveness of mind "training" for older adults and raises doubts about whether it has any long-term impact on intellectual processing. According to research psychologist Arthur Kramer of the University of Illinois, Urbana, "There is no doubt that older people can improve their performance on these tasks through training. What we don't know is whether this transfers to real-world skills and cognitive function."[5] Thus, activities designed to improve clients' intellectual QOL need to be deeply stimulating and engaging, such as visits to museums, reading interesting books or articles, or learning new skills or knowledge.

Benefits of Activities That Promote Physical QOL

It seems obvious to state that research shows the importance of regular physical activity in promoting holistic QOL. However, with clients who have moderate to severe physical limitations, GCMs may inadvertently overlook physical activities that go beyond goal-oriented physical therapy to support more overall functioning. Recent research about the effects of physical activity specifically focused on older adults gives compelling new reasons why this element of holistic QOL cannot be neglected in addressing an older adult's well-being, no matter what limitations may exist.

Researchers at the University of Illinois at Urbana-Champaign found that previously sedentary seniors who incorporated physical activity into their lifestyles not only improved physical function, but experienced psychological benefits as well. Kinesiology professor Dr. Edward McAuley, who led the study, notes, "The implications of our work are that not only will physical activity potentially add years to your life as we age, but the quality of those years is likely to be improved by regular physical activity."[6]

In addition to promoting psychological well-being and better health, physical activity also appears to help preserve brain functioning for older adults. According to the *Wall Street Journal*, interventions that indirectly target intellectual fitness through physical conditioning show promise for brain preservation. In a 2003 review of 18 studies, Professor Kramer and his colleagues of the University of Illinois, Urbana, found that strength training and aerobics keep high-level brain functions, such as planning, remembering, and multitasking, sharp. Professor Kramer notes, "Cardiovascular fitness training improves cognitive function in the elderly in as little as six months. It increases the volume of gray matter [neurons] and white matter [which connects neurons] in regions that handle executive functions. It also improves the efficiency of networks that underlie some forms of memory and attention."[5]

Researchers are finding, however, that all physical activity is not the same; some types of activities have more benefits than others do. Although walking and other cardiovascular activities are wonderful for older adults, there is new information about the positive effects of strength training for this population. If the idea of an older adult lifting big barbells seems outlandish, consider the evidence about the benefits of strength training, no matter how low the weight or how adapted the activity is to accommodate physical limitations. Weight training not only helps prevent deterioration of the musculoskeletal system (something that aerobic exercise does not accomplish), but it has also been proved to help older adults build new muscle. Weight training has other positive physiological and psychological outcomes. A Harvard University study showed significant psychological improvements when older adults engaged in strength training programs. After 12 weeks of strength exercise, 14 of 16 previously depressed elders in the study no longer met the criteria for clinical depression.[7]

The wonderful part about focusing on physical QOL is that it can have a ripple effect on the other factors that affect a client's well-being. As documented earlier, physical conditioning can improve mental acumen and functioning. With improved mental and physical health, an older adult can also more fully participate in group activities (emotional QOL), continue learning (intellectual QOL), and pursue endeavors that give him or her meaning and purpose in life (spiritual QOL).

Benefits of Activities That Promote Spiritual QOL

Given the myriad ways that individuals may interpret the term *spiritual*, it is difficult to find empirical research that "proves" the importance of a focus on spirituality for older adults. Undaunted, researchers have been trying to tackle this dilemma to better support the case for spiritual practice in elder care.

There is much rich, ethnographic research about the ways that older adults respond to and appreciate connecting with a larger spiritual purpose, whether it is through a church or temple, volunteer work, or time with pets or nature. Nurturing spirituality may be as simple as encouraging gratitude and taking stock of life's blessings. According to Eugene Bianchi, who works with elder adults in Atlanta, Georgia, "A strong trait among creative elders is a spirit of gratitude toward life. They are able to receive the small and large gifts along the way as blessings that evoke thankfulness. . . . These elders do not deny the pain and hardship of negative events, but they seem to be able to learn from them or at least to accept them as they turn back toward life."[8]

■ HOW GCMs CAN IMPROVE HOLISTIC QUALITY OF LIFE

There are so many ways that GCMs can promote emotional, intellectual, physical, and spiritual QOL for their clients; the key is to find the unique formula that gives meaning for each client and to build a plan from there. There are four steps to addressing a client's holistic QOL: assessing his or her needs and interests, prioritizing these needs, developing and implementing an activity plan that will address these needs; and evaluating success and refining the plan. Although this may seem complex and time-consuming, in reality it is a fairly intuitive process.

For example, one GCM focused her holistic QOL efforts for one client on gardening:

> My client, Mrs. J, was an avid gardener until she had a massive stroke with frontal lobe damage. When Mrs. J became distressed that she could no longer tend to her garden, I worked with the family to put in raised beds with wide edges so she could still get her hands dirty and experience the beauty and wonder of growing flowers, despite her stroke. While Mrs. J may have planted some of her flowers upside down, her ability to still do the thing she loved—gardening—gave a tremendous boost to her quality of life
>
> —Michelle Boudinot,
> NorthBay Eldercare Solutions

■ ROADBLOCKS TO ADDRESSING HOLISTIC QUALITY OF LIFE

There are many, real roadblocks that can prevent care managers from focusing on holistic elements of QOL. Care managers are often brought in when a client is experiencing more urgent health matters, such as compliance with prescriptions, recovery from surgery, or deteriorating physical and/or mental capacity, which need immediate attention and leave little room for any other kind of care in the short term. In addition, there are baseline physical and mental health issues, including depression, decreased physical or cognitive functioning, social isolation, and client apathy, which can cause care managers to inadvertently ignore the client's holistic QOL needs.

Also, the general public is largely unfamiliar with how an older adult's holistic QOL can improve physiological ailments. As a result, GCMs have had to educate family members and medical practitioners about the importance of QOL in overall care planning and about the value of spending care management dollars on QOL issues. Although these impediments are sometimes difficult, they are not insurmountable, and by using creativity and drawing on community resources, care managers can adapt activities and adjust expectations to facilitate emotional, intellectual, physical, and/or spiritual stimulation for almost any client. The best way to get started on creating a QOL plan is to figure out what will provide the client with an enhanced sense of purpose, meaning, or connectedness.

■ STEP 1: ASSESS THE CLIENT'S HOLISTIC QUALITY OF LIFE

Assessing a client's needs in terms of holistic QOL can be done either formally, informally, or through a combination of the two approaches.[1] Unlike other kinds of health assessments, understanding an individual client's "recipe" for enhancing holistic QOL is far from scientific. Although the GCM using an assessment tool is helpful, ultimately it is a nuanced, relationship-driven process that will enable the care manager to figure out what gives each client meaning and purpose. In this chapter, there are examples of both formal and informal assessments that can be used to identify both how well a client's holistic QOL needs are being met and which elements are still missing. However, each care manager will probably develop his or her own unique way of assessing this very personal, individual question for clients. Ultimately, it does not matter how GCMs explore

the elements of emotional, intellectual, physical, and spiritual well-being with their clients; what matters is that they find a way that works for each person.

Formal Assessment of Holistic Quality of Life

Geriatric care advocates and researchers now propose that assessing QOL for older adults should include an evaluation of the older adult's mind, body, spirit, environment, and life experiences.[9] In terms of formal assessment, Rosalie Kane and her colleagues at the University of Minnesota have developed an assessment for QOL in nursing homes that focuses on 11 outcome domains that constitute "psychosocial" QOL, including individuality, enjoyment, meaningful activity, and spiritual well-being. For purposes of this focus on holistic QOL, this assessment has been adapted and shortened as Exhibit 19-1.

Some care management practices have their own ways to assess holistic QOL and may be able to provide care managers with useful tools for determining where to focus QOL activities. Sage Eldercare Solutions, based in San Francisco and San Mateo, California, has developed the assessment shown in Exhibit 19-2 to help GCMs better understand their clients' holistic QOL needs as part of a therapeutic activities program they offer to their clients.

Informal Assessment of Holistic Quality of Life

Conducting a formal assessment of a client's holistic QOL is helpful for establishing a baseline of the client's current situation and needs. This baseline will be useful when evaluating progress and refining the holistic QOL plan for the client. However, care managers also build rich relationships with their clients and assess their clients' needs through more informal observations and conversation. This type of informal assessment can

Exhibit 19–1   Formal Assessment for Holistic Quality of Life

Holistic QOL Area	QOL Outcome	Outcome Indicators	How to Assess Client QOL in This Area
Emotional	Relationships	Clients engage in meaningful person-to-person interchange where the purpose is social.	• Ask client to list the people in his life that are important to him. • Check his schedule and/or ask him when he last saw any/all of these people. • Interview caregivers and family members to assess how often the client has social interactions.
Intellectual	Autonomy	Clients take initiative and make choices for their lives and care.	• Ask client to name one decision she has made in the last month. • Interview caregivers and family members to assess how much they engage client in decision making.
	Enjoyment	Clients express or exhibit pleasure and enjoyment, verbally and nonverbally. Conversely, they do not express or exhibit unhappiness, distress, or lack of enjoyment.	• Ask client what brings him enjoyment and to identify activities that have been enjoyable in the past month. • Interview caregivers and family members to find out what brings pleasure and enjoyment for client. • Determine how often the client gets to do the things he finds enjoyable.
	Meaningful activity	Clients engage in discretionary behavior, either active activity or passive observation, which they find interesting, stimulating, and/or worthwhile. Conversely, they tend not be bored with their lives.	• Ask client to name at least one thing she enjoyed doing in the past. • Ask client to name at least one thing she enjoys doing now. • Ask client to describe the last time she engaged in an activity related to her past or present interests. • Interview caregivers and family members about the client's interests and the types of activities she does that match her interests.
Spiritual	Spiritual well-being	Clients perceive that their needs and concerns for religion, prayer, meditation, moral values, and meaning in life are met.	• Ask client about his religious background and the level he is/was engaged in a religious community, for example, church, temple, mosque. • If he no longer attends any regular services in his religion, probe for the reason why, assessing whether it is a logistical issue or true choice. • If the client is not affiliated with any formal religion, ask what gives him meaning in his life. Is it time with friends/family? Nature? Volunteering? Pets/animals? • If client is religious, ask what aspects of the religion are most meaningful to him. • Interview caregivers and family to explore what may give the client deeper meaning in his life.

Source: Reproduced with permission from Oxford University Press.

Exhibit 19–2   Sage Awakenings Therapeutic Program Assessment

Personal Interest Inventory

Name: _____

Address: _____

Place of Birth & Past Residences: _____

Current Living Status: ❑ Single   ❑ Married   ❑ Separated   ❑ Divorced   ❑ Widowed

Titles Held: _____   Dates of Marriage/Divorce/Death: _____

Past Occupations: _____   Special Achievements: _____

Hobbies: _____   Interests: _____

Social Activities Enjoyed: _____

Sports Played/Forms of Exercise Enjoyed: _____

Veteran: ❑ Yes   ❑ No   If so, dates served, posts and branch of military? _____

Dreams: _____

Work/Volunteer: _____   Pets (past and present): _____

Birth Family Structure: _____   Nuclear Family Structure: _____

Primary & Languages Spoken: _____   Education (highest grade level)
                                          & Field of Study: _____
                                          Religious Preference: _____

Culture / Ethnicity: _____   Literacy: ❑ Reads English   ❑ Writes English
                                                  ❑ Reads / Writes in Spoken Language

Favorite Foods: _____

Family Traditions: _____

Daily Rituals: _____

Sensory Limits: _____

Functional Limits: _____

Most Memorable Experiences:

1. _____
2. _____

Three things I enjoy the most:

1. _____
2. _____
3. _____

Three Things You Should Know About Me (Values, Beliefs, Traditions, Achievements):

1. _____
2. _____
3. _____

Exhibit 19-2   Sage Awakenings Therapeutic Program Assessment (continued)

ACTIVITIES CHECKLIST: (Care Manager to fill in based on information provided below; may also be helpful to read off several items to gauge client's interest level for each)

- Brain Aerobics
- Crosswords
- Memoir creation
- Quizzes
- Documentaries
- Scrapbook creation
- Memory exercises
- Life review
- Reminiscence
- Creative writing
- Exercise
- Yoga
- Tai chi
- Historical review
- Painting, drawing
- Flower arranging
- Dancing
- Singing
- Playing instruments
- Sculpting

- Collage
- Gardening
- Poetry
- Cooking
- Shopping
- Sending and receiving mail
- Computer research
- Listening to music; types of music

  _____

- Social engagements:

  _____

- Philosophical inquiry
- Animals, pets; specify area of interest:

  _____

- Performances; mediums of interest:

  _____

- Arts and lectures; topics of interest:

  _____

- Lifelong learning; topics of interest:

  _____

- Nature walks and hikes

Source: Sage Awakenings Therapeutic Services, Sage Eldercare Solutions. www.sageeldercare.com.

yield excellent information from the client and the client's caregiver and/or family because the care manager can weave questions and inquiries into the conversation in a way that may be less threatening than a formal evaluation.

If the goal of a formal assessment is to determine the "when" and "how" in terms of integrating a focus on a client's QOL, then the informal assessment will help determine the "what"—which activities will resonate with the client and are most likely to bring him or her meaning and fulfillment. This "what" information will come into play during the next step, creating the plan for improving the client's holistic QOL. Exhibit 19-3 provides a framework for informal assessment of holistic QOL.

Exhibit 19-3 Questions to Use for Informal Assessment

Emotional

- How satisfied are you with the frequency of social interactions (with friends, family, neighbors) in your life?

- How do you feel when you are getting ready to see family members? How do you feel afterward?

- Is loneliness an important problem in your life?

- Do you cultivate friendships as one remedy for loneliness?

- Are friends more or less meaningful in your life than immediate family members are?

- If you have friends of long standing, to what do you attribute the success of these relationships?

- Do you seek out groups or organizations where you might meet new friends?

- How do you feel when you are getting ready to see friends? How do you feel afterward?

Intellectual

- What was your career when you were working? Are you involved in this profession in any way now? Would you like to be?

- How important was work to you? Was it more important than other, nonwork activities or relationships?

- Please describe some of your greatest achievements.

- What kinds of activities do you or did you engage in to use your mind and intellect? Reading? Crossword or other word puzzles? Political discussions?

- When was the last time you learned something new (new game, new kind of information, new way to do something)? How did this feel?

- What are some interests that you haven't yet had the opportunity to pursue?

Physical

- Looking back on your life, what were the things you did to foster your physical health? How can you retrieve and adapt these activities for the sake of your health today?

- If you were physically active in earlier stages of your life, what did you enjoy most about it?

- Do you have any fears or stereotypes that are holding you back from engaging in physical activity?

Spiritual

- Do you consider yourself a spiritual person? If so, what were the most influential factors (persons, teachings, institutions, events) in shaping this spirituality?

- If the words *spiritual* or *religious* have no meaning or have negative connotations for you, how do you express your deepest philosophy of life? What are its principles, its virtues, its goals, and its actions?

- What are you grateful for? Can you make a brief list of the things for which you are most thankful—either small happenings (for example, the warm sun through the window) or major items (for example, a loving family).

- How important is being in nature to you? What places, elements, or environments (beach, mountains, parks, or birds) bring you the most enjoyment?

Source: Crossroad Publishing Company (1994). Bianchi, Eugene. pp. 199–222. Used with permission.

■ STEP 2: ANALYZE ASSESSMENT RESULTS AND PRIORITIZE CLIENT NEEDS

After the GCM conducts formal and/or informal assessments, the GCM will have gathered a lot of information about the client's needs and interests in the areas of emotional, intellectual, physical, and spiritual QOL. In all likelihood, a few themes or key areas will emerge in looking through these data. Perhaps the GCM noticed many photos of pets and the client mentioned a love of animals during their conversations. Or maybe the client is completely sedentary, yet described in great detail the wonderful camping and hiking trips he took in his youth. Or maybe the care manager learned that the client was a teacher for many years and yearns to work with children again in some capacity. Or it could just be that the client is lonely and needs to see other people, including family and potential friends, more often.

The point is for the care manager to prioritize the client's needs based on the information gathered and to create a holistic QOL plan based on these priorities. Given limited time and resources, this prioritization process should help the care manager rank the various areas of holistic QOL in order of importance for the client and give a clear understanding of which should be addressed first, second, and so forth.

■ STEP 3: CREATE A PLAN FOR ADDRESSING THE CLIENT'S HOLISTIC QUALITY OF LIFE

Now that the care manager has a concrete understanding of *what* brings the client joy or sparks interest or boosts his or her energy and which areas are most likely to bring the client fulfillment and improved well-being, the question is *how* to get there. This next section includes examples of activities and programs designed to engage older adults in the areas of emotional, intellectual, physical, and spiritual well-being, along with stories of how GCMs have successfully affected their clients' lives in these areas.

A. Explore Ideas and Resources Related to Each Element of Holistic QOL

The list that follows is just the beginning of learning how to address holistic QOL. GCMs can gather other ideas by talking with colleagues, visiting local community or senior centers, or using the Internet. Ultimately, each care manager will utilize her own creativity, along with all the resources and ideas she has gathered (including input from other professionals—art therapists, recreational therapists, care providers—and community opportunities), to tailor a plan that meets her clients' needs.

Emotional Quality of Life

When care managers work to address a client's emotional QOL, they tend to focus on social interactions, whether it is time with family and friends, or participation in programs that forge intergenerational relationships or provide structured social opportunities with other elders. If the client's family is nearby, it could be as simple as working to arrange a regular schedule for visits and marking the visits on the calendar or having visitors sign a guestbook when they arrive so the client knows when to expect company and can look forward to these interactions instead of not knowing when or if someone is going to arrive.

If family is far away or unavailable for other reasons, the focus may turn to friendships, helping the client nurture or rekindle relationships by arranging the transportation or other logistics necessary for the client to see his or her friends on a regular basis. Senior centers, which provide drop-in opportunities and structured events, can provide other occasions for older adults to have social interactions that may lead to friendships. Many schools and day care centers also have intergenerational programs, where older adults can spend time with children, each enjoying the special gifts the other brings to the exchange.

One care manager put together an extraordinary event for the clients in her care, which honored their wisdom and beauty and provided a big boost to the emotional quality of their lives.

> As a Mother's Day event and gift, I planned a ladies tea and called it "Les Grandes Dames Tea." The party (complete with formal invitations) was held at one of the nicest senior communities in the area, where we arranged for wait staff to serve petits fours and fancy cookies and pour coffee and tea from silver tea services. The care managers and our "ladies" all dressed up in all manner of finery, including big picture hats, treasured wraps, and lace gloves. Each Grande Dame even received a wrist corsage and even a glass of champagne. We also enlisted the services of a tuxedo-clad handsome young man who played the piano and sang oldies to each and every lady. A film crew and photographer caught all of this on tape and each lady had a personal filmed interview session. It was the best of care management—a celebration for those Grande Dames whose lives are no longer filled with very many high spots.
>
> —Marsha R. Foley, RN, MBA,
> ElderCare Options, Ltd.

Another care manager organized a social occasion in her client's assisted living facility, which evoked the client's past history as a very social person in her community:

> When Mrs. R, a former garden club lady, was moved into an apartment in an upscale assisted living facility, I decided to help her host a Christmas tea to meet her new neighbors. I arranged for some furniture from her old house to be delivered, sent out invitations to all of the residents, and took her shopping to buy a

nice outfit for the occasion. Mrs. R. was thrilled to play hostess again and it really helped her feel comfortable in her new living situation.

> —Sally Gold, MSW,
> Geriatric Resource Services

Sometimes the relationship between the care manager and the client itself can produce measurable improvements in the client's emotional QOL (and, as in the following anecdote, for the care manager, too):

> When I first started working with Mrs. D, she had advanced dementia, was striking her care providers and refused to take her medications. To assist her, I decided to accompany her on outings around the city—something I love to do. We began walking around her lively San Francisco neighborhood, talking with interesting people we met, and pausing to entertain onlookers. These experiences provided socialization outside of her residential facility and enriched her daily life. During my time with her, Mrs. D has transformed from threatening other residents in her facility to creating collages in expressive arts groups with a smile on her face. Her anti-anxiety medications have also been reduced to their lowest level in years. Our relationship has helped Mrs. D re-ignite with her inner spark, and has allowed me to do the same.
>
> —Tara Bradley, MA, MFTI,
> Sage Eldercare Solutions

These are wonderful examples of social interactions for clients, but there are other ways to positively affect a client's emotional QOL, such as through pet or massage therapies. One care manager had tremendous success in helping address her client's loneliness through the adoption of a pet cat:

> We had one client, Mrs. N, who was 90 and had been widowed for over 25 years. Since the passing of her husband, Mrs. N had few constants in her life; family was far away and many of her friends were

gone too. She loved to feed the squirrels and birds in front of her house, and spoke fondly of her neighbor's cat. After discussing the idea with her, we brought Mrs. N to the SPCA on her birthday, where a volunteer spent several hours helping her select an older cat that had been waiting for the right owner. The new pet was named "Penny," and she became Mrs. N's closest relationship, a loving lap cat who could sit for hours on her owner's knees. Penny gave Mrs. N a sense of responsibility for another creature and helped motivate her to keep living. Her connection to Penny also mitigated the loss of control Mrs. N experienced as her body changed over time.

—Nina Pflumm Herndon, MA, CMC
Sage Eldercare Solutions

Touch therapy or massage is another innovative way to help clients feel emotionally connected and improve their physical well-being. According to national statistics, about one-third of massage patients are adults age 55 and older, and this growing popularity is helping to dispel some of the negative misconceptions about massage among seniors. Elmer "Lee" Manning, an 81-year-old man who has been getting regular massages for two years, has become a convert to the healing benefits of the practice. "It sure helps me sleep. It helps me move," he said. "It helps about everything." Massage and other forms of touch therapy can also provide clients with tangible emotional well-being. Anita Booth, a massage therapist who works with many older adults, sees the impact of touch for her senior clients. "The elderly don't get loving touch. They might get medical attention, but they don't get loving touch," she says. "Massage therapy is very special. It's a much more sustained and loving connection between human beings."[10]

Intellectual Quality of Life

The informal assessment data gathered in step 1 are essential in helping the GCM figure out how to foster intellectual QOL for a client. Some clients, who were very attached to their careers, will resonate most closely with activities and events that provide an opportunity to utilize their professional skills, such as talking with a former colleague or reading (or being read to/from) books or articles related to their professions.

For example, one care manager tried countless strategies to mitigate her client's sometimes disruptive behavior until she tapped into his background as an architect:

> One client was a man with Alzheimer's who had major agitation but was also wheelchair-bound. He was in a facility and was always pulling things apart and driving the staff crazy. We tried several interventions—nothing worked. Then we recalled that he used to be a draftsman and bought him an Etch-a-Sketch. The device reminded him of his former career and he was so content playing with all those lines!
>
> —Michelle Boudinot, MA,
> NorthBay Eldercare

The role of creativity is also very important for intellectual QOL. This category is not limited to traditional art activities; anything that inspires an older adult to engage with mind and spirit and to enthusiastically participate can be seen as "creative." Creative activities include cooking, hobbies, interesting conversation, or even community work. Creative activities not only help bolster the intellectual QOL for clients, but they may also improve their physiological health. According to researchers, "Experimental studies indicate that creative activities and their consequent positive effect on mood and morale can lead to an increased production of protective immune cells."[11] Many senior centers and community colleges offer low-cost cooking, art, or writing classes for older adults, where they can pursue their creativity in a supportive, low-risk setting.

One care manager tapped into her client's creativity to stimulate her intellectual QOL through the photographs the client had taken throughout her life:

> One client had been an accomplished photographer who took many pictures, but none were in photo albums. I arranged for a high school student to get credit in her class for community service by working with this client. The student visited twice weekly to talk about the photos and put them in albums where she could show the client the pictures. Some days, the client couldn't tell anything about a picture, but she always recognized the image and loved seeing the photo again. This activity also connected back to the client's career as a teacher and her love of working with students.
>
> —Martha J. Brown, MSW, LISW, RG,
> Geriatric Care Management, LLC

Travel to new or familiar places is another way for clients to stimulate past interests and improve their intellectual QOL.

> I had a client who was devastated when his wife died of Alzheimer's. He didn't want to leave the nursing home where the two of them had lived, and became completely passive, refusing to even get dressed without assistance. As he grew increasingly complacent at the nursing home and depression loomed, we suggested that maybe it would be fun for him to take a trip, as he had once been an avid traveler. He researched his options and chose New York City so he could take in a Broadway show and go to some great restaurants. Not long after, he decided to go to Las Vegas, where he saw "girlie shows" and Cirque du Soleil, stayed at the Bellagio, and ate wonderfully. These trips recharged his interest in life and he now uses a laptop computer, talks on his cell phone and reads voraciously, despite his low vision. He's very frail and uses a walker, but he's planning his next trip to Paris and taking French lessons to get ready. Despite his age and the loss of his dear companion, this

client is reinventing his life and in the process is stimulating his intellectual, emotional and spiritual quality of life.

> —Sally Gold, MSW,
> Geriatric Resource Services

Reminiscence and Storytelling

The role of storytelling and reminiscence is very important for older adults, and especially powerful for clients that are beginning to experience memory loss and dementia. There has been much documented success with writing programs for Alzheimer's patients, where the participants come together regularly to write down and share their life stories with one another. Alan Dienstag, who documented the group's work, notes, "The writing group gave memory back to its members. They transformed in the experience of writing from people who forget to people who remember."[12] Although the members of the group struggled to continue to write and read their stories as time progressed and their illnesses worsened, they still found dignity and solidarity in the process of sharing their lives with each other.

A similar program for more independent older adults, the Illuminated Life workshop is a comprehensive, structured life review program designed to help improve participants' psychological functioning.[13] Through the workshop, participants look retrospectively at their lives to consider creative postretirement roles and integrate the learning they have gathered throughout their lives. Created in 1987 by Dr. Abe Arkoff, the workshop has been presented at its home base, the University of Hawaii's Osher Lifelong Learning Institute, and in other venues, including retirement residences, senior centers, churches, Elderhostel, and several mainland sites. At each weekly session, the participants discuss a predetermined life question and work in small groups to share their answers. Research with older women completing the workshop in 2000 showed significant gain on a measure of psychological well-being in contrast to a control group that showed no change.[13]

Similarly, the Autobiographical Studies Program, at the University of California, Los Angeles, helps participants become aware of the lives they have lived and more confident and optimistic about facing the future.[13] By utilizing five different courses, including Guided Autobiography and Family History, the program equips participants to use the gift of long life in productive ways. According to the program's research, participants report feeling empowered in their self-knowledge and use their newly honed empathetic skills to forge new friendships and pursue new interests.[13]

Time Slips is a program being replicated around the country that encourages older adults with dementia to tap into creativity and share their stories.[13] Using hour-long, group storytelling sessions with up to a dozen people in the middle stages of dementia, care manager facilitators encourage creative responses that downplay the importance of memory. Using an image to prompt responses, a facilitator asks open-ended questions and weaves together all the answers, from the poetic to the nonsensical, into a story. The participants are encouraged to laugh, sing, and move as they tell their stories, which are often difficult to capture in words.

Even if a formal group is not available nearby, care managers can foster the act of reminiscences through writing prompts that begin with phrases such as, "I remember. . . ," "The house where I grew up . . . ," or "The last time I saw . . ." If the client is unable to write, the care manager can record his or her words in a special journal and can read these words back to the client periodically as a way of preserving these memories for him or her and honoring the life that the person has lived.[12]

One care manager utilized poetry to help her client connect with past memories:

One client had been an English and biology high school teacher, who wrote many poems. We copied them and put them in page protectors and in a three-ring notebook so visitors and staff at the care home could look at and read her the poems and on good days (she also has dementia), she can read the poems herself. She also illustrated them. Having someone read them and refer to them honors and validates this client, and gives her extra attention.

—Martha J. Brown, MSW, LISW, RG,
Geriatric Care Management, LLC

Another care manager worked with an art therapist and the client's caregivers to help the client develop a scrapbook of family memories:

For one client, who had a moderate degree of dementia, I worked with both an art therapist and the client's caregivers to create a family history scrapbook. The art therapist, who started the scrapbook project and met with the client once a week, also trained the caregivers so they could continue the process between visits. The client's aides were able to facilitate reminiscences while they worked with her on the scrapbook by learning about her family members and reading letters from different periods of her life. These activities had a calming effect for the client, and helped her connect to her family's rich history. Within six weeks after working on the scrapbook, the client had improved remarkably. She had amazing eye contact and had totally changed from agitated mumbling to having lucid moments with greater clarity of speech. She was also more connected to her past interests, more calm and could relate better to her care providers.

—Leonie Nowitz, MSW, BCD,
Center for Lifelong Growth

The scrapbook activity, where the caregivers pick some of the client's favorite photos and letters, is an excellent way to begin building an individualized therapeutic activity kit or "toolbox" to improve intellectual QOL for clients with dementia. This type of box (or basket, bin, etc.) contains activities that can be implemented by the GCM, caregivers, or family members to stimulate mental processing and ease the side effects of dementia for the client. Examples of items that might go in a therapeutic activity kit include letters in plastic coverings that can be read and reread regularly, music CDs, art supplies, postcards from places where the client has traveled, playing cards, balls or fabrics with different textures to help stimulate touch, and photos or other items that trigger pleasant memories and cognitive response.[14]

Of course, some clients may not resonate with or have the capacity to engage in activities related to past careers, reminiscences, or creativity. For these clients, who need some form of intellectual QOL activity, traditional "mind exercises," such as jigsaw, crossword, or other word puzzles or other activities, may work best. There may even be a level of comfort for clients in the repetition of mind activities and in working to meet new challenges in the exercises as they become familiar with the process.

Physical Quality of Life

As described earlier, there is a great deal of new research about the benefits of physical exercise for older adults, and about the different kinds of exercise that this age group can continue to practice. Common forms of exercise for older adults include walking, yoga, tai chi, gardening, and specially designed exercise classes that focus on cardiovascular, stretching, and/or weight training. Senior day care and senior centers are wonderful resources for exercise classes and activities for elders, as are local recreation centers, YMCAs, and community colleges.

Physical engagement is an area where care managers often encounter resistance from some clients. After all, by age 75, about one in three men and one in two women do not engage in

any physical activity,[15] so encouraging older adults to be physically active may require creativity and persistence from care managers and other care team members. One approach is to focus on a particular activity and how fun/interesting it may be rather than on the health or physical benefits of it. For example, if a client mentions that she used to love to dance with her husband, the care manager can probe about what kind of music they enjoyed while dancing. Then, on the next visit, the GCM can bring some samples of that music and encourage the client to get up and dance along. Once the client has connected back to her love of dancing with her husband, the care manager can then explore senior dance programs (e.g., at a local community center), where the client can get physical exercise while she has fun.

One care manager worked with a client's caregivers to use music and dance to encourage the client to walk to the bathroom, which she had been refusing to do:

> Since the client was a world traveler, we tried out a range of music. The aides started using jazz music to motivate her to get up and "dance" to the bathroom, which helped the client overcome her refusal to use the facilities.
>
> —Leonie Nowitz, MSW, BCD,
> Center for Lifelong Growth

Spiritual Quality of Life

When a care manager focuses on a client's spiritual QOL, he or she has an opportunity to explore what gives the client deeper meaning and purpose. For some people, "spirituality" may mean traditional religion, and, for these clients, care managers can help encourage contemplation about the role of religion and about the client's interest in rekindling or renewing an interest in religious faith. The care manager can also help tackle the logistics (e.g., transportation, wheelchair access), which may be preventing the client from participating in regular services, whether they are at a church, temple, mosque, or other house of worship.

For homebound clients, traveling to a religious service may seem overwhelming, but for those who still wish to connect with a larger spiritual community, the care manager may be able to connect to alternative ideas. Perhaps a minister or chaplain could visit the client in his or her home or care facility, or maybe there is a small chapel or scaled-down service available through a local assisted care facility designed for people of the same faith, such as a Jewish community center. Religious services that are broadcast via television or radio can also provide a way for clients with limited mobility to bond with rituals and prayers that carry significance and meaning.

One care manager worked for over a year to help her client reconnect with her faith community because, despite her advancing dementia, the manager knew how important this community was to her:

> One client was very involved in her church and had been part of a Sunday school group for more than 25 years. For a while, the Sunday school group used to visit her, but once her dementia progressed, the visits stopped. Knowing how important this connection was for my client, I provided information to the church about her dementia. Eventually, the group finally started visiting the client again, coming back for her birthday party. The client really responded and rose to the occasion. The visitors from the church enjoyed it too and saw that the residential care home was a welcoming place with really caring staff. Now, individual members of this group visit her regularly.
>
> —Martha J. Brown, MSW, LISW, RG,
> Geriatric Care Management, LLC

For some clients, the topic of faith may provoke some fear, especially for older adults who are unresolved about their feelings or memories of organized religion, and may be afraid of facing the end of life without clear beliefs about what will happen after death. If care managers encounter fear when discussing faith or spirituality with a client, it is important to not back away, but to let the client discuss and work through whatever feelings arise.

With other clients, for whom traditional religion does not have a lot of meaning, the care manager may need to use conversation and reminiscences to discover what activities, places, or people may provide each individual with a sense of deeper purpose.

One care manager in New Mexico found a way for one client to connect with the mountains, which had been a source of inspiration during his younger years:

> In our practice, we try to focus on what matters or mattered a lot in a person's life—especially for those clients with dementia. For example, we had a client who used to live in Alaska; he was a bush pilot and he loved the mountains. We arranged for a companion service with a wheelchair van to take him on drives twice a week where he could see the sky and the mountains. His dementia was advanced to the stage where he couldn't talk, but the staff said that after the drives, he was calm and content, and whenever the driver arrived, he would break out in a huge smile. By bringing this client close to the mountains, the sky, and to nature, we honored the elements that gave him meaning and improved his spiritual quality of life. While the landscape may not have been as dramatic as Alaska, it offered a hint of what this man knew and loved and lived all those years.
>
> —Martha J. Brown, MSW, LISW, RG,
> Geriatric Care Management, LLC

Another care manager used a "soft" approach to help a client reignite an interest in his religion and participate in meaningful rituals:

> I heard that my client had once been an Orthodox Jew, but was no longer practicing

his religion. When I went to visit him during Hanukah, the caregivers had put up Christmas decorations all around the living space, but I did notice a Menorah tucked away on a shelf. I visited him at the time of day when a candle is normally lit, brought down the Menorah, and offered to read the accompanying prayer. He said, "You know I am agnostic." When I was quiet in response, he continued, "I was an orthodox Jew at one time." After a brief conversation, he asked me to proceed with reading the prayer, and I could tell that he was definitely tuned in. At the Passover holiday, he insisted that the care providers light the Menorah each evening for eight nights. While this is not a traditional way of celebrating Passover, it was his way of acknowledging the passing of time and reaching out for a ritual that had previously been a source of meaning for him.

—Leonie Nowitz, MSW, BCD,
Center for Lifelong Growth

Rituals, Traditions, and Music

This example also illustrates the importance of ritual and traditions, which can promote spiritual QOL, either as part of or outside of religious practices. For the preceding client, just lighting the candles was enough to evoke a sense of calm and well-being, even though this ritual was not officially designated by the religious holiday he was recognizing. Similarly, setting the table a certain way, eating or preparing certain foods, or singing songs can help older adults to connect with rhythms and routines from their past lives that bring comfort and meaning. Sometimes a client will be able to request these kinds of rituals when asked, but other times the care manager and/or care providers will need to make suggestions or even initiate these rituals (for example, beginning to sing a Christmas carol or Hanukah song) before the client will be able or willing to participate.

For example, one care manager advocated tenaciously to ensure that her client, an elderly Japanese woman, could enact an important ritual by brewing green tea in her room each afternoon:

My client was yearning to brew and serve tea, which was important for her culture and also for her health. However, her assisted care facility told her she could not have a hotplate in her room for safety reasons. I negotiated with the care facility managers for months until they allowed her to have an electric teapot with a safety mechanism. My client was thrilled to once again participate in a daily ritual that had deep significance for her.

—Sally Gold, MSW,
Geriatric Resource Services

Other care managers have had great success with using food as a ritual that can be curative and restoring for clients by bringing pleasure and cultural connections:

We had a French client with whom we celebrated Bastille Day by making crepes and also arranged for the care provider to bring her to local French restaurants. Despite having lived in the U.S. for more than 50 years, she had a close connection to her native France. She often talked of moving home to France, so we facilitated her making a visit. A few months after returning home, she decided to move back to France, where she could share an assisted living apartment with a cousin. Similarly, we had a client who was born in Italy, but who had stopped going to the local park for bocce ball matches when he could no longer drive. We worked with the family to hire a care provider who could bring him back to the park, accompany him on long-forgotten Wednesday lunches at the Italian American club, and take him out for a cappuccino in the afternoons. These simple rituals seemed to mean the world to him, and resulted in marked improvement in his demeanor and helped mitigate the behavioral problems we were brought in to help address.

—Nina Pflumm Herndon, MA, CMC
Sage Eldercare Solutions

Another care manager found that music, particularly war songs, were helpful to her client in reducing the effects of his advancing dementia:

When I began music therapy sessions with Mr. Y at the local Veteran's Hospital, I was told that he could not communicate verbally and that he had a history of striking care providers. I quickly found that Mr. Y was able to sing old war songs clearly and that his agitation seemed to be immediately eradicated through the use of music and sound. I experimented with practicing scales, movement exercises, energy work, and acupressure, and engaging him in music therapy techniques. These approaches reduced his body twitches and improved his clarity of speech. The music also seemed to evoke something deeper in Mr. Y, as he would often close his eyes and cry when we would terminate a session. I trained his care providers in these techniques and they reported the same positive results.

—Tara Bradley, MA, MFTI,
Sage Eldercare Solutions

Improving a client's spiritual QOL takes creativity and perseverance, but can have tremendous impact on his or her physical and psychological well-being. To address spiritual QOL, the care manager must be open to helping the client explore whatever gives him or her meaning and must not be afraid to delve into the feelings that may arise from this exploration, both joyous and troubling. It is a highly individual, unique process, and one that has almost infinite permutations. As Victor Frankl wrote in his unforgettable book about surviving the concentration camps in Nazi Germany, "What matters, therefore, is not the meaning of life in general, but rather the specific meaning of a person's life at a given moment."[16]

B. Tap into Informal Networks: Caregivers' and Family Members' Information, Talent, and Willingness to Help

A client's caregiver (either at home or in a facility), neighbors, friends, volunteers, assisted living community staff, adult children, and grandchildren are all excellent resources for both understanding what the client needs in terms of holistic QOL as well as for implementation of ideas for addressing these needs.

Before beginning the process of assessing the client's holistic QOL, the care manager should meet with the caregiver(s) and family members to explain the assessment process and to clarify the goals of the process. The GCM can explain how the caregivers and family members will be part of the assessment, and how important their ideas will be when creating the plan for addressing the clients' needs and, later, implementing them. As mentioned earlier, both parties may have some conscious or unconscious preconceived ideas about what the client needs, wants, and is interested in, which may or may not be accurate, so it will be important to also utilize an assessment process to really get to know what makes the client "tick," beyond what others say or believe about him or her.

Once the assessment process is complete, the care manager can go over the results with caregivers and family members and start to gather their ideas about how to address some of the areas that the client needs the most, whether it is emotional, physical, or another aspect. Family members may have great ideas about activities that may evoke pastimes the client used to enjoy in his or her younger years, and caregivers will have experience about what kinds of activities tend to engage the client. It is paramount to engage the client's larger network (family, friends, neighbors, etc.) and care providers in implementing a holistic QOL plan because of budget limitations (it is not cost-effective to have the care manager carry out many of the interventions) and to ensure that the care providers are engaged in making an impact during all the hours that the client's specialists are not there.

One care manager, whose client had advanced dementia and was experiencing a great deal of agitation, worked closely with the client's aides to create activities that would improve her emotional, intellectual, and physical QOL:

> Through these conversations, the aides became incredibly interested in the client; they understood that they had an opportunity to develop their own special interactions and generated a range of ideas about things to do with her. One aide counted blackberries with her and they were able to reach number six (a big milestone). Because the client was once a school teacher, the aides also decided to take her to nearby parks, where she could watch the children play. By collaborating with the caregivers, I was able to help them learn how to use the client's environment as a tool for stimulation, and to develop ideas for outings and stimulating activities that meshed with her interests and past history.
>
> —Leonie Nowitz, MSW, BCD,
> Center for Lifelong Growth

C. Develop an Action Plan for Addressing Holistic Quality of Life

When putting together the actual plan for how to improve a client's holistic QOL, it can be helpful for care managers to keep in mind the 3 Rs:

- *Respectful:* It is essential to respect the client's comfort level with any given activity and to honor his or her desire to do it or not. It may take many attempts before a client will be willing to try something that he or she perceives as "risky" and it is only through gentle, respectful communication that the care manager will be successful in overcoming these feelings.
- *Realistic:* The domains of holistic QOL—emotional, intellectual, physical, spiritual—may touch on some very charged and difficult issues for clients. As a result, care managers can expect a fair amount of resistance when introducing activities related to QOL and may need to take baby steps to help clients get past their negative feelings in some of these areas.
- *Responsive:* Although care managers need to keep an eye on their goals in terms of holistic QOL, it's also important to be responsive to the client, and follow his or her lead when planning activities. It is an interactive process, and the care manager will have a better chance of success if she keeps an open mind, adjusting plans and ideas in tune with the client's needs and desires.

There is no one right way to create a good QOL plan, and each care manager may develop an approach that works best for her. However, there are a few elements that should be included in any QOL plan, including the following:

- Specific QOL area focus
- Evidence from the assessment that supports the need to address this area
- Feedback from family and caregivers about the client's needs and interests
- Activities to try, with a range from introductory to more advanced, along with space to record client response and potential next steps

Exhibit 19-4 provides a sample plan for addressing intellectual QOL.

Exhibit 19–4   A Sample Action Plan for Addressing Intellectual Quality of Life

---

Client Name: Mr. G

QOL Area to be Addressed: Intellectual

Evidence from Assessment:

- Family members said he used to paint when younger
- Paintings he did are around the apartment
- Caregiver said she suggested painting, but Mr. G said his hands shake too much
- Mr. G listed art and museums as two of his favorite things

Activities to Try	Response	Next Step
1. Bring in some "coffee table" art books for Mr. G to look at, note level of interest and which types of art seem to engage him		
2. Plan outing to art museum—choose type depending on response to different art books		
3. Bring materials for painting at home with GCM and caregiver		
4. Enroll client in senior art class at local recreation center		

■ STEP 4: EVALUATE AND REASSESS

Implementing a plan for improving a client's holistic QOL is an iterative process—the care manager will try an activity, gauge its success, try something else, and keep going until he or she sees positive change for the client. The goal is to be respectful, realistic, and responsive throughout the process and to continually adapt to the client's needs, reactions, and physical and cognitive condition.

After a care manager has been implementing the holistic QOL plan with a client for a reasonable amount of time—six weeks or so— it is time to reassess the plan and revise it depending on the outcomes through a care monitoring visit. Reassessing the plan involves talking with caregivers and family members to see what kinds of changes they have noticed and conducting an informal assessment with the client, which includes conversation and observation. During this process, the care manager is looking for signs that the client's QOL has improved in any/all of the areas targeted in the original plan, and if not, to rethink the activities and approach that has been used.

It's important to reconsider not only the "what" of the plan (i.e., which specific activities), but also the "how" (who has been working with the client on these activities? where?). Perhaps the reason a particular activity has not succeeded or the client experienced a negative reaction was because of how the activity was delivered. For example, if the client didn't want to work with the care manager on a reminiscence project, the care manager doesn't need to rule out this type of activity, but instead might see if it can be done with a caregiver who might have a closer relationship with the client, or with an art therapist who specializes in this type of work. Similarly, a client might resist going for a walk or engaging in other physical activity with his caregivers, but might be open to an outing with other older adults that is planned by a local senior center.

■ CONCLUSION

Addressing a client's holistic QOL is a process that does not have a specific end goal. There are almost endless ways that care managers can improve a client's emotional, intellectual, physical, and spiritual QOL and almost endless ways that clients may respond to these activities. For the care manager, the caregivers, and the client's family members, the process of considering these elements may itself provoke new understanding of the client and new respect for his or her unique and special gifts. As demonstrated in the examples throughout this chapter, holistic QOL activities can also be fun and can add a dimension of playfulness and joy to the work of geriatric care for all parties involved.

Most GCMs already have the skills they need to be successful in this area; it just takes willingness and a conviction to prioritize holistic quality of care concerns at the same level with more traditional care management objectives. Although it may require a shift in thinking for the care manager, family, and client to focus on holistic care, the benefits for clients are potentially enormous. Improving emotional, intellectual, physical, and/or spiritual QOL has been shown not only to improve a client's affect and attitude toward life, but also to literally improve physical health. To be successful in addressing holistic QOL, care managers need only draw on the attributes that probably brought them to the field of geriatric care in the first place: creativity, resourcefulness, and respect for the humanity of older adults.

Indeed, a focus on QOL can be a win for all parties involved: improved well-being for the older adult, measurable and positive impact from the care manager, and relief and support from the older adult's family members and caregivers. This focus is also life-affirming for clients, who still yearn to connect with their whole selves. As one 90-year-old woman said, "The invisible part of me is not old. In aging we gain as well as lose—our spiritual forces expand. A life of the heart and mind takes over as our physical force ebbs away."[17]

■ NOTES

1. Frytak J. Assessment of quality of life in older adults. In: Kane R, Kane R, eds. *Assessing Older Persons*. New York: Oxford University Press; 2000:200–237.

2. Centers for Disease Control and Prevention. Social support and health-related quality of life among older adults—Missouri, 2000. *MMWR*. May 6, 2005. Available at: http://www.cdc.gov/mmwr/preview/mmwrhtml/mm5417a4.htm. Accessed June 5, 2006.

3. Brickel CM, Brickel GK. A review of the roles of animals in psychotherapy and the elderly. *Int J Aging Hum Dev*. 1980;12:119–128.

4. National Institutes of Health. Use it or lose it? Senior Net; February 12, 2002. Press release. Available at: http://www.seniornet.org/php/default.php?PageID=6796. Accessed June 7, 2006.

5. Begley S. Dementia studies confuse causes with effects. *Wall Street Journal*. April 28, 2006.

6. News Bureau, University of Illinois, Urbana. Exercise adds years to life and improves quality, researchers say. November 19, 2005. Available at: http://www.news.uiuc.edu/NEWS/05/1110exercise.html. Accessed June 1, 2006.

7. Westcott WL. Strength training for older adults. Healthy Net; 1998. Available at: http://www.healthy.net/scr/Column.asp?id=228. Accessed June 13, 2006.

8. Bianchi EG. *Elder Wisdom: Crafting Your Own Elderhood*. New York: Crossroad; 1994.

9. Kane R. and Associates, 1999, from Frytak J. p. 214.

10. Baker S. Massage therapy for seniors provides a "loving touch." Copley News Service. *Jewish News Bulletin of Northern California*. January 25, 2002. Available at: http://www.jewishsf.com/content/2-0/module/displaystory/story_id/17615/edition_id/349/format/html/displaystory.html. Accessed June 29, 2006.

11. Cohen GD. *The Creative Age: Awakening Human Potential in the Second Half of Life*. New York: HarperCollins Publishers; 2001:61.

12. Dienstag A. Lessons from the Lifelines Writing Group for people in the early stages of Alzheimer's disease: forgetting that we don't remember. In: Ronch J, Goldfied J, eds. *Mental Wellness in Aging*. Towson, MD: Health Professions Press; 2003:350.

13. MetLife Foundation. MindAlert Awards 2004. Available at: http://www.asaging.org/awards/mindalert.cfmm. Accessed June 29, 2006.

14. Conedera F, Mitchell L. Therapeutic activity kits. Try This. 2004;1(4). Available at: http://www.hartfordign.org/publications/trythis/theraAct.pdf. Accessed October 3, 2006.

15. Department of Health and Human Services. *Physical Activity and Health: A Report of the Surgeon General*. Centers for Disease Control and Prevention; 1996. Available at: http://www.cdc.gov/aging/info.htm. Accessed June 15, 2006.

16. Frankl VE. *Man's Search for Meaning*. New York: Washington Square Press, Simon and Schuster; 1963:171.

17. University of Kentucky Cooperative Extension Service. Aging gracefully: quotes for aging wisely. Available at: http://www.ca.uky.edu/fcs/aging/pdf/Quotes_for_Aging_Wisely.pdf. Accessed October 3, 2006.

PART 4

Clinical Issues

Chapter 20

Dementia and the Older Adult: The Role of the Geriatric Care Manager

Peter S. Belson

■ INTRODUCTION

For the geriatric care manager (GCM), dementia and the attendant physical, social, and familial issues are at the core of most of the work with the elderly and their families. As the number of GCMs in the United States has grown throughout the last two decades, geriatric care management has begun to be taught as a specific body of knowledge and practice in a number of schools and programs. New practitioners still bring with them, however, the skill set and knowledge base of their primary discipline. Whether the primary discipline is nursing, social work, psychology, occupational therapy, counseling, law, or medicine, the presence of a core body of knowledge provides the GCM with a base to build on and integrate new information, theory, and technique. GCMs from all disciplines need a thorough understanding of the effects, symptoms, and types of dementia they will encounter in practice. Additionally, they need guidelines for assessment, diagnosis, and strategies for conveying complex information to families. This chapter provides an overview of the definition and diagnosis of dementia and discusses, from case information, the GCM role in dementia care and work with other professionals.

The statistics on dementia, and Alzheimer's disease (AD) in particular, are well known to the GCM. By age 65, 1% to 2% of the population has dementia; 50% to 60% of people in their 90s will suffer from dementia, most of which will be AD.[1] There are more than 70 identified causes of dementia, with AD being the largest cause (50–60%).[1]

According to the 2005 fact sheet from the Alzheimer's Association:

- 1 in 10 Americans said that they had a family member with AD, and 1 in 3 knew someone with the disease.
- From the time of diagnosis, people with AD survive about half as long as those of similar age without dementia.
- National direct and indirect annual costs of caring for individuals with AD are at least $100 billion.
- More than 7 out of 10 people with AD live at home, where family and friends provide almost 75% of their care.
- Half of all nursing home residents have AD or a related disorder.[2]

Currently, an estimated 4.5 million Americans have AD. The number of Americans with AD has more than doubled since 1980, and those numbers will continue to grow—by 2050, the number of individuals with AD could range from 11.3 million to 16 million.[3] Although some of the relative increase can be ascribed to improved diagnostic capability, an additional factor is the increase in lifespan of the U.S. population. As the population has aged, people are living long enough to develop dementias.

GCMs operate both from within families, exercising and supporting executive decision making, and from without, providing expertise and counsel to the variety of stakeholders in an elder's life and community. During the course of the preparation of this edition of this book, the chapter author was involved in the assessment and eventual placement of a parent in an assisted living memory disorder unit. The experience has contributed to a revised understanding of the pressures on the family, who must hear and integrate information about dementia, as well as the experience of the affected elder.

■ DEFINING DEMENTIA: WHAT IS DEMENTIA?

One of the gravest roles of the GCM is that of educator to the family in the arena of explaining the diagnosis of dementia, differential diagnosis, test findings, and logistical and placement issues. The GCM is often the first professional to begin to interpret the family observations of memory loss and other findings and begin to move the family toward further assessment.

Most elderly people experience some degree of age-related memory loss. For those elderly, their cognitive performance is essentially unchanged, but they may require some prompting or additional time to complete tasks. Those with age-related memory loss continue to be able to learn new information and recall that which has been learned previously, albeit with some prompting or assistance. Elders who experience age-related memory loss are often more aware of, and embarrassed about, it than their families are.

One woman with the disease once offered to attend a GCM conference wearing a signboard that read "specimen." Despite her acute awareness of age-related memory loss, the elderly person has been able to learn to use complicated computer applications, keep up with her friends (and all of their ailments) via e-mail, manage a considerable financial picture, and travel extensively. Most of those with age-related memory loss show little effect on their daily functioning.

In contrast, dementia is characterized by significantly impaired functioning with progressive cognitive decline in a broader range of areas. The International Statistical Classification of Diseases and Related Health Problems (ICD–10) lists dementia under organic disorders classified into 9 categories with 40 subcategories ranging from multi-infarct dementia to the more rare Creutzfeldt-Jakob disease (CJD).[4] The fourth edition of the *Diagnostic and Statistical Manual of Mental Disorders (DSM–IV)* divides dementia into 12 categories.[5] Both the ICD–10 and *DSM–IV* classifications agree that the progressive decline is categorized into mild, moderate, and severe levels of dementia, although the rate of decline varies significantly from person to person, and progression frequently takes place within a 10-year span.[6]

Of critical importance to the GCM is consideration and evaluation of the role that depression plays in dementia. In mild and moderate phases of dementia, it is estimated that up to 40% of elders experience vegetative signs of depression, including sleep and appetite disturbance, reduced attention and concentration, decreased interest in self-care and activities, decreased energy, decreased production of language, and sometimes confusion.[7] Differential diagnosis becomes vitally important because depression can both exacerbate existing dementia symptoms, leading to a diagnosis of more advanced dementia, and can also suggest dementia where symptoms do not yet exist, as in "pseudo-dementia."

An additional issue in differential diagnosis is the issue of weight loss. Many people who become demented lose significant amounts of weight prior to the appearance of other signs and symptoms of dementia. Because depression often manifests with appetite disturbance, the GCM is left to discern whether the weight loss is from depression, deficits in planning and organization resulting in fewer and less substantial meals, suppression of appetite, or changes in metabolic rate related to changes in the brain.

■ TYPES OF DEMENTIA

As noted earlier, there are close to 70 identified causes of dementia. The ICD-10 lists dementia under organic disorders classified into 9 categories with 40 subcategories, ranging from multi-infarct dementia to the more rare CJD.[4] *DSM–IV* divides dementia into 12 categories.[5] Both the ICD-10 and DSM-IV classifications agree in tracking the diagnostic progression through mild, moderate, and severe stages.[4]

Degenerative and vascular dementias account for nearly 80% of all dementing illness. Other smaller cohorts include frontotemporal dementias (FTDs), dementias with parkinsonism, either primary or secondary, and other sources including tertiary syphilis, Huntington's chorea, acquired immune deficiency syndrome (AIDS)-related dementia, Fragile X linked dementia, and CJD and the new "mad cow" variant. Figure 20-1 illustrates the relative percentages and categories of dementia.

Degenerative Dementias

Alzheimer's Disease

AD is the most common degenerative dementia, accounting for up to 60% of all dementia diagnoses.[8] Increasing numbers of plaques and tangles, composed of nerve components, surround amyloid and tau proteins and eventually interfere with neurotransmission. Most people have some degree of plaques and tangles in their brain as they age, but those with AD have excessive numbers. Recent research suggests that the degree of dementia is highly correlated with tangles as opposed to plaques.

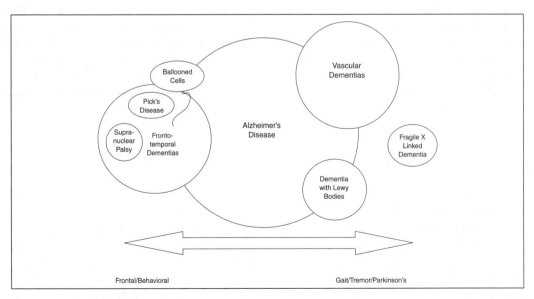

Figure 20–1   Venn Diagram

The classic picture of AD is one of insidious progression, characterized by increasing lack of orientation, significant short-term memory impairment, disturbance in attention and concentration, disturbance in expressive and receptive language, and profound mental status changes centered around the erosion of personality, increased paranoia, and disintegration of social skills.

Dementia with Lewy Bodies/ Parkinson's Disease

Named after Frederich Lewy, the physician who first described them in 1913, Lewy bodies are abnormal developments of the protein alpha -synuclein inside certain cells of the brain.[9] Lewy bodies have a strong relationship with Parkinson's disease, and frequently diagnosis is made of dementia with Lewy bodies with parkinsonism. In dementia with Lewy bodies, Lewy bodies occur in the cerebral cortex and other areas of the brain. In Parkinson's disease, Lewy bodies occur in selected subcortical structures, most notably the substantia nigra. Dementia with Lewy bodies, Parkinson's disease, and AD overlap considerably. For example, patients who have Parkinson's disease may develop dementia with Lewy bodies; patients who have AD may have a modest number of Lewy bodies, and patients who have dementia with Lewy bodies may have plaques and tangles.

Initial cognitive deterioration resembles that of other dementias. Patients may have well-defined visual hallucinations (often threatening), fluctuations in cognitive function, and mild parkinsonism. Periods of being alert, coherent, and oriented may alternate with periods of being confused and unresponsive to questions, usually over a period of days to weeks, but sometimes during the same interview. Paranoia and falls are common. Delusions occur in 50% to 65% of patients and are often complex and bizarre, compared with the simple persecutory ideation common in AD.

Dementia with Lewy bodies also causes daytime drowsiness and sleeping (often for more than 2 hours before 7 PM); patients tend to stare into space for long periods. Cognitive impairment affects visuospatial and visuoconstructional function more than it affects memory. These features also may help distinguish this dementia from AD.[10] An extreme sensitivity to antipsychotic drugs offers an additional opportunity for differentially diagnose dementia with Lewy bodies from AD.

Memory is impaired, but impairment appears to result more from deficits in alertness and attention than from deficits in memory acquisition. Patients who have dementia with Lewy bodies or who have Parkinson's disease may act out dreams.

Frontotemporal Dementias /Pick's Disease

FTD describes a clinical syndrome associated with shrinking of the frontal and temporal anterior lobes of the brain.[11] Clinically, it often presents with changes in personality, restlessness, disinhibition, and impulsiveness, and the clinical features can be complicated by neurological signs, such as motor neuron signs, parkinsonism, and gait disturbances. As it is defined today, the symptoms of FTD fall into two clinical patterns that involve either (1) changes in behavior—fixated primarily in the frontal lobe, or (2) problems with language—fixated primarily in the temporal lobe. The first type features behavior that can be either impulsive (disinhibited) or bored and listless (apathetic) and includes inappropriate social behavior; lack of social tact; lack of empathy; distractability; loss of insight into the behaviors of oneself and others; an increased interest in sex; changes in food preferences; agitation or, conversely, blunted emotions; neglect of personal hygiene; repetitive or compulsive behavior; and decreased energy and motivation.[12] The second type primarily features symptoms of language disturbance, including difficulty making or understanding speech, often in conjunction with the behavioral type's symptoms. Spatial skills and memory remain intact. There is a strong genetic component to the disease; FTD often runs in families.

Fragile X Linked Dementia

Fragile X is caused by expansion of the *FMR1* gene, located on the X chromosome. It was discovered in 1991 that expansion of the allele for the *FMR1* gene beyond 200 units leads to the mental retardation and characteristic physical features of Fragile X syndrome, which affects young boys. Hagerman et al. reported in 2001 that a small group of men, all of whom were grandfathers of one or more boys with Fragile X syndrome, had shown evidence of progressive intention tremor, ataxia, and dementia.[13] Within this group, dementia was seen to develop some years after the detection of the movement disorder. Further research is ongoing with implications for other genetically linked dementias, including "early Alzheimer's."

Vascular Dementias

Approximately 10% to 15% of dementia cases in the elderly are caused by vascular disease, with another 10% or more caused by the combined effects of vascular and degenerative disease, that is, mixed dementia. Ott and Grace[14] have developed a listing of vascular disease that is associated with dementia, as shown in Exhibit 20-1. Although the GCM may encounter some of the more rare forms of vascular dementia, this chapter focuses on the two most commonly identified forms.

Multi-Infarct Dementia

The risk of developing dementia increases after stroke. However, not all stroke victims become demented. Cummings estimates that 25% to 50% of stroke patients eventually develop vascular dementia.[15]

Following a stroke, patients often suffer acute, multiple cognitive and functional

Exhibit 20-1   Vascular Diseases Associated with Dementia

Thromboembolic dementia: cardiac and vascular sources
    Multi-infarct state
    Single "strategic" infarcts

Dementia associated with primary cerebrovascular disease
    Atherosclerosis
    Lipohyalinosis of small vessels
        Lacunar dementia
        Binswanger's disease
    Cerebral amyloid angiopathy
    Granular cortical atrophy
    Other arteriopathies, including inflammatory

Radiation-induced injury

Hypoxic-ischemic encephalopathy

Hyperviscosity syndromes
    Myeloproliferative disorders
    Proteins, such as IgM
    Lipoproteins

Hypercoagulable states
    Malignancy
    Deficiency states, such as protein S, C, antithrombin III
    Lupus anticoagulant

Intracranial hemorrhage
    Chronic subdural hematoma
    Hemorrhagic infarcts
    Intracerebral hematomas
    Amyloid angiopathy with multiple lobar hemorrhages

Hereditary diseases
    Amyloid associated vasculopathy
    CADASIL

Mixed type dementia
    Alzheimer's disease plus discrete infarctions
    Alzheimer's disease with central white matter involvement

impairments. These impairments result from the effect of hemorrhagic events that damage specific cortical and/or subcortical regions.

As part of the natural history of stroke, patients usually steadily and spontaneously recover physical and cognitive function until reaching a plateau 3 to 6 months post stroke. This course of acute cognitive and functional decline followed by partial or complete recovery does not necessarily constitute a dementia because there is not a continuing, progressive decline of cognitive and functional status. In contrast to this typical course, some stroke victims show progressive cognitive and functional deterioration over time. A single massive stroke may result in dementia, but the clinical course is not progressive.

Unlike AD, short-term memory is sometimes relatively preserved. Neurological deficits are often present that may be apparently unrelated to the short-term stroke-related deficit. Weakness or neglect in an extremity and visual neglect or disturbance that is otherwise unexplained are common. Patients with vascular dementia tend to be more aware of their deficits than are patients with AD, and consequently the prevalence of depression may be higher.

Cerebral Amyloid Angiopathy

Cerebral amyloid angiopathy is one of the primary features of AD when there is a vascular component.[16] It is often a precursor to the development of AD. As discussed earlier, one of the cellular components of AD is the presence of plaques containing the amyloid protein surrounded by neural elements. The presence of the amyloid protein in the capillaries or microvasculature causes small punctures or tears that cause small hemorrhages or microbleeds. The repeated assault on the microvasculature eventually leads to a larger hemorrhage or stroke, often in the cortex or subcortex.

Clinical features of cerebral amyloid angiopathy show elements of degenerative dementias in the early stages until AD symptoms become pronounced. The presence of vascular dementia

symptoms may become apparent following larger hemorrhagic episodes.

Other Etiologies

On an occasional basis, GCMs see elders with dementias from sources other than those discussed earlier. A brief discussion of some of the less frequently seen etiologies follows.

Neoplastic Dementias

Cancer can be causative of dementia both as a primary cause, as in cancers of the brain, as well as secondary, when there is involvement in the liver.

AIDS-Related Dementia

The human immunodeficiency virus, which causes AIDS, attacks the brain cells and creates enlargement, producing dementia. AIDS secondarily contributes to dementia because of the lowered immune threshold, thereby exposing the patient to infection.

MS and Other Sclerotic Diseases

As in Parkinson's disease, sclerotic diseases such as multiple sclerosis (MS), amyotrophic lateral sclerosis, Huntington's chorea, and myasthenia gravis eventually produce dementia symptoms.

Poisoning

The GCM should be alert in taking a thorough work and social history. Lifetime exposure to organophosphates in the form of fertilizers and weed and pest controls in a farmer or industrial worker should suggest a laboratory battery. Those in occupations such as mining, jewelry manufacture, storage battery manufacture, electronics manufacture with long-term exposures to heavy metals such as lead, cadmium, mercury, and antimony are at risk for dementia for dementia.

Long-term exposure to radiological sources in employment such as health care, mining, waste management, and manufacturing also represents a risk for dementia.

Traumatic Brain Injury

Traumatic brain injury is not limited to catastrophic events involving workplace injury or motor vehicle accidents. In taking the patient's history, the GCM needs to be aware of events that could possibly represent traumatic brain injury caused by surgery, repeated falls, or episodes of loss of consciousness as a result of violence. A classic form of dementia caused by this type of noncatastrophic brain injury is pugilist's Parkinson's. The great boxer Muhammad Ali shows evidence of this form of dementia clearly caused by repeated blows to the head without one identifiable catastrophic event.

Normal Pressure Hydrocephalus

Senior GCMs have reported increased referrals for elders with normal pressure hydrocephalus,[17] an abnormal increase of cerebrospinal fluid in the brain's ventricles, or cavities.[18] If the normal flow of cerebrospinal fluid throughout the brain and spinal cord is blocked in some way, it causes the ventricles to enlarge, putting pressure on the brain. Possible sources are hemorrhage, head trauma, infection, tumor, or complications of surgery. Surgical correction with an implanted ventricular shunt can show positive effects in reducing the gait difficulties, tremor, and dementia associated with this disorder.

Substance Abuse and Alcohol

Although brain trauma induced by use of stimulants resulting in hypoxia or stroke should properly be categorized in vascular dementias, long-term use of recreational drugs can produce symptoms that dramatically resemble dementia.

Long-term excessive use of alcohol as the result of alcoholism can produce alcoholic dementia or Korsakoff's dementia.

■ OBSERVABLE EFFECTS OF DEMENTIA

The effects of progressive dementia change throughout the course of disease. The GCM is frequently in the position of both interpreting observed effects in the elder for the family as well as conducting more formalized assessments (discussed in more detail later).

Cognition Effects

Orientation

Elders with mild dementia may experience loss of orientation. Initially, there may be some loss of orientation to date and time, and following that, to surroundings. When visiting a friend's home or the home of a grandchild, the elder may become disoriented in the infrequently visited location while remaining able to be oriented to place in his or her own home, local market, and familiar surroundings.

With the progression to moderate dementia, elders may lose orientation to familiar surroundings and have difficulty orienting to persons. They may mistake people for others, and behavioral problems may ensue as a result of this mistaken identity. A patient with moderate dementia recently visited the hospital where she has been treated all of her adult life and was asked by a nurse to identify where she was. She responded by stating that she was "at a place, a nice place, the food's not bad, but it's not home." When pressed further to see whether she understood that she was in a hospital, she was surprised and frightened to discover that she was in the hospital.

In severe dementia, there is a lack of orientation in all spheres.

Higher-Order Cognition

Although the degree to which higher-order cognition is affected varies significantly between FTDs and vascular dementias, there is clear degradation of cognitive functioning in all dementias.

In mild dementia, initial word-finding difficulty may progress to aphasia, either expressive aphasia or receptive aphasia or both in the latter stages of moderate and severe dementia. The patient referred to previously, complaining that she was being deprived of access to a telephone in the memory disorder unit where she resides, stated, "There isn't one of those things that go next to the bed." Some vascular dementias result in acalculia, the inability to manipulate and use numbers. When presented with a restaurant bill, a woman with mild dementia asked her dining companion to take care of the bill, handing over three $100 bills while being unaware of their value or the cost of the meal, which was less than $30.

The impaired ability to identify objects despite being able to handle them appropriately from a sensory perspective (agnosia) becomes more pronounced during the course of dementia. A patient was observed attempting to unlock a door to her home with a pair of glasses.

Coupled with agnosia, apraxia, the impairment in the ability to perform previously learned motor activities, can have profound impact on a demented person's inability to perform activities of daily living and instrumental activities of daily living. Additionally, impairment in the ability to plan, organize, sequence, and execute—the so-called executive functions—affect the elder's safety and independence in both mild and moderate stages. As briefly mentioned earlier, weight loss is a marker, often appearing before other frank symptoms are visible. With the appearance of agnosia and apraxia, and the degradation of executive functioning, it is easy to imagine an elder with mild to moderate dementia having difficulty working in the kitchen. Opening a can of tuna fish or cat food, making coffee, operating a microwave or toaster oven, or taking food out of the freezer to defrost prior to heating or attempting to eat it can be increasingly out of reach as the dementia progresses, leading to weight loss.

In the latter stages of moderate dementia, the inability to sequence tasks can have disastrous consequences. A patient known to the author was lighting a match in the bathroom in a deeply ingrained (and therefore somewhat resistant to the inroads of apraxia) ritual. He accidentally dropped a lit match into his underwear around his ankles, and was unable to sequence and organize to either pick up the match or, failing that, take one step into the shower in front of him and turn it on, thereby putting out the fire. He died some time later of complications of third-degree burns.

Spatial and Kinesthetic Orientation

As patients progress, there is increased risk of falls as a result of confusion over the elder's body in space. As the surroundings become more unfamiliar, scanning of the environment becomes more frequent, leading to agitation and anxiety. This, in turn, heightens confusion and disorientation, which makes the elder more prone to falls.

In latter stages, this spatial confusion coupled with the impact on neurotransmission, which can affect voluntary musculature, can reduce the elder's ability to walk and eventually to move.

One of the diagnostic signs for dementia with Lewy bodies is frequent falls.

Attention and Concentration

It almost goes without saying that attention and concentration are impaired in dementias. An important distinction for the GCM to discriminate between are short-term memory deficits and attention and concentration. Although attention and concentration and short-term memory are inextricably linked, there are also other contributing factors affecting attention and concentration. Anxiety over self-perceived decline in cognition and depression, as mentioned earlier, can contribute significantly to impairments in attention and concentration, possibly suggesting more impairment in short-term memory than actually exists. Impairments in sequencing, referred to previously, also can affect performance on assessments of concentration and attention.

In latter stages, attention and concentration are significantly affected. Hospitalized patients with moderate dementia may be unable to retain the concept of having a Foley catheter in place and will constantly cry out that they need to urinate, even though they may have been told a moment ago that they have a catheter in place.

Recall, Fund of Knowledge, and Cognitive Reserve

Longer-term memory or recall can have peculiar manifestation in dementia. In mild dementia, recall can offer the elder an opportunity to form connections to others by discussing common or shared events. A patient who had been a pediatrician to the interviewer remarked that he had enjoyed the opportunity to treat her and now "the shoe is on the other foot." The patient was able to access general records of events and link them to his current fund of knowledge.

This patient also points to important issues in overall assessment and planning. The "cognitive reserve" available to a former physician who was a professor of medicine and had an active practice and teaching appointment until the development of AD affords this patient a larger vocabulary, experience with language, and adaptability not available to a less educated person. The issue of cognitive reserve becomes important in using mental status assessment tools, creating care plans, and engaging the client in the plan.

Recent research suggests that those patients with higher cognitive reserve are more likely to experience concomitant depressive symptoms, possibly caused by being placed in situations where more complex cog-

nitive tasks are required or where a higher degree of self-awareness is present.[7]

As the dementia progresses, frequently there is an interaction between the availability of recalled events and a developing psychosis in terms of orientation to current reality, and the elder can appear "stuck" in a prior experience or context.

A patient, prior to her placement in a memory disorder unit, would call her son frequently to announce that she had "just heard that your father died. Why hasn't anyone told me before this? Did you know about it?" The patient was present when her husband died some six months before.

Mental Status Effects

A patient appeared to be reliving the anguish of the discovery of her now many-years-dead husband's affair. She was convinced that her daughter was "the other woman" and refused to see her. Oddly enough, the GCM was aware of two important facts. The husband had indeed had a long-standing affair that was known by both now-adult children. The daughter does look strikingly like both the "other woman" *and* her mother.

Hallucinations

In the patient mentioned just previously, was she experiencing an hallucination, perceiving her daughter with the face of the hated "other woman," or was she merely "tangled" up in the earlier context? For the GCM, clinical experience can be invaluable in discerning the context in which the elder's perceptions take place. In advancing dementia, psychotic symptoms, including hallucinations and delusions, occur in approximately 25% of patients.[1] Sometimes, what appear to be reported hallucinations are the elders' inability to recognize their own face in the mirror, producing panic and a report that "there is someone else in the house." The presence of hallucinations can also serve the GCM as additional diagnostic information. For example, a report of definitive visual hallucinations embodying bizarre features with only mildly reduced attention and concentration might suggest Lewy body dementia as opposed to AD.

Delusions

Delusions are common in advancing dementia. Ironically, in the context of the patient discussed earlier, a common delusion is that one's spouse is or has been unfaithful. Other common delusions are that people are stealing from them. This delusion can be linked to the cognitive difficulties discussed previously such as acalculia and executive processing. Losing track of objects, not recognizing those objects as one's own, and being unable to understand the denominations of money can contribute to delusional thinking about theft. In contrast to the relatively simple delusions seen in AD, delusions in Lewy body dementia are complex and often bizarre, offering additional clues to a differential diagnosis.

Agitation and Behavioral Manifestations

Some frontotemporal dementias are well known for disinhibition and hypersexuality. Other behavioral effects can include agitation and assaultiveness in certain contexts. Patients can be easily frustrated looking for "safe" places from recall that may not or no longer exist. After being picked up by the police and brought to the emergency room in a confused and panicked state, a patient reported to a GCM that he had been trying to get to his date at the Norumbega Ballroom, a once well-known dance hall that had burned down more than seven decades ago. Another patient, nearly 90 years old and busily spitting, swearing, and assaulting the police when brought to the emergency room was apparently reliving his experience of being picked up by the Gestapo in Germany during the Holocaust. He was so vehement in his rage that the police reported that they had rarely encountered someone so dangerous. When it was pointed out to the police that the patient was almost 90 years old,

the senior officer of the group noted that "hell, somewhere in there is a very dangerous 20-year-old, that's who we're afraid of."

Mood and Affect

Affect is often labile in the mild forms of dementia. In latter stages, apathy can set in with rapid progression to flat affect and social withdrawal. Some FTDs appear to have a "manic" tone to the affect picture.

Depression and Suicidality

A patient reports that she is "happy" to have been recently diagnosed with bladder cancer. The GCM wonders whether she has a complicated expressive language disorder related to her prior diagnosis of vascular dementia. "No," she clarifies under further questioning, "I know I can't think clearly anymore, I can't take care of [her husband, who is moderately demented]. I can't cook. I can't enjoy the soaps. So, yeah, I'm happy that I'm going to die. It's a load off."

Many of the current elderly generation have grown up with a strong spiritual, cultural, and religious imperative against suicide. Many members of this cohort do not have the experience of being sufficiently aware of their internal lives to acknowledge that what they feel is depression or suicidal ideation. It is the work of the GCM to discern the nature of the depressive thinking and possible suicidal ideation and to place it in context with an understanding of the elder's spiritual, cultural, and emotional life.

Physical Effects

Tremor and Gait

Recently it has been reported that late-onset tremor, gait unsteadiness, and dementia can be associated with brain atrophy in males of normal intelligence and the premutation carrier state of the Fragile X syndrome.[19]

Parkinson's dementia and Lewy body disease with Parkinson's are among the dementias that evidence difficulties with walking and in the upper extremities.

Seizures

The incidence of seizures, both focal and tonic-clonic, appears to increase as dementia symptoms progress.

Swallowing

In severe dementia, along with general physical deterioration, there is often decline in the ability to swallow. This can cause aspiration of food and liquids, leading to pneumonia.

■ ASSESSMENT OF DEMENTIA

The GCM can and will play a large role clarifying a diagnosis and interpreting that diagnosis for the family. A degree of familiarity with diagnostic criteria, routine and specialized examinations, and assessment tools contributes to the skill set of the GCM.

Laboratory and Diagnostic Tests

Although there are no current laboratory tests specific to the diagnosis of AD, a thorough laboratory workup can assist in determining whether other dementias can be ruled in or out. A blood-chemistry panel, complete blood count, tests of thyroid function, measurement of vitamin B_{12} levels, and screening for inflammatory and infectious disease are recommended. Computed tomography or magnetic resonance imaging (MRI) of the brain can rule out structural lesions indicative of vascular dementia, neoplastic disease (cancer), and other acute brain abnormalities. If indicated, lumbar puncture to rule out central nervous system infection or heavy metal screening may be performed. The blood tests and neuroimaging studies listed in Table 20-1 are important in the differential diagnosis to rule out metabolic and structural causes.

Assessment for Dementia

GCMs need to be able to offer clear and understandable information to the families they work with. If at all possible, the expectation is to have the elder receive a thorough medical evaluation, including the diagnostic tests referred to earlier. Objective data are then collected through direct observation and utilization of functional assessment instruments. Direct observation of the client experiencing dementia is important because the elder with suspected dementia will not, by definition, be able to accurately assess his or her own status. Families as well, even those with nurses, physicians, or GCMs, will have

---

Table 20-1   Dementia Workup

Test	Rationale
Urinalysis	Rule out kidney dysfunction, toxic encephalopathy
CBC, sedimentation rate, electrolytes	Rule out anemia, electrolyte imbalance
Blood Urea Nitrogen (BUN)/ creatinine, liver function tests	Rule out liver dysfunction
Thyroid function	Rule out thyroid dysfunction
Serum B_{12}	Rule out vitamin deficiency
Syphilis serology	Rule out syphilis
HIV test	Rule out AIDS dementia
Neuroimaging studies: CT or MRI	Rule out tumor, subdural hematomas, abscess, stroke, or hydrocephalus

Source: Adapted with permission from J. Corey-Bloom et al., Diagnosis and Evaluation of Dementia, *Neurology*, Vol. 45, pp. 211–218, © 1995, Lippincott, Williams & Wilkins.

difficulty accurately interpreting data about their family members.

Assessment Instruments

Standardized assessment instruments that have been rigorously evaluated for consistency and accuracy are critical tools for the GCM. They provide additional objective information in the overall assessment process that ultimately will lead to a diagnosis and development of a care plan. Appendix 20-A evaluates some of the more commonly used functional assessment instruments and their usefulness when assessing dementia. Familiarity with the strengths and weaknesses of the various assessment instruments will help the GCM select the most appropriate instruments for the individual client.

Assessment of Mental Status

As discussed earlier, dementia has observable effects on orientation, language, cognition, higher-order functioning, mental status, and spatial and kinesthetic capabilities. Two well-known and respected instruments, the Mini-Mental State Examination[20] (MMSE; Exhibit 20-2) and the Short Portable Mental Status Questionnaire[21] (SPMSQ; Exhibit 20-3) both assess orientation, attention and concentration, recall, and language. The limitation of the SPMSQ is that it is entirely language-based in comparison to the MMSE, which includes items on registration and tests both expressive and receptive language. The MMSE also tests comprehension, sequencing, and visuospatial abilities. Scoring and diagnostic criteria are available on the SPMSQ instrument itself. The MMSE administration and scoring, as originally delineated by Folstein and elaborated upon by Knutson and Gross, is described as follows.[22]

> *Orientation (10 items):* Orientation is assessed on the MMSE by asking the client questions about time (year, season, month, day of the month, and day of the

week) and place (if the client's residence: state, county, town, home address, room; if a hospital: building, floor of the building, part of the city, city, state). The season should be correct within a day either way of the season change. One point is given for each correct response.

> *Registration (3 items):* Registration is measured on the MMSE by asking the client to name three unrelated objects. The first attempt to say the three words is used in scoring. One point is given for each object. After completing the task, the client is asked to remember the objects and repeat them 5 minutes later.

> *Attention and Calculation (5 items):* Attention refers to the ability to focus and concentrate on a particular task and is measured by asking the client to say digits or letters forward and backward, with backward repetition providing greater information about attention. Attention is assessed on the MMSE by asking the client to perform the Serial 7s, a test that also measures calculation ability. The GCM says, "I'd like you to count backward from 100 by 7. What is 100 take away 7?" The GCM does not give further reminders once the client has started. Then the GCM has the client spell *world* forward and then backward. For the latter count, the score is the number of letters that are in the correct order (DLOW = 4, DLDRW = 3, DLOLD = 2). The GCM uses the higher of the two scores (either the Serial 7s or the *world* backward score).

> *Recall (3 items):* Recall is often impaired in dementia, and impaired recall is the most noticeable symptom in AD. Memory is measured on the MMSE by asking the client to repeat the three objects that were said 5 minutes earlier during the Registration section of the test. The score is the number spontaneously recalled without a cue. One point is given for each correct answer.

Exhibit 20-2   Mini-Mental State Examination

Maximum Score	Score	
		ORIENTATION
5	( )	What is the (year) (season) (date) (day) (month)?
5	( )	Where are we: (state) (county) (town) (hospital) (floor)?
		REGISTRATION
3	( )	Name 3 objects: 1 second to say each. Then ask the patient all 3 after you have said them. Give 1 point for each correct answer. Then repeat them until he learns all 3. Count trials and record. Trials _____
		ATTENTION AND CALCULATION
5	( )	Serial 7s. 1 point for each correct answer. Stop after 5 answers. Alternatively, spell *world* backward.
		RECALL
3	( )	Ask for the 3 objects repeated above. Give 1 point for each correct answer.
		LANGUAGE
9	( )	Name a pencil, and watch (2 points)
		Repeat the following "No ifs, ands, or buts." (1 point)
		Follow a 3-stage command:
		"Take a paper in your right hand, fold it in half, and put it on the floor" (3 points)
		Read and obey the following:
		CLOSE YOUR EYES (1 point)
		Write a sentence (1 point)
		Copy design (1 point)

Total score _____

ASSESS level of consciousness along a continuum _____

Alert   Drowsy   Stupor   Coma

Language (9 items): The Language section covers key functions and includes assessing aphasia (difficulty expressing or comprehending language) and apraxia (difficulties where the client with intact motor and sensory pathways forgets motor skills [e.g., how to walk]). Language is measured on the MMSE by naming everyday objects, repeating, understanding a three-stage command, reading, writing, and copying. Naming is measured by holding up a watch and pencil one at a time and asking the client to name the objects. One point is given for each correct name. Repetition is measured by asking the client to repeat "No ifs, ands, or buts." One point is given for the completed repetition. The three-stage command is measured by asking the client to take the paper in

Exhibit 20–3   The Short Portable Mental Status Questionnaire

Scoring: Count the number of correct and incorrect responses

Question	Correct Responses	Incorrect Responses
1. What are the date, month, and year?	_____	_____
2. What is the day of the week?	_____	_____
3. What is the name of this place?	_____	_____
4. What is your phone number?	_____	_____
5. How old are you?	_____	_____
6. When were you born?	_____	_____
7. Who is the current president?	_____	_____
8. Who was the president before him?	_____	_____
9. What was your mother's maiden name?	_____	_____
10. Can you count backward from 20 by 3s?	_____	_____

SCORING
0–2 errors: normal mental functioning
3–4 errors: mild cognitive impairment
5–7 errors: moderate cognitive impairment
8 or more errors: severe cognitive impairment

*One more error is allowed in the scoring if a patient has had a grade school education or less.
*One less error is allowed if the patient has had education beyond the high school level.

Source: Pfeiffer E. A short portable mental status questionnaire for the assessment of organic brain deficit in elderly patients. *Journal of the American Geriatric Society* 1975 Oct; 23(10):433–441.

his or her dominant hand, fold the paper in half, and throw the paper on the floor. One point is given for each command. (The three-stage command should not be repeated.) Reading is measured by asking the client to read "close your eyes" and to do what the phrase says. One point is given when the client performs that task, not when the client reads the phrase. Writing is measured by asking the client to write a spontaneous sentence. The sentence should be legible, but spelling and grammar errors should be ignored. One point is given when the client writes a sentence. Copying is measured by asking the client to copy intersecting pentagons so that they are about the same size as the first example drawn. The GCM should give the client a point if each pentagon has five clear sides, the overlapping angles form a diamond-like shape, and a complete side is not part of the overlap. The GCM should ignore rotation or tremor.

Scoring (range 0–30). For college-educated individuals, scores of 25 or under are suspect.[23]

Neuropsychological Assessment

The GCM, having completed the MMSE of the elder and received a score that suggests there is significant cognitive impairment, may want to schedule a more thorough assessment by a neuropsychologist to gain differential diagnostic information about specific deficit areas and continued strengths.

Visuospatial Assessment

A common follow-up to the administration of a test of mental status is a test of visuospatial ability such as the Clock Drawing Test[24] shown in Exhibit 20–4. The patient is given a piece of clean paper and a pen or pencil. The patient is instructed to draw a clock showing the hours, and then to draw the hands to indicate 2:45.

An assessment of visuospatial ability provides the GCM with a broader understanding of the elder's ability to move throughout space and understand the function of objects.

Emotional Functioning

An example of the many screening tests for depression is the Yesavage Geriatric Depression Scale (GDS).[25] Further discussion of the use of the GDS can be found in Chapter 21 on the subject of depression in the elderly. As discussed previously, depression can be a result of awareness of limitations imposed by dementia, and it can mask or simulate symptoms of depression as well. Coupled with data gained from the assessment of mental status, an assessment of the elder's level of depres-

Exhibit 20-4   Clock Drawing

Ability to Follow Instructions and Draw a Clock	Score
Either no attempt or an uninterpretable effort is made	1
Drawing reveals some evidence of instructions being received but only a vague representation of a clock	2
Numbers and clock face no longer obviously connected in the drawing. Hands are not present	3
Distortion of number sequence. Integrity of clock face is now gone (numbers may be missing, placed outside of boundaries of clock face, etc.)	4
Crowding of numbers at one end of the clock or a reversal of the numbers. Hands may be present in some fashion.	5
Inappropriate use of clock hands (use a digital display circle numbers despite repeated instructions)	6
Placement of hands is significantly off course	7
Noticeable errors in the placement of hours and minute hands	8
Slight errors in the placement of the hands	9
Hands are in correct position to indicate 2:45	10

Interpretation:
- A score from 1 to 5 reflects an inability to draw a clock face with numbers.
- A score from 6 to 10 reflects that the ability to draw the clock face with numbers intact.
- A low score correlates with dementia.

Score	Interpretation
10	Normal
8 or 9	Probably normal; may have mild dementia
6 or 7	Indeterminate (either normal or demented)
5	Probably demented; a few normal
1 to 4	Demented

Source: Reprinted with permission from T. Sunderland et al., Clock Drawing in Alzheimer's Disease, A Novel Measure of Dementia Severity, *Journal of the American Geriatric Society,* Vol. 37, pp. 725–729, © 1989, Trey Sunderland, MD.

sion can indicate the need for antidepressants, psychotherapy, increased stimulation, or a combination of solutions.

Degenerative versus Vascular

A scoring system has been developed that has shown significant accuracy and validity in assisting in the differential diagnosis between primary dementias such as AD and vascular dementias, such as those caused by stroke. When neuroimaging or neuropsychological testing are unavailable, the Hachinski Ischemic Score[23] (see Exhibit 20–5) can assist the GCM in determining the most likely source of dementia. Identifying the category of dementia can provide the GCM and the family with valuable information about the course of the disease process, available support, and treatment options.

Exhibit 20–5
Hachinski Ischemic Score

Abrupt onset	2
Stepwise deterioration	1
Fluctuating course	2
Nocturnal confusion	1
Relative preservation of personality	1
Depression	1
Somatic complaints	1
Emotional incontinence	1
History of hypertension	1
History of strokes	2
Associated atherosclerosis	1
Focal neurological symptoms	2
Focal neurological signs	2
Maximal Score	18
Vascular range	7–18
Mixed range	5–6
Degenerative range	0–4

Source: Reprinted with permission by Hachinski, V.C., Iliff, L.D. et al. Cerebral blood flow in dementia. *Archives of Neurology.* 1975; 32:632.

■ THE ROLE OF THE GCM IN DEMENTIA

During the period when the revision of this chapter was undertaken, the author became a client and purchaser of professional geriatric care management services for his mother. For the writer, the experience has served to solidify the concept of essential knowledge for the GCM, has confirmed what is important about geriatric care management practice, particularly interacting with the identified client, and perhaps most valuable, changed perspective on the emotional issues attendant on assessing and diagnosing dementia and developing an appropriate care plan in response.

Case Information

The chapter author's mother is an 80-year-old left-handed former attorney who suffered the loss of her spouse of 55 years, 7 months before the writing of this chapter. She has maintained a number of friends throughout her lifetime and had traveled extensively with both friends and her husband and family throughout the world. She has been a cigarette smoker for close to 60 years. Until very recently, she has been very active, playing singles tennis weekly with players two and three decades younger than she, and participating in a walking partnership with a much younger woman, averaging 10 to 12 miles once or twice a week. Always in robust health, she had never been hospitalized other than for childbirth. Never overweight in her adult life, she appeared to be getting thinner, but when asked about this, she reported that she was "just the same." She had been evaluated by a neurologist two years earlier for "dizziness" but related to her children and her husband that she was "found to be all right." She was on no medication. She drank alcohol moderately throughout her life with some increase in volume and rate of consumption in the last 10 years. She reported a high degree of stress in the past 29 years of her life caring for her husband who had cancer.

During the last two years of his life, the father increasingly complained that his wife was "getting impossible, she can't remember a thing and her cooking is getting inedible." In contrast, the mother would report, "Your father is so difficult to take care of, he doesn't listen." Their adult children rarely had visits with them individually outside of their home, and so the couple were almost always observed together or in close proximity.

Approximately 4 months prior to his death, the father fell while at home alone and was unable to reach the telephone. Upon discovering him, the mother asked her husband, who was partially conscious, to wake up and help her figure out what to do. He told her to call the police and she asked him how to do that. He said, "Go get the cordless phone and I'll do it." She brought him the phone and he called 911 and requested an ambulance.

Discussion

The case information to this point provides the GCM with observations in a number of areas.

- The GCM faces a dilemma every time he or she begins the process of interviewing family members. Reports of incidents and shared experiences can be dramatically at odds from one family member to another. The addition of multiple generations as reporters further compounds the problem. The GCM needs to collect complete histories from all of the relevant family members and then synthesize his or her impressions into a uniform history that is understandable and internally consistent. The risk for the GCM is to place too much weight on one report over another before having the opportunity to use his or her professional judgment based on all reports.
- In addition to evaluating and synthesizing information about events, the GCM also needs to be aware of the context from which each of the family members comes.

In this case, the GCM needs to be aware that the patient is a college-educated professional who worked in an environment requiring extensive use of language, had traveled extensively, and may have spoken multiple languages. As such, the patient can be expected to have a significant cognitive reserve. For the GCM, this presents a number of issues. The patient on interview may refer to something in his or her own experience that may be outside of the experience or awareness of the GCM or use words from another language that is completely unfamiliar to the GCM. Is it fantasy or delusion, or a reference to traveling by camel across Afghanistan? Is it a neologism, or an insult to the GCM in Farsi? Integrating the history of the patient and family and an awareness of the cultural context in which the assessment is being completed will significantly improve the GCM's work.

- The GCM, working with dementia patients who are part of a couple, needs to have clinical skills working with couples. In addition to the capacity to draw on his or her own experience and understanding of relationships, the GCM needs a background in theory that will place the knowledge about how couples of long standing develop mechanisms that support one another and cover inadequacies in the appropriate context. Couples contribute according to their ability, and, during the usually long period of homeostasis, receive according to need. A colleague reported on a case involving a couple, who when together, the husband was always the one to give a response, "Lady Di says we can't do that next week as we're having company." Only after the husband's sudden death was it discovered that "Lady Di" had been expressively aphasic and essentially mute for the prior six years. (See the section titled "Assisting Spousal Caregivers and Working with Couples" in Chapter 17 for more information.)

- In the course of taking a history, the report to the GCM of deteriorating quality of food preparation and weight loss are signals, but until connected to other data, remain just signals. They could represent a depressive response to the ongoing stress of caregiving. They could be changes in the sensorium, such as decline in the ability to smell or taste, or decline in the visual sphere, making it difficult to read recipes and preparation instructions. They are also, seen in the context of later information, marker events for the development of dementia.

- The Chinese adage about crisis and opportunity is very pertinent to the GCM. A crisis event, while distressing and calamitous to the participants, represents for the GCM an opportunity to collect information that may have been hidden, to observe the behavior of family members under stress, and often, to move a "stuck" family beyond a previously held position. Crisis events invariably bring out the best and worst in people, often simultaneously. The mother's response to the father's fall could be seen as a panic response, a freeze-up of sorts. Alternatively, seen in the context of the mutually supportive dyad, the father had clearly been the one who was making sure that the intellectual and cognitive activities central to the couple were being completed while the mother was accomplishing the physical activities. When it became necessary for the mother to execute activities beyond her capabilities, she was at a loss.

Case Information (continued)

During the months prior to the father's death, the mother's family began to become concerned about her repetitive questions and apparent inability to comprehend the termi-

nal nature of her husband's illness. She also began to ask for rides to the various facilities where her husband was, offering that she was "too tired to drive" or needed gas in the car. She had always been an intensely private person, particularly about her health. Questions about how she was doing were invariably met with the response, "I'm fine, there's nothing wrong with me, I'm just tired. I'm worried that they're not doing enough for your father, shouldn't we call _____?" Opinions within the family systems were mixed. Some felt that the mother was depressed from the caregiving experience. Some were concerned that there was evidence of the beginning of significant memory loss, and some agreed with the mother that she was just tired and agreed with her concern about the care the father received. It was decided to send an e-mail to the mother's primary care physician reporting on the observed behavior and asking him to take a look at these issues.

The primary care physician was thankful for the communication and had his patient care coordinator call the mother and schedule an appointment. The mother asked for a ride because "her eyes were tired from sitting in that room with your father all day." The physician requested neuropsychological testing and scheduled a visit to the mother's ophthalmologist.

The neuropsychological testing was completed, as was the ophthalmologic evaluation. Again the mother was insistent that nothing be shared with her children regarding the results of the neuropsychological testing. The ophthalmologic exam was essentially normal with the exception of a slight cataract in the right eye. The neuropsychologist recommended that the mother be seen in the Memory Disorder Clinic by the senior behavioral neurologist because of her concerns about the findings of the testing. When asked about the results of the testing by the writer, the mother reported, "We had a nice chat, she asked me things and I asked her things." A week later, when the neuropsychologist called her house to inform her about the appointment with the behavioral neurologist, the mother was unable to recall whom the neuropsychologist was.

The father died in the intervening period before the appointment with the neurologist. At the neurologist appointment, the mother was unable to recall when her husband had died, reporting, "he's been dead for years" even though it had only been a few weeks. When the neurologist asked to speak to the children, the mother did not object. The neurologist noted that because of the level of seriousness of his findings, he felt it necessary to speak with the children about the mother despite the issues of privacy and confidentiality. The neurologist reported that he felt that the results of his exam, the neuropsychological testing, and review of the mother's health care record showed findings consistent with cerebral amyloid angiopathy. Specifically, he referred to deficits in executive processing and short-term memory. He noted that she remained most unaware of the level of deficit. He also noted that she had had a stroke at the time she was evaluated for what she had reported as an episode of dizziness. He ordered an MRI to follow up on the status of the stroke and to assess whether there were visible changes from the cerebral amyloid angiopathy. The MRI showed new evidence of a very recent hemorrhage. Additionally, he ordered Aricept (donepezil) to attempt to slow the progression of memory loss and an anxiolytic. Consistent with her lifelong behavior, the medications were refused.

The family elected to hire a GCM to assist in beginning to provide consultation and guidance to the family as a whole. The son felt that he was not in a position to be sufficiently objective about diagnostic issues, strategy, and ongoing planning in the face of differences of opinion about diagnosis.

A local GCM was engaged and began to work with the family. There were significant differences of opinion about the source of the mother's difficulties. These ranged from the perception that the mother was moving rapidly toward moderate dementia as the result of multiple infarcts and cerebral amyloid angiopathy to the mild dementia being transient and related to stroke to that it was not dementia but an extended grief reaction. The GCM listened to all of the opinions and helped the family focus on concrete steps that could be taken regardless of an agreed-upon diagnosis. An attempt was made to add staffing to the mother's home, which caused the mother to become agitated and was rejected.

Family members attended the follow-up appointment with the neurologist two months later. At that time, the neurologist noted that he observed increased evidence of dementia and was now comfortable in adding AD to his diagnosis on the basis of symptoms. He stated that in his professional opinion the mother was not competent to make significant decisions on her own behalf and expressed concern about her continued safety in the home and in the community because she had continued to drive.

Discussion

- For the GCM, assessment and reassessment are an ongoing process. Data about the patient rarely remain constant, and frequently, data are made available to the GCM that change the perspective on symptoms or care planning. For example, in reporting to the GCM, one of the mother's closest friends recalled events from their walking tour of Sicily five or six years prior. She reported that the mother would frequently pack and unpack her bag at night, was resistant to reading menus, and often asked the friend to take care of the check, sometimes offering her large amounts of cash or credit cards. Information such as this provides the GCM with valuable insight. Without these data, it would be easy to assume that the dementia symptoms had begun around the time of the father's last months. The information, however, serves to suggest to the GCM that the prodromal phase was much longer than had been thought. This, in turn, has implications for reevaluation of the assessment data as well as contributes to the care-planning phase.

- As health care professionals working with large volumes of information on elders and their families, the GCM must not only be fully aware of Health Insurance Portability and Accountability Act requirements, confidentiality restrictions, and privacy issues, but needs to formulate and be conversant with policies regarding these issues for the professionals with whom they work. The GCM must be prepared, from the initial meeting with family members, to discuss his or her policies on safeguarding critical information as well as to define for them the circumstances under which information needs to be shared and with whom. As a "team leader," the GCM must also be prepared to work with other professionals on a case whose rules and regulations regarding these issues are significantly different. Interestingly, many of the professionals involved in the mother's care in this case were more than willing to work around privacy restrictions in the mother's best interest.

- Earlier in the discussion of the case, it was suggested that the GCM have experience in working with couples. Experience and grounding in the theory of work with families is also of great value to the GCM. The GCM doesn't merely work in a therapeutic context with the family but as an educator, advocate, internal consultant, and coach. In this context, the GCM brought in to work with the family deliberately ignored the fact that one of the client family members was a GCM. In doing so, she was able to put the rest of the family at ease and in a better position to hear assessment and diagnostic information and to better work toward consensus. The GCM also made the family aware of the important role that the mother continued to play in the decision-making process. By placing the mother's wishes in the context of education around the cognitive limitations of dementia, the GCM helped the family to understand which of the mother's wishes were unrealistic and which could be embraced. (See Chapter 17.)

- The work of the GCM encompasses not only health care but legal, financial, vocational, home management, and often employment and logistics areas. In addition to a knowledge base in these areas, the GCM needs to be able to recognize when there are issues with the elder or family that cross over between the subject areas. Part of the leadership responsibilities for the GCM working with families with a demented member is to discuss necessary legal and financial instruments, gain consensus about decision making, and when possible ascertain the elder's wishes about care. In this case, the neurologist's statement about the mother's competence served a number of purposes. It brought home to other family members the degree of impairment and it helped them to begin to focus more on specific issues such as home safety, driving, and planning. Additionally, the statement served to activate the mother's health care durable power of attorney.

Case Information (continued)

By hearing and focusing on the most outlying opinions in the family, the GCM was able to propose novel solutions. One family member felt that the mother should only be told "the truth" about her behavior and the family's concerns. When a family member was insistent that the mother's problem was one of grief and loneliness, the GCM used that opinion to introduce the concept of a "friendly visitor" who could come by and have dinner with the mother. The GCM introduced the family to the idea of using some degree of fiction to get the mother to accept a visitor in her home where she had been resistant and hostile to "official" staff. A carefully selected companion (one who spoke multiple languages, had traveled, and had another interesting job) was introduced as a friend of the GCM. Under the guise of being lonely and alone herself, she asked if she could drop by and share dinner sometimes with the mother. The fact that she had never met the children enabled the visitor to put the mother's suspicions about "managers" to rest.

During this period, the family became increasingly concerned about the mother's cigarette smoking and her continued driving. Of additional concern, but one that was not shared by all members of the family, was the fact that some but not all of the children were called frequently by the mother when she was home alone. Often these calls consisted of requests for cigarettes, money, food, or to fix something. Over time, these calls increased to where one of the children was receiving up to 50 calls a day. During times of frustration, such as when the car was removed overtly, many family members were exposed to repeated dialing. This led to the temporary return of the car. Only when the mother was occupied with the friendly visitor or her friends or family would the calls cease. On many occasions, a child would have just left the house, having dropped off cigarettes and ice cream, and be only a few doors away before the calls would begin again asking the child if he was going to stop by and whether he could bring some cigarettes.

The GCM recommended that the family begin to think about alternatives to the mother remaining at home and scheduled visits to a select group of assisted living facilities that had memory disorder units. Some family members had difficulty with the idea of removing the mother from the home and placing her in what was referred to as "lockdown." Other family members were pressing for placement as soon as possible to avert a perceived future catastrophe involving smoking.

Also at this time, the GCM assisted the family in creating another fiction to assist in the removal of the car after the mother was observed driving by a family member. The car was disabled and the mother was allowed to discover that the car did not work. A note was left under to the hood for the AAA explaining the situation and asking for their help in maintaining the fiction. Eventually, the family offered to have the car towed to "the garage," in reality a family member's driveway, and the battery was reconnected. Some time thereafter it was reported from "the garage" that the car was a total loss and could not be repaired. This time was easier because family members who had been committed to only telling the truth about the mother's situation had been on the receiving end of many phone calls during the prior loss of the vehicle.

As the family members continued to visit memory disorder units, the GCM provided the family with education about what qualities were important from a clinical point of view to enhance their understanding of the wide range of facilities.

After the family had come to consensus about placement and a selection was made, the GCM readied the family by creating a checklist of activities, the game plan that needed to take place. Selection of what items, including furniture and art, to bring from home to the apartment in the memory disorder unit, selecting clothes, and assigning tasks in the move were discussed and approved. The GCM stressed that only those who could fully participate in the process without showing emotion inappropriate to the necessary fiction could participate. With the help of the program director of the facility, a fiction and move day game plan was developed. One family member would take the mother out for a Mother's Day outing, including hair, nails, shopping, and luncheon. A team of other family members would arrive at the mother's house shortly after departure with a truck, move the designated items out, transfer to the facility, set up the apartment, and then all but one, the "designated hitter," would leave. A call would be made to the Mother's Day escort, reporting that there had been a flood at the house, the power was out, and the electric company was not allowing anyone in because of the danger. Ironically, there *had* been serious flooding in the area in the week prior to the move, but the game plan had been developed well in advance of this; for the family, fortuitous coincidence served to bolster the fiction.

The mother was informed of "the crisis" and was told that she should come to where the designated hitter was because he had arranged for a temporary apartment. The Mother's Day escort dropped her off and, pleading being late for work, left. The mother was introduced to a "friend" (in actuality the program director of the memory disorder unit), who had been visiting when he had heard about the flood, and fortunately, the friend had a spare apartment. Keeping up a stream of chat, they walked into the unit. After a while, the family member also had to go back to work and left, promising to return soon.

Discussion

- Following the interpretation and integration of findings, the next large task for the GCM is the formulation of a strategic plan for the family. In this case, the GCM recognized that a number of family members were health care professionals so that it was less important to bring everyone "up to speed." By encour-

aging the less emotionally contaminated members of the family to explain to others about assessment results, definitions, and diagnosis, the GCM could proceed to think about concrete tasks as well as formulate a strategy to address the conflicting views of the mother and her problems. Care managers with a background or prior training in family therapy or counseling have the benefit of theory and practice to assist them in situations such as these. Best practices would suggest that GCM practice needs to include some exposure to theory and technique in this area.

- The GCM needs to think carefully about how much is the correct amount of activity in the delivery and execution of the strategic plan. In this case, the GCM elected to function primarily in the consultative role, encouraging and supporting the family to create roles within the plan that fit with temperament, skill set, and choice. In other settings and with other families, the GCM might choose to take a more active stance.

- The ability of the GCM to provide leadership and consultation to families, acknowledging the emotional strain without engaging in overt therapeutic effort, is a critical role and one that defines the future profession of professional geriatric care management.

- In general, all work the GCMs do, but work with dementia in particular, raises the specter of emotional stress and countertransference phenomena as GCMs think about not only their own families but themselves.

- Many people have strong objections to the use of fiction in the service of outcomes. In her thorough and excellent review on the moral and ethical issues encountered in the use of "therapeutic fiblets," Cress[26] speaks about filial maturity and the GCM's ability to help the adult child accept the present parent.

- Is it responsible of a GCM to allow a moderately demented person, one who is acknowledged to have significant deficits, to continue to make larger-scale decisions such as this when they are, by definition, unable to understand that they are impaired? GCMs frequently come into contact with family and some GCMs themselves who feel that demented elders should be "told the truth" about their dementia, where they are, and how they got there. GCMs need to become comfortable with the idea that the use of fiction is in the service of safety and security. Drilling down into the core information in this case, the mother has moderate dementia of both degenerative and vascular types, rendering her abilities in higher-order cognition and executive functioning to be significantly impaired. She would be unable to follow the logic contained in an argument that she requires a facility that provides increased stimulation, structure, regular meals, high foot-candle lighting, and controlled egress, even if she were able to acknowledge that she needs one because she is demented. Telling her the "truth" (i.e., that she is being held against her will, that there is nothing wrong with her house, because her children think that she is incapable of living at home) would only serve to make her extremely upset, and she would then forget *why* she was upset, but would remain physiologically stressed.

- Invariably, the question of substituted judgment becomes another issue in practice methodology for the GCM. It is of critical importance for the GCM to be cognizant of his or her own feelings on the issue and actively seek out and create consensus on this issue within the family

and consultation where the ethical issues are complex. This, however, was not a legal problem in this particular case because there was a durable power of attorney for health care that had been executed more than a decade ago.

■ CONCLUSION

The advancing age of the baby boomer generation inevitably means that there will be a steady increase in the numbers of clients seeking the services of a GCM. Of that increasing number, there remains the potential for an even larger increase in the percentage of geriatric care management cases involving dementia. This chapter has discussed the manifestations and symptoms of dementia, provided a review of types of dementia, and included a discussion of assessment instruments. Case information and discussion of relevant issues within the case were reviewed. This information is important in developing the GCM's knowledge about dementia. It remains important, however, for the new GCM to gain supervised experience and an opportunity to know his or her position on the complex moral and ethical issues raised by dementia.

■ NOTES

1. Beers MH, Berkow R, eds. *The Merck Manual of Geriatrics*. 3rd ed. Whitehorse Station, NJ: Merck Research Laboratories; 2000.

2. Hebert LE, Scherr PA, Bienias JL, Bennett DA, Evans DA. Alzheimer disease in the US population: prevalence estimates using the 2000 Census. *Arch Neurol.* August 2003;60(8):1119–1122.

3. Brookmeyer R, Gray S, Kawas C. Projections of Alzheimer's disease in the United States and the public health impact of delaying disease onset. *Am J Pub Health.* 1998;88(9):1337–1342.

4. World Health Organization. The ICD-10 classification of mental and behavioral disorders: diagnostic criteria for research. Geneva, Switzerland: World Health Organization; 1993.

5. American Psychiatric Association. *Diagnostic and Statistical Manual of Mental Disorders.* 4th ed. Washington, DC: American Psychiatric Association; 1994.

6. Keady J. The experience of dementia: a review of the literature and implications for nursing practice. *J Clin Nurs.* 1996;5:275–288.

7. Spitznagel M, Tremont G, Brown L, Gunstad J. Cognitive reserve and the relationship between depressive symptoms and awareness of deficits in dementia. *J Neuropsych Clin Neurosci.* 2006;18:186–190.

8. McKhann G, Drachman D, Folstein M, Katzman R, Price D, Stadlan E. Clinical diagnosis of Alzheimer's disease: report of the NINCDS-ADRDA work group. *Neurology.* 1984;34:939–944.

9. Bonanni L, Thomas A, Onofrj M. Diagnosis and management of dementia with Lewy bodies: third report of the DLB Consortium. *Neurology.* May 9, 2006;66(9):1455.

10. Guidi M, Paciaroni L, Paolini S, DePadova S, Scarpino O. Differences and similarities in the neuropsychological profile of dementia with Lewy bodies and Alzheimer's disease in the early stage. *J Neurol Sci.* June 16, 2006; 10:1016.

11. Mendez MF, Perryman KM. Neuropsychiatric features of frontotemporal dementia: evaluation of consensus criteria and review. *J Neuropsych Clin Neurosci.* 2002;14:424,425 (Table 1).

12. Neary D, Snowden JS, Gustafson L, et al. Frontotemporal lobar degeneration: a consensus on clinical diagnostic criteria. *Neurology.* 1998;51:1546–1554.

13. Hagerman RJ, Leehey M, Heinrichs W, et al. Intention tremor, parkinsonism, and generalized brain atrophy in male carriers of Fragile X. *Neurology.* 2001;57:127–130.

14. Ott R, Grace M. Vascular dementia. *Med Health R I.* May 1997;80(5):150–154.

15. Cummings J. The one-minute mental status examination. *Neurology.* February 24, 2004; 62(4):534–535.

16. Paul R, Cohen R, Moser D, et al. Clinical correlates of cognitive decline in vascular dementia. *Cog Behav Neurol.* March 2003;16(1):40–46.

17. Saltz E. Private communication, June 21, 2006.

18. Diagnosing idiopathic normal-pressure hydrocephalus. *Neurosurg.* 2005;57(3 suppl): S2-4–S2-16.

19. Rogers C, Partington MW, Turner GM. Tremor, ataxia and dementia in older men may indicate a carrier of the Fragile X syndrome. *Clin Genetics.* July 2003;64(1):54–58.

20. Folstein MF, Folstein S, McHugh PR. Mini-Mental State, a practical method for grading the cognitive state of patients for the clinician. *J Psychiatr Res.* 1975;12:189–198.

21. Pfeiffer E. A short portable mental status questionnaire for the assessment of organic brain deficit in elderly patients. *J Am Geriat Soc.* October 1975;23(10):433–441.

22. Knutson K, Gross P. Advanced assessment: integrating the biopsychosocial needs of client and family. *Geriatric Care Manage J.* 2000;10:4–13.

23. Hachinski VC, Iliff LD, Zilhka, E, et al. Cerebral blood flow in dementia. *Arch Neurol.* 1975;32:632.

24. Sunderland T, Hill JL, Mellow, AM, et al. Clock drawing in Alzheimer's disease. A novel measure of dementia severity. *J Am Geriat Soc.* 1989;37:725–729,726 (Table 1).

25. Yesavage J, Brink TL, Rose T, et al. Development and validation of a geriatric depression screening scale: a preliminary report. *J Psychiatr Res.* 1983;17:37–49.

26. Cress C, Boudinot M. Geriatric fiblets—necessary white lies or bad therapeutic technique? How to do an ethical query for your own practice. *Geriatric Care Manage J.* Spring 2006;16:2.

Appendix 20–A
Evaluating Functional Assessment Instruments

▪ ACTIVITIES OF DAILY LIVING AND INSTRUMENTAL ACTIVITIES OF DAILY LIVING INSTRUMENTS

Many of the activities of daily living (ADLs) and instrumental activities of daily living (IADLs) instruments came out of research studies and were designed as lengthy self-report questionnaires. Although they can be given to family members, they cannot be successfully administered to clients with dementia and may not provide as much information about physical functioning as the professional geriatric care manager (GCM) requires. Performance-based assessment is preferred. In performance-based assessment, the GCM can observe the client doing certain tasks rather than having to ask whether the client can do the tasks. Although reliable and valid in discriminating those who can do the function from those who cannot, the ADL and IADL scales are not sensitive to changes in condition, especially in the highest-functioning clients.[1,2] GCMs using ADL and IADL scales will want to complement them with other measures of function that better establish a baseline and assess change from one visit to the next. The instruments listed here are commonly used in assessing basic activities of self-care.

Katz ADL Scale

The Katz ADL Scale assesses basic activities of self-care and is not sensitive to small changes. It is useful in rehabilitative settings.[1,3] The weakness of the instrument is that it assesses a limited range of activities and the ratings are subjective.

Physical Self-Maintenance Scale (ADL)

The Physical Self-Maintenance Scale assesses self-care, mobility, and transfers.[1,3] It allows direct observation of a range of functions and is useful in a variety of settings. The weakness of the instrument is that it is time-consuming to administer and difficult to use with seriously ill or cognitively impaired older adults.

Scale for Instrumental Activities of Daily Living (IADL)

The Scale for Instrumental Activities of Daily Living assesses more complex activities, including food preparation, shopping, and housekeeping.[1,3] It has a higher range of performance than the Katz ADL Scale does but is not sensitive to small changes. The weakness of the instrument is that it is subjective and difficult to use in cognitively impaired older adults.

▪ COGNITIVE FUNCTION INSTRUMENTS

Although mental status instruments cannot establish that a person has dementia, they are important in identifying the client who needs further evaluation. Screening tests for mental status remain the cornerstone of documenting suspected cognitive impairment.[4,5] The client's age, education, ethnicity, and language have been shown to influence responses to mental status screening, all factors the GCM must consider in selecting the most appropriate instruments. Although there are several instruments for staging and following the progression of dementia, they have been used primarily in Alzheimer's disease, and their value in other dementias is less clear.[6] It is best to use the staging instruments after a formal dementia workup is completed and diagnosis of Alzheimer's disease is made. Cognitive function instruments can also be used to follow the progression of change in dementia. Another method for following the progression of change after a differential diagnosis of Alzheimer's disease is made is to combine the standard mental status tests with staging instruments. Future reassessments can then be compared to the baseline assessment to document changes in cognition. The instruments discussed here are commonly used in assessing cognitive function.

Folstein Mini Mental State Examination

The Folstein Mini Mental State Examination assesses a broader range of functions than the Short Portable Mental Status Questionnaire and is particularly useful in screening for moderate impairment.[1,7] It is a fairly quick and sensitive instrument and has been validated over time. The weakness of the instrument is that it will not detect mild cognitive impairment and is not designed to grade progression. Also, clients with primary expressive aphasia may appear more impaired because of difficulty with language.

Clock Drawing Test

The Clock Drawing Test assesses visuospatial difficulties and basic executive functions such as planning and simple abstraction.[8] Studies have demonstrated that clients with normal mental status draw normal clocks and that clients with Alzheimer's disease draw abnormal clocks. Visuospatial skills may be the primary deficit in some clients in the early stages of Alzheimer's disease.

Global Deterioration Scale

The Global Deterioration Scale assesses seven stages in the course of dementia with well-specified observed criteria: mild Alzheimer's disease is stage 3 or 4; moderate is stage 5 or 6; and severe is stage 7.[6,9] The Global Deterioration Scale gives an overall picture of the disease process and assists the GCM in accurately placing the client at the appropriate stage of dementia. Language performance is not used to stage the dementia. The weakness of the instrument is that it has been used primarily in Alzheimer's

disease and its value in other dementias is not clear. It provides information on the general progression of the disease and does not take into account individual variations.

Functional Assessment Staging Tool

The Functional Assessment Staging Tool (FAST) is for distribution to the family and provides specific information on the order in which various functions are lost.[9] FAST also provides the family members with an estimated time frame so they have an approximate idea of how long a given level of functioning will last. Along with the Global Deterioration Scale, FAST helps the GCM to understand each stage of Alzheimer's disease and make suggestions to clients and families regarding appropriate decision making (e.g., decision making about level of care and care needs). The weakness of the instrument is that it has been used primarily in Alzheimer's disease and its value in other dementias is not clear. It is an informational table about the general progression of the disease and does not take into account individual variations.

Short Portable Mental Status Questionnaire

The Short Portable Mental Status Questionnaire assesses a narrow range of basic mental functions, including memory, attention, and orientation, and is capable of detecting gross cognitive dysfunction only. The weakness of the instrument is that it is insensitive to small changes.[1,10]

Wechsler Memory Scale

The Wechsler Memory Scale assesses a broad range of memory functions and is sensitive to more subtle changes.[1,11] The weakness of the instrument is that it takes a long time to administer and has inadequate norms for the older adult population. The latest version, WMS–III, has norms to age 89.

■ DEPRESSION INSTRUMENTS

Functional assessment instruments for depression do not establish a diagnosis of depression but are important in identifying the client who needs further evaluation. Most of the depression scales are reasonably valid, reliable, and useful for screening and provide an assessment of the effects of therapy. Most of these scales have difficulty differentiating the effects of physical illness from those of depression because they include questions about physical symptoms such as fatigue and pain. Their usefulness may be limited in clients experiencing severe dementia.[1] The instruments discussed here are commonly used in screening for depression.

Geriatric Depression Scale

The Geriatric Depression Scale is designed for older adults, assesses symptoms of depression, and includes a broad range of questions about mood.[1,12] It is quick and reliable and avoids an excess of physical symptom questions. The weakness of the instrument is its limited usefulness in clients with severe dementia.

Beck Depression Inventory

The Beck Depression Inventory is a self-rating scale that assesses symptoms of depression and includes a broad range of questions.[1,13] It is validated in older adults and medical patients. The weakness of the instrument is that it relies too heavily on physical symptoms, making it less useful in older adults with physical impairments. It is also difficult for cognitively impaired clients to use.

Hamilton Depression Inventory

The Hamilton Depression Inventory assesses objective symptoms of depression and can estimate severity of depression.[1,14] The weakness of the instrument is that it relies on physical symptoms, thus making it less useful in older adults.

■ NOTES

1. Applegate W, Blass J, Williams T. Instruments for the functional assessment of older patients. *New Engl J Med.* 1990;322:1207–1213.

2. Johnson J, Mezey M. Functional status assessment: an approach to tertiary prevention. In: Lavizzo-Mourey, R., ed. *Practicing Prevention for the Elderly.* Philadelphia, PA: Hanley & Belfus; 1989:141–152.

3. Guralnik J, Branch L, Cummings S, Curb J. Physical performance measures in aging research. *J Gerontol.* 1989;44:141–146.

4. Mercer B. Evaluating memory loss in older women. *Wom Health Primary Care.* 1998; 1:785–797.

5. McKhann G, Drachman D, Folstein M, Katzman R, Price D, Stadlan E. Clinical diagnosis of Alzheimer's disease: report of the NINCDS-ADRDA work group. *Neurol.* 1984;34:939–944.

6. Corey-Bloom J, Thal L, Galasko D, et al. Diagnosis and evaluation of dementia. *Neurol.* 1995;45:211–218.

7. Folstein MF, Folstein S, McHugh PR, et al. Mini-Mental State, a practical method for grading the cognitive state of patients for the clinician. *J Psychiatr Res.* 1975;12:189–198.

8. Sunderland T, Hill J, Mellow A, Lawlor B, Newhouse P, Grafman J. Clock drawing in Alzheimer's disease: a novel measure of dementia severity. *J Am Geriatr Soc.* 1989; 37:725–729.

9. Reisberg B, Ferris SH, deLeon MJ, Crook T. The Global Deterioration Scale for assessment of primary degenerative dementia. *Am J Psychiatry.* 1982;139:1136–1139.

10. Dalton JE, Pederson SL, Blom BE, Holmes NR. Diagnostic errors using the portable mental status questionnaire with a mixed population. *J Gerontol.* 1987;42:512–514.

11. Wechsler D. A standardized memory scale for clinical use. *J Psychol.* 1945;19:87–95.

12. Yesavage J. Development and validation of a geriatric depression scale: a preliminary report. *J Psychiatr Res.* 1983;17:37–49.

13. Beck A. *Beck Depression Inventory.* San Antonio, TX: Psychological Corporation; 1987.

14. Hamilton M. Development of a rating scale for primary depressive illness. *Br J Soc Clin Psychol.* 1967;6:278–296.

Chapter 21

Depression and the Older Adult: The Role of the Geriatric Care Manager

Miriam K. Aronson

Depression is not a normal part of aging, despite common misconceptions. Rather, it is a serious but very treatable illness with associated physical, emotional, social, and financial burdens. This chapter discusses the phenomenology of depressive illness in older persons and the role of the geriatric care manager (GCM) in its assessment and management.

Approximately 15% of Americans over the age of 65 report clinically significant depressive symptoms, but only approximately one-fifth of these individuals meet the criteria for major depression. The rest suffer from depression-related clinical and subclinical states. Prevalence rates are the highest among those in nursing homes and in primary care settings and lowest (less than 3%) among healthy community-residing older people.[1,2] Older women are more likely to report depressive symptoms than are men: although 16% of women aged 65 to 69 reported depressive symptoms, only 10% of men did. The prevalence of these reports rises with increasing age, 20% for those 85 and over as compared to 13% of those ages 65 to 69.[3]

Risk factors for depression in older persons are similar to those for younger populations; namely, it is more likely to affect women, per-sons who are unmarried or widowed, individuals experiencing stress, and persons with poor social support systems. But comorbid medical illness is the hallmark of depression in older persons, the major difference between depression in older persons and depression in younger persons. The predominant comorbid disorders are personality disorders and substance abuse in younger persons.

Symptoms of major depression, as defined by the fourth edition of the *Diagnostic and Statistical Manual of Mental Disorders* of the American Psychiatric Association, include a pervasive sad mood that lasts for more than two weeks or markedly decreased interest or pleasure in all activities plus at least three or four of the following symptoms: sleep disturbance, decreased energy, poor concentration, appetite disturbance or problems, psychomotor retardation or agitation, feelings of worthlessness or guilt, and suicidal ideation.[4] Crying may be part of the depressive symptom complex. However, in and of itself, crying does not mean depression. It may be an involuntary poststroke phenomenon or a manipulative strategy. Expressions of guilt are less prevalent in older than in younger depressed individuals.[5] In older persons, there may be a range of physical complaints, as in the case of Mrs. W.

CASE STUDY

The Case of Mrs. W

Mrs. W was an 89-year-old widowed woman who had resided in an upscale assisted living facility for several years. She had a part-time private-duty aide to assist with bathing, grooming, and mobility. Mrs. W had been a controlling matriarch most of her life. She had a husband whom she dominated and three very devoted children. She had experienced episodic bouts of depression throughout her life and had exaggerated complaints of pain at various times. Her medical care was fragmented and resulted in polypharmacy. Most recently, a pain practitioner had prescribed strong drugs for osteoporosis-associated pain. The drugs were not taken as prescribed; in fact, Mrs. W developed a "stash" of pills that became a concern to her family and physicians and a tool for her to manipulate her family. She had alienated her primary care physician and was dissatisfied with her current medical care.

Over the past few months, she had become increasingly unhappy. She withdrew from her accustomed activities and became more isolated. In addition, she complained of sleeplessness, fatigue, loss of appetite, inability to concentrate, pain, and loneliness. Despite treatment with pain medication and anxiolytic drugs (in addition to her blood pressure, heart, and osteoporosis medications), her depressive symptom complex did not abate. The more unhappy she was, the more demanding she became of her children, who were concerned about her but frustrated by her lack of improvement despite the medications and physician visits, the beautiful environment in which she lived, and all of their efforts. They sought a consultation from a GCM.

Although Mrs. W lived in an assisted living facility where there were opportunities for socialization, she was isolated and felt very alone. She had limited her activities to watching television, listening to music, and playing a very occasional bridge game. She did not attend any facility activities regularly and rarely ventured outside of the facility, despite her children's invitations and willingness to transport her.

The role of the GCM here was to assess Mrs. W in her facility and to develop a care plan. The GCM identified fragmentation of medical care, polypharmacy, and depression as areas of immediate concern in this cognitively intact woman. Additionally, her loneliness and social isolation were prominent. The GCM recommended that Mrs. W have a comprehensive medical evaluation by a geriatrician and that she engage the geriatrician to be her primary care physician. The geriatrician recommended an antidepressant and also set about addressing the pain and polypharmacy. The GCM also recommended emotional support for Mrs. W and her children and consultation with facility staff, with goals of improving her affect and increasing her socialization and physical activity. Mrs. W was resistant to suggestions about nonpharmacologic interventions such as physical therapy, exercise, increased socialization, and a later bedtime.

The high comorbidity of medical illnesses and late-life depression and the infinite combinations of medical and mood symptoms pose diagnostic and classification challenges to clinicians across all settings. Anxiety is associated with depression but also with other medical and psychiatric disorders. With depression and anxiety, older persons tend toward expressing their problems as somatic complaints, which they perceive as less stigmatizing than psychiatric illness.[6]

Because of the complex nature of late-life depression and the multisystem involvement, there is a need for flexible and multidimensional approaches to treatment; thus, it has been proposed that late-life depression be considered a geriatric syndrome rather than a single categorical disease.[7] This suggested classification may also be applied to other prevalent conditions, including cognitive impairment, incontinence, falls, and malnutrition.

Unexpected changes in life circumstances are common in the lives of older persons and are social and demographic risk factors for late-life affective disorder. There are also losses of roles and losses of function. Feelings of grief over these losses are not uncommon. There are disease-related losses of physical function. Losses of friends and relatives are frequent, and the social support network inevitably shrinks. Changes in living arrangements may become necessary and these changes exacerbate feelings of loss and unhappiness. In fact, recently admitted nursing home residents are an at-risk population for depression (Exhibit 21–1).[8]

Exhibit 21–1   Sociodemographic Situations Associated with Depression

- Retirement
- Multiple role losses
- Bereavement
- Deaths of family members and friends
- Loneliness and isolation
- Responsibility for care for an older person with a disability
- Residence in a nursing home
- Elder abuse
- Neglect
- Substance abuse

■ BEREAVEMENT

Bereavement is common for individuals of advanced ages. Grieving is a normal process and does not always require intervention; however, for some individuals, grief becomes pathological and requires psychological and pharmacologic intervention. Little information is available regarding when "normal grief" becomes "pathological grief," when treatment is required, and which interventions are most appropriate. Older adults are more likely than younger adults to develop a major depression following bereavement.[7]

■ DEPRESSION AND MEDICAL ILLNESS

Evidence about the relationship between depression and medical illness is increasing.[9-11] Depressive disorders may themselves cause or contribute to medical illnesses. Conversely, medical illnesses may cause or contribute to depression (Exhibit 21–2).[12] And each condition complicates recovery

Exhibit 21–2   Medical Conditions Associated with Late Life Depression

Cardiac and vascular conditions
Myocardial infarction
Cerebrovascular accident

Other medical conditions
Acute pain
Chronic pain

Neurological conditions
Dementia
Parkinson's disease
Cancer

Physical disabilities
Hip fracture
Loss of mobility
Trauma

Sensory Impairments
Vision problems
Hearing decrements

from the other. Unfortunately, most clinical drug studies involving depressed older people have excluded persons with significant medical illness.[13]

Depression negatively affects quality of life, functionality, physical health, longevity, and family and other interpersonal relationships. Depression causes "excess disability," complicating the course of illnesses, slowing recovery, and compromising the impact of interventions such as rehabilitation. Depression is often a "silent partner" responsible for resistance to care, inconsistency of course, and negativity. It also can cause added pain and suffering.

In addition to its social, psychological, and physical toll on affected individuals, depression is associated with significant costs to the health care system because of increased health resource utilization. Medical outcome studies have revealed that only serious heart disease had a greater negative influence on functional status and bed days than did depression and only arthritis had a greater association with pain.[14] Depression also confers an added risk for mortality.[15,16]

■ PAIN

Pain may interfere with mood, function, appetite, sleep, energy level, and body image and may cause helplessness and hopelessness. These symptoms can mimic or overlap with those of depression and anxiety. Persistent pain can cause depression and anxiety and, conversely, depression and anxiety can worsen pain. Thus, management of pain is an important mental health issue for older adults.[17]

■ SUICIDE

Suicide is the extreme and life-threatening potential outcome of depression. Studies of depressed people have shown that their risk for death by suicide is approximately 30 times greater than the risk for the general population.[14] Individuals with major affective disorder have been estimated to have a lifetime suicide mortality rate of 19%. Other research suggests that there is an increased risk of suicide in late-life affective illness. Americans older than age 65 have a suicide rate that is 50% higher than that of the general population. Older men have the highest suicide rate (38 per 100,000, but 50 per 100,000 near age 85).[18] Although more women attempt suicide, more men succeed. The most significant risk factor for suicide is a previous suicide attempt. This and other risk factors are listed in Exhibit 21–3. Most suicides have multiple causes.[19]

A study of primary care patients revealed that relatively few suicide completers had been treated by mental health professionals. In a study of suicide completers age 75 or older, about three-quarters had seen a physician within one month and 35% within one week of death. Although a substantial number of these persons were determined, by psychological autopsy, to have substantial psychopathology, many were not treated at all. Among those whose psychopathology was recognized by their physicians, treatment was inadequate.[13] Thus, suicide prevention is a very important role for the primary care physician.[20]

Exhibit 21–3   Risk Factors for Suicide in Later Life

- Previous suicide attempt
- Prior depression or other psychiatric diagnosis
- Advanced age
- Poor social support
- Delirium
- Advanced medical disease
- Lifelong alcohol abuse
- Substance abuse
- Poorly controlled pain
- High level of hopelessness
- Loss of independence

■ SELF-NEGLECT

Self-neglect may also be an indication that an older person is at risk for self-injurious behavior. It is often hidden and likely very much underreported. It is incumbent on the GCM to look for and report signs of self-neglect. These may include unexplained weight loss, poor hygiene, poor housekeeping, hoarding, resistance to seeking or accepting any ameliorative services, and lack of compliance with medical regimens. Dementia and/or depression are often present. Whether self-neglect is part of other psychiatric conditions or a discrete geriatric syndrome is a matter of current debate.[21] Self-neglect can be frustrating for professionals trying to intervene and is the most common reason for referrals to adult protective services agencies. It may be necessary for the GCM to make a protective services referral in more serious cases.

■ SCREENING INSTRUMENTS

Standardized screening tools can be administered easily to identify depressive symptoms as a potential problem. Some of the more commonly used screening tools are the Geriatric Depression Scale, the Zung Self-Rating Depression Scale, the Depression Inventory, and the Hamilton Depression Inventory. Some of these instruments are described elsewhere, including in an article by Aronson and Shiffman.[22] These instruments are not diagnostic, but abnormal scores indicate a need for medical or psychiatric evaluation and further follow-up. Which tool is selected is not as critical as the need for the GCM to include depression screening in the clinical assessment. This procedure will be 10 or 15 minutes very well spent. A history of other psychiatric conditions must be obtained as well.

Although the depression screening instruments are sensitive to major depression, minor depression and anxiety disorders may be missed. Thus, the GCM must look not only at the score but the appearance, manner, and function of the elder. Unexplained declines in grooming, hygiene, interest in leisure activities, and interactions with family and friends may indicate possible depression.[23] Also the GCM must be alert to inconsistencies.

Getting a depressed older person to agree to medical evaluation and treatment may be easier said than done. Resistance may manifest itself as denial, a struggle for power, nastiness, or fear. The GCM must always keep in mind that most older persons do not consult psychiatrists. Rather, they are treated for psychiatric symptoms by their primary care physicians, if at all. Thus, the GCM must establish rapport with the client, his or her family, and his or her primary care physician. It may take substantial time and effort to get the client to agree to an evaluation, let alone treatment. A substantial proportion of individuals may never agree to evaluation or treatment.

■ DIAGNOSING DEPRESSION

As noted earlier, depression is not a normal part of aging and can cause unnecessary discomfort and diminished quality of life. It is important that younger persons not impose their fears and stereotypes about old age on older persons.[24] Depressive illness covers a spectrum of conditions, including dysthymia, minor depression, situational depression, and major depression. Because of depressive illnesses' high comorbidity with medical illness in later life, a comprehensive assessment is recommended for differential diagnosis. Elements of a diagnostic workup are listed in Exhibit 21–4.

The GCM plays a very important role in the diagnosis and management of depression. He or she is on the front line and must recognize the presence of depression and initiate the diagnostic and treatment processes. In older persons, depressive symptoms may be present

Exhibit 21–4 Diagnostic Workup for Late Life Depression

- Psychosocial history
- Mental status (cognitive) screen
- Depression screen
- Assessment of activities of daily living and instrumental activities of daily living
- Assessment of sleep and activity patterns
- Assessment of severity of depressive symptoms
- Assessment of suicidal ideation and history of prior attempts
- Medical history
- Review of prescription and over-the-counter medications
- Physical examination
- Routine diagnostic tests (e.g., electrocardiogram), laboratory tests, or imaging (e.g., computed tomography scan or magnetic resonance imaging), if indicated to clarify diagnosis
- Psychiatric consultation, if needed for clarification
- Neuropsychological testing, if needed for clarification

as physical complaints such as pain, fatigue, appetite changes, or sleep problems. A comprehensive psychosocial evaluation by the GCM includes obtaining information about changes in relationships and activity patterns, severity of depressive symptoms, alcohol or other substance abuse, suicidal ideation, plans for suicide, prior suicide attempts, impulsivity, and hopelessness.[25]

The GCM must work collaboratively with the physician to obtain a differential diagnosis and develop and implement a feasible care plan. The GCM can be an important resource for the physician because he or she is able to offer insights into the client's living arrangement, family relationships, social network, functional abilities, beliefs, compliance, coping style, and other factors that must be taken into account in determining appropriate treatment and management strategies.

◼ DEPRESSION AND DEMENTIA

Symptoms of depression and dementia may overlap or occur as comorbidities with other medical conditions as well as with each other.[26] For example, vitamin deficiencies may present with depression as well as dementia. Hypothyroidism may present with symptoms of decreased interest and energy, symptoms that are common to both depression and dementia. On close review, many symptoms are similar but not identical (Table 21–1).

For example, the sad affect of a depressed individual may often be confused with the blank affect of an individual with dementia. The lack of response to questions or slow responsiveness of the depressed individual caused by poor concentration may superficially appear to be similar to the loss of memory of the individual with dementia. Poor hygiene and self-neglect may be common to both conditions. These similarities are confounded by the fact that depression occurs concurrently in about 35% of dementia cases.[27] The presence of depression often causes excess disability, worsening the dementia symptoms. Evaluation and treatment of both the dementia and the depression are warranted.[28]

CASE STUDY

The Case of Mrs. C
Mrs. C presented to the GCM with early dementia after her husband and family had consulted with the GCM regarding care planning on several occasions. They were heartbroken by the diagnosis and fearful of the future. Mrs. C had been diagnosed with an "Alzheimer-type dementia" and was on no medication or other active treatment. An attractive, physically active, and extremely social woman in her early sixties, Mrs. C verbalized anxiety about her condition and fear about her future. She described having "night terrors" with a recurrent

Table 21–1   Symptoms of Depression and Dementia

	Depression	Dementia
Affect/mood/demeanor	Pervasive sadness, dourness, negativity	Blank matter-of-fact expression Possible overlay of sadness
Memory	Poor concentration and temporary memory decrease	Progressive impairment of short term memory, eventually long-term memory
Function	Functional ability diminished by lack of motivation	Functional ability (activities of daily living and instrumental activities of daily living) diminished by declining abilities
Organization	Impaired decision making	Impaired executive function (e.g., organization, prioritization)
Orientation	Intact or impaired orientation	Impaired orientation
Language	Slowed language	Trouble finding words and naming things
Motivation	Impaired motivation	Possible impaired motivation
Appetite/Weight	Either decreased appetite and weight or increased appetite and weight	Trouble remembering to eat Decrease in weight with no obvious explanation
Sleep	Possible problems falling asleep, staying asleep, or waking up	Possible sleep problems or no sleep problems
Thinking/reasoning; Ability to learn	Slow thinking and reasoning Ability to learn is retained Inability to learn new things	Impairment
Danger	Possible suicide	Safety concerns because of impaired judgment
Somatic complaints/pain	Possible multiple or exaggerated somatic complaints Fatigue	Complaints that are under-reported or perseverated upon Fatigue
Depression screening tool	Possible high scores	Possible high scores or low scores

dream about being in a coffin. She described crying spells and stated that she also was unable to enjoy activities as much as she had previously. She had loved entertaining family and friends but had withdrawn from this activity. She also had started napping in the afternoon, which had never been part of her daily routine.

The GCM believed that this individual had a comorbid clinical depression and guided the family into obtaining a psychiatric evaluation and active treatment for the depression. Additionally, the family was urged to seek the pharmacotherapies that were available for the cognitive impairment. The client's depression was brought under control and the overlay of "excess disability" was diminished. The family was advised to have her discontinue driving the car and to hire a companion, who would help Mrs. C participate in activities and would ensure mobility and socialization. These comprehensive interventions helped to stabilize her and enable her to participate in a range of daily activities. Mrs. C remained on a plateau for at least a year but then experienced a gradual but noticeable deterioration. Her activities were adjusted and readjusted as her cognitive and functional abilities changed.

The overlay of depression in Mrs. C had eluded several physicians, including the primary care physician, who allegedly knew Mrs. C well. This is not uncommon.[29] The GCM was able to step in and facilitate the needed medical intervention. The treatment of the depression unquestionably improved the quality of life for both the client and her family. In the course of the GCM's work with this family, there had been care planning, entitlement counseling, advocacy, counseling about available programs and resources, training of formal caregivers, and emotional support for the client, spouse, and family. The spouse developed a clinical depression in response to the worsening of his wife's condition, which he had difficulty accepting and for which he resisted treatment.

In this case, the client was quite verbal and there were reliable historians to query, so needed historical information was available to the GCM to suggest that the client was depressed. Depression may be difficult to assess in individuals who live alone because they may be poor historians and there may be no one available to objectively report changes in socialization, motivation, sleep, anxiety, performance of activities of daily living, and nutritional status. In these situations, the GCM may have to locate an informant—a relative, friend, or neighbor who sees the client frequently and is familiar with his or her day-to-day life. Additionally, several observations over a period of weeks or months may be required to ascertain the existence and persistence of depressive symptoms.

■ DELIRIUM

In the course of determining a differential diagnosis, there is a third "D," delirium, that must be taken into account along with depression and dementia.[30] Delirium is a state of acute confusion to which older persons with dementia are more vulnerable than are older persons without dementia. The onset of delirium is sudden and may occur in any setting, hospitals and nursing homes included. Depression, dementia, and delirium are compared in Table 21-2.

The GCM, who follows clients regularly and knows their behaviors and routines, may be the first to identify a precipitous change in condition such as the development of a delirium. If a delirium is suspected, it is important that medical intervention be obtained immediately, because delirium may be a manifestation of a serious medical condition and can be life-threatening.

■ DEPRESSION AND FAMILY CAREGIVERS

Approximately 80% of the care of older persons is provided by family caregivers; spouses, who may be older and frail themselves; or adult children, most commonly daughters and daughters-in-law. Caregiving is a demanding

Table 21-2   The Three D's: Depression, Dementia, and Delirium

	Depression	Dementia	Delirium
Onset	Usually within a period of weeks	Slow, insidious, over a period of months/years	Abrupt, may be within hours or days
Symptoms	Pervasive sadness or loss of pleasure, plus vegetative signs	Gradual decline in functioning, including recent memory loss	Fluctuation in consciousness and attention Possible hallucinations, delusions
Course	Episodic, treatable resolvable	Progressive, manageable	Treatable, usually resolvable
Consequences	May complicate course of other illnesses May lead to decrease in self-care May lead to suicide and various safety problems	Results in decrease in ability to perform activities of daily living, poor judgment, and decreased ability to learn	May be harbinger of medical illness Can flag life-threatening emergency Requires prompt medical intervention
Phenomenology	Can coexist with other Ds, causing "excess disability, and may complicate course of other illnesses	May make depression and delirium harder to recognize	Is more prevalent in persons with dementia and hospitalized patients
Treatment	Multiple simultaneous interventions	Multiple simultaneous interventions	Medical intervention first, to address underlying illness

job that often becomes overwhelming. For this reason, depression is quite prevalent among caregivers. Studies of caregivers of individuals with dementia indicate that the prevalence of depression is approximately 35%. The GCM must be sensitive to this possibility and must consider it in the assessment and care planning process. The depression of the caregiver affects both caregiver and care recipient. Research has indicated that depressed persons were less likely to recover when their caregivers reported more psychiatric symptoms, more difficulties in providing care, and poorer physical health themselves.[31] Unfortunately, caregivers resist seeing themselves as people who themselves need interventions, which have been shown to be effective.[32]

CASE STUDY

The Case of Ms. A

Ms. A, a 55-year-old widow and only child, had been the primary caregiver to her 84-year-old mother for 15 years. For most of this time, she also held a responsible full-time job. When she was forced to retire because of corporate reorganization, she became a full-time caregiver. As hard as Ms. A worked as a caregiver, her mother's dementia progressed, the incontinence worsened, and so, too, did her mother's propensity to fall. After about a year of full-time caregiving, Ms. A was considering placing her mother in a nursing home because the physical and emotional demands of caregiving had become overwhelming.

As she deliberated over the decision to place, she herself began to cry frequently, had difficulty making decisions, had sleep problems, and had other classic signs of clinical depression. She became increasingly isolated and lonely. She became immobilized in the face of the need to make a decision and was unable to make the placement. With much encouragement from a GCM, she joined a caregiver support group and was advised to seek psychiatric evaluation and treatment for her depression. With group, individual, and psychopharmacologic interventions, she was able to make the placement successfully. This enabled her to mobilize herself to re-enter the work force, to rebuild her personal life, and to decrease her isolation and loneliness. In this case, the caregiver's immobility and inability to make the placement decision caused her pain and suffering and also denied her mother the level of care she truly needed. Once the caregiver responded to the interventions she required, the placement of the parent with dementia was able to occur.

The tasks of the GCM in this case were to assess both client and caregiver and to develop a care plan—in this case, placement of the older person with dementia and intervention for the overwhelmed caregiver. The GCM had to work with the caregiver, nursing home, and physician to facilitate the placement. She also had to recommend and support appropriate treatment for the caregiver's depression and provide emotional support. It is incumbent on the GCM to educate and advise family caregivers about available resources for themselves as well as for the person for whom they are caring. In this case, the GCM was instrumen-

tal in supporting Ms. A through the difficult process of placing her mother and the subsequent rebuilding of her life and her career and witnessed the resilience of this caregiver.

Caregivers may themselves be resistant to following an appropriate care plan. This is especially true when it comes to making tough decisions such as taking over the finances or placing a loved one in a nursing home. Deciding to place a loved one is one of the hardest decisions a caregiver may ever have to make. The case of Ms. A illustrates the painfulness of the placement decision and how caregivers can get stuck in a vicious cycle of depression, guilt, martyrdom, and neglect of their own needs.[33]

CASE STUDY

The Case of Ms. H

Ms. H, a 60-year-old widow, cares for her ailing father, who lives with her in a housing arrangement that is unsuited to her father's mobility limitations. Her father has severe cardiovascular disease with a history of stroke and a mixed (vascular and Alzheimer's) dementia. Access to their apartment involves a steep flight of stairs that her father is physically incapable of navigating. Ms. H holds a full-time job and uses a combination of part-time in-home caregivers and day care to get through the days. Both the client and the caregiver have limited incomes and assets.

Although her father can be very pleasant at times, he is generally difficult to manage and resistive to personal care. He has intermittent sleep disturbance, which leaves Ms. H perpetually tired, frustrated, and angry. When she yells at him, she feels guilty; yet she cannot contain her anger.

Ms. H is an only child and is estranged from her children. She had a difficult upbringing, and so did her children. The family issues remain unresolved. She gets no help from her children, only criticism when she sees them occasionally. Ms. H cries easily, is anxiety ridden, and is frustrated. Physically, the caregiving is getting more difficult, and she is "maxed out" on the amount of help she can afford to hire to supplement what is supplied under the benefits entitlement system.

While her own health was deteriorating with potentially serious conditions she tried to ignore, she was struggling with the idea of placing her father in a nursing home. Her ambivalence prevented her from acting. She felt guilty even thinking about placement, although she was overwhelmed and her father was not getting as much care as he needed. Although placement would allow her to break the vicious cycle she was in and become free enough to begin rebuilding her own life, she remained overwhelmed and immobilized. It took more than a year before she was able to accomplish the placement. She became clinically depressed after placement and refused to visit her father for several weeks.

The GCM worked with Ms. H and supported her emotionally through this difficult time. The GCM also urged Ms. H to seek medical evaluation for pharmacotherapy to treat her depression so she could cope with the placement and begin the process of rebuilding her own life. Placing an older person in an institutional setting is often traumatic and increases emotional distress, which may require crisis intervention.

■ RECENT TRENDS

In the 1990s, rates of diagnosis of depression in Medicare beneficiaries increased dramatically, with concomitant increases in treatment. The number of prescriptions for anti-depression medications has risen. How-

ever, there remain significant disparities by age, ethnicity, and insurance coverage in the treatment of those who were diagnosed.[34] "Older minorities and the old-old are less likely to access depression treatments."[35] And there is little information regarding the quality of care. Thus, despite better recognition by health providers and increased treatments, elderly patients may still not be receiving effective care for depression.

■ TREATMENT

Treatment for depression is available in outpatient settings, inpatient settings, and in day hospital programs—also called partial hospitalization or intensive outpatient programs. Although hospitalization may be necessary in severe cases, it is not always the best setting for frail older persons. Unfortunately, however, Medicare reimbursement favors inpatient hospitalization. For inpatient services, Medicare reimburses treatment for psychiatric illness as it would medical illness. For outpatient treatment, however, there are financial disincentives, including a large copayment (50%) and an annual limit for physician reimbursement. With the introduction in 2006 of prescription drug coverage under Medicare Part D, older persons have greater access to expensive psychotropic medications and this will likely affect practice patterns.

Pharmacologic and nonpharmacologic interventions have been shown to be effective in treating depression.[36-39] When pharmacotherapy is utilized, doses must be therapeutic and clients must be closely followed.[40] Pharmacotherapies may not be sufficient in and of themselves, but may make depressed individuals more amenable to other interventions. Supportive therapy is often effective in helping those older persons with adjustment disorders or difficulties in adaptation to losses or other stressors. Electroconvulsive therapy is often an effective modality. Problem-solving therapies have been reported to be a suitable modality. Group or individual sessions may be utilized.[41] Positive outcomes have been reported with the use of physical exercise, yoga, and activities.

There is no evidence that any one therapeutic modality is better than another, and an eclectic approach is usually warranted. Social and family support is integral to recovery, so it is incumbent on the GCM and other involved clinicians to mobilize, educate, and support the members of the afflicted individual's family and social network. Although loss and infirmity are common, depression must be seen as an illness, separate from sadness over illness or loss. Therapeutic goals must be realistic. Older persons need to be treated so they can find meaning in their lives, despite their limitations, and can enjoy and maintain remission of their depressive symptoms.

There is a dearth of well-designed outcome studies on treatment of depression in older persons in general and frail older persons in particular. Most of the existing studies have been done on inpatient populations, which are not necessarily a representative sample of older depressed individuals. The data suggest that there is a higher degree of recidivism than for younger depressed persons. Clinical trials of pharmacologic agents have intentionally included subjects without significant comorbidities. Often, they have had an upper age limit as well. Thus, little is known about outcomes of treatment of medically ill older persons and the oldest among them, who are actually the most affected by depressive illness.

Hospitalization is indicated in severe or clinically complex cases or for those persons with no available at-home caregiver. However, for many older persons, hospitalization disrupts the routine of life and can be disorienting. Intensive outpatient treatments such as day hospitals and day treatment programs are good alternatives to hospitalization because they enable depressed persons to maintain their familiar surroundings and social ties.

■ SAFETY ISSUES

Severely depressed individuals are always at risk for suicide and should not be left alone. Where supervision cannot be provided by family or paid caregivers, movement to a sheltered setting is indicated. Monitoring the person and making the home safer are important when dealing with a depressed person. This is essential, even upon the return of a previously hospitalized person to the community. The GCM can be instrumental in this process and should be proactive. The family should be instructed to remove the following items from the home: weapons such as guns and knives and potential weapons such as axes, hammers, razors, and scissors. Poisonous household products such as cleaning solutions and solvents should be removed or locked up. Matches should be kept out of reach. Unused medications must be discarded, and available medications should be kept only in small quantities that are not lethal.

■ DEPRESSION AND THE ROLE OF THE GCM

The GCM should serve as the linchpin in the process of recognition, diagnosis, and management of depression, not only by working directly with the client, family, and physician but also by working with other health providers and formal and informal caregivers, providing emotional support and training.

Recognizing depression in older persons can be a challenge to professionals and laypersons alike. Professionals are not necessarily immune from ageism and therapeutic nihilism and all too often hold negative stereotypes that delay prompt diagnosis and treatment of depressive symptoms in older persons. This is confounded by the fact that older persons may not tell their health providers or their families directly about their feelings or physical symptoms because of a fear of being labeled "mental" or otherwise stigmatized. Rather, older persons with depression may look, act, or express themselves differently or may demonstrate a generalized "failure to thrive."[42] These changes may be quite apparent to those who know the older person well but vague or inconclusive to others, including health providers. It may take time and patience to identify and sort out the symptoms, and many health providers do not spend this time. In some situations, there may be economic disincentives toward spending the time needed to obtain an adequate history, do a comprehensive assessment, and provide carefully monitored and effective treatment. Thus, there is an ongoing search for a quick fix—perhaps a "magic pill."

■ THE GCM AS EDUCATOR AND TRAINER

How can the GCM promote recognition of depression in frail older persons? Informal and formal caregivers must be taught to observe and assess the usual behavior patterns and activity level of the frail older person, so that they will be able to recognize physical, mental, and emotional changes if they occur. Changes can occur quickly and may have significant consequences. The GCM must make older persons themselves and their caregivers aware that they must not merely accept unexplained changes in mood and function, ascribing them to aging, illness, or loss; rather, they must report these changes to their health providers. It must be emphasized that depression is an illness and occurs in addition to social losses and physical infirmities. It is treatable and manageable, with the potential outcome of treatment being an improvement in quality of life for the individual and those around him or her. All depressed individuals, including frail older persons, deserve competent assessment and appropriate treatment.

The GCM must present basic strategies for identifying and managing depression. The starting point in identifying depression or other mood changes is to determine how the client feels and how he or she functions. The GCM will use a combination of techniques to assess the client. Basic assessment techniques include observation and listening. The assessor must listen carefully to what the client says and must get a good history from a reliable informant, if necessary for clarification. Screening tools may also be used.

As an individual becomes clinically depressed, his or her appearance changes and the assessor must look for these changes. While the changes may be subtle at the beginning and difficult for an individual who sees the client daily to detect, they will probably be apparent to the trained eye of the GCM. Possible changes are listed in Exhibit 21–5.

As a clinical depression develops, there will also be changes in behavior and activity level. The GCM must gather this information as well. Some more common behavior and activity level changes are described in Exhibit 21–6.

The affected individual may make statements indicative of hopelessness or self-deprecating comments during the assessment or

Exhibit 21–5
Changes in Appearance

- Newly stooped posture
- Slowing of movement
- Slowing of thought processes
- Unexplained weight loss or weight gain
- Clothing that does not fit
- Poor grooming
- Poor maintenance of clothing
- Poor hygiene
- Diminished energy level
- Unexplained fatigue
- Sad affect

Exhibit 21–6   Changes in Behavior and Activity Level

- Decrease in social participation
- Increase in isolation and social withdrawal
- Decreased interest in things
- Difficulty with decision making
- Difficulty concentrating
- Unusual negativism

these types of statements may be reported by the caregiver. Exhibit 21–7 contains some of these statements.

In working with depressed individuals, caregivers need to use various strategies for interaction and communication. The GCM can serve as a role model in this regard. Suggestions are contained in Exhibit 21–8.

Exhibit 21–7   Statements That May Be Indicative of Depression

- I'm not the person I used to be.
- I can't manage to get anything done.
- I'm awake all night and then get to sleep in the morning.
- Nobody can do anything for me.
- I don't care if I die.
- Things are hopeless.
- I don't want to be a burden to anyone.
- I've heard that medicines have too many side effects, so I don't want any.
- I may be nervous, but I'm not mental.
- Who cares?
- Nobody wants me.
- I'm too poor to afford that.

Exhibit 21–8   Strategies for Communication with and Outreach to a Depressed Person

- Listen.
- Recognize changes—trust your eyes, ears, sense of smell, and general intuition.
- Remain calm—do not panic.
- Acknowledge the person's feelings. Do not try to talk the person out of the feelings.
- If the person expresses suicidal ideas, refer the person for immediate psychiatric evaluation and treatment.
- Be reassuring. The person is ill, and things will get better.
- Don't be judgmental. Depression is an illness and not something the person has chosen.
- Provide positive reinforcement, as appropriate.
- Acknowledge positive steps toward recovery.

■ CONCLUSION

Depression is a prevalent and perplexing problem in the older population. Although there has been a dramatic increase in depression diagnosis and treatment in the last decade or so, significant attitudinal, financial, and system barriers remain. Given the Baby boomers' greater knowledge and concern regarding health and mental health issues, tomorrow's elderly persons will be more likely to seek diagnosis and treatment than are today's elderly and will demand more from the system.

The projected explosion of the older population and their increasing longevity make it necessary to address the gaps in information, training, and practice regarding depression in older persons to promote a better quality of life for those who are afflicted.

■ NOTES

1. Unitzer J, Simon G, Belin TR, Dott M, Kayton W, Patrick D. Care for depression in HMO patients aged 65 and older. *J Am Geriatr Soc.* 2000:48:871–878.

2. Hughes CM, Lapane KL, Mor V, et al. The impact of legislation on psychotropic drug use in nursing homes: a crossnational perspective. *J Am Geriatr Soc.* 2000;48:931–937.

3. Federal Interagency Forum on Aging–Related Statistics. Older Americans 2004: key indicators of well-being. Washington, DC: U.S. Government Printing Office; 2004.

4. American Psychiatric Association. *Diagnostic and Statistical Manual of Mental Disorders.* 4th ed. Washington, DC: American Psychiatric Association; 1994.

5. U.S. Department of Health and Human Services. *Depression in Primary Care.* Vol 1. Washington, DC: U.S. Department of Health and Human Services; 1993. AHCPR Clinical Practice Guideline Number 5.

6. Smith SL, Sherrill KS, Colenda CC. Assessing and treating anxiety in older persons. *Psychiatr Serv.* 1995;46(1):36–42.

7. Kennedy GJ. The geriatric syndrome of late-life depression. *Psychiatr Serv.* 1995;46:43–48.

8. Hagans E, Hanscom J. Assessment of depression in a population at risk: newly admitted nursing home residents. *J Gerontol Nurs.* 1998;24:21–29.

9. Bisschop MI, Kriegsman DMW, Deen JH, Beekman AT, VanTilburg W. The longitudinal relation between chronic diseases and depression in older persons living in the community: the longitudinal aging study. Amsterdam. *J Clin Epidemiology.* 2004:57(2):187–194.

10. Schnittker J. Chronic illness and depressive symptoms in late life. *Soc Sci Med.* 2005: 60(1):13–23.

11. Szegedy-Maszak M. Reason to be happy. *US News and World Report.* April 10, 2006:41–43.

12. Lyness JM, Bruce ML, Koenig HG, et al. Depression and medical illness in late-life: report of a symposium. *J Am Geriatr Soc.* 1996; 44:198–203.

13. Caine ED, Lyness JM, Conwell Y. Diagnosis of late-life depression: preliminary studies in primary care settings. *Am J Geriatr Psychiatry.* 1996;4:S45–50.

14. Conwell Y. Outcomes of depression. *Am J Geriatr Psychiatry.* 1996;4:S34–44.

15. Takeshita J, Masak K, Ahmed I, et al. Depressive symptoms are risk factors for mortality in elderly people, particularly in those who are physically healthy. *Am J Psychiatry.* 2002; 159(7):1127–1132.

16. Adamson JA, Price GM, Breeze E, et al. Are older people dying of depression? Findings from the Medical Research Council Trial of the assessment and management of older people in the community. *J Am Geriatr Soc.* 2005;53:1128–1132.

17. Aronson MK. Management of pain: an important mental health issue for older adults. *Dimensions* (Newsletter of the ASA Mental Health and Aging Network). 2005;12:5.

18. Conwell Y, Lyness JM, Duberstein P, et al. Completed suicide among elder patients in primary care practices. *J Am Geriatr Soc.* 2000;48:23–29.

19. Arbore P. Dangerous behavior: assessment, intervention and treatment of suicidal ideation in older adults. Presented at: The American Society on Aging/NCOA Joint Conference; Anaheim, CA: March 2006.

20. Wittenberg JS. Interventions for older suicidal patients. *Geriatr Consultant.* 1993;12:24–27.

21. Pavlou MP, Lachs MS. Could self-neglect in older adults be a geriatric syndrome. *J Am Geriatr Soc.* 2006;54:831–842.

22. Aronson M, Shiffman JK. Clinical assessment in home care. *J Gerontol Soc Work.* 1995;24: 213–231.

23. Kennedy GJ. *Geriatric Mental Health Care.* New York: Guilford Press; 2000.

24. Rimer S. Gaps seen in treating depression in the elderly. *New York Times.* September 5, 1999:1.

25. Szanto K, Reynolds CF, Conwell Y, Begley AE, Houck P. High levels of hopelessness persist in geriatric patients with remitted depression and a history of attempted suicide. *J Am Geriatr Soc.* 1998;46:1401–1406.

26. Merriam A, Aronson, MK, Gaston P, Wey S, Katz I. The psychiatric symptoms of Alzheimer's disease. *J Am Geriatr Soc.* 1988;36:7–12.

27. Katz I, Aronson MK, Lipkowitz R. Depression secondary to dementia presents an ongoing dilemma. *Generations.* 1982;7:24.

28. Aronson MK, Gaston P, Merriam A. Depression associated with dementia. *Generations.* 1984;9:49–51.

29. Katz IR. What should we do about undertreatment of late life psychiatric disorders in primary care? *J Am Geriatr Soc.* 1998;46:1573–1575.

30. Breitner JCS, Welsh KA. Diagnosis and management of memory loss and cognitive disorders among elderly persons. *Psychiatr Serv.* 1995;46(1):29–35.

31. Hinrichson GA, Zweig R. Family issues in late-life depression. *J Long-Term Home Health Care.* 1994;13:4–15.

32. Mittelman MS, Ferris SH, Shulman E, et al. A comprehensive support program: effect of depression on spouse-caregivers of AD patients. *Gerontologist.* 1995;35(6):792–802.

33. Aronson MK, Weiner MB. *Aging Parents, Aging Children: How to Stay Sane and Survive.* New York: Rowman & Littlefield; 2007.

34. Crystal S, Sambamoorhi U, Wakop ST, et al. Diagnosis and treatment of depression in the elderly Medicare population: predictors, disparities and trends. *J Am Geriatr Soc.* 2003;51:1718–1728.

35. Arcan PA, Unitzer J. Inequities in depression management in low-income, minority and old-old adults: a matter of access to preferred treatments? *J Am Geriatr Soc.* 2003;51:1808–1809.

36. Schneider LS. Pharmacologic considerations in the treatment of late-life depression. *Am J Geriatr Psychiatry*. 1996;4(1):S51–S65.

37. Zistook S. Depression in late-life: special considerations in treatment. *Postgrad Med*. 1996; 100(4):161–167.

38. Zarit SH, Knight BG, eds.. *A Guide to Psychotherapy and Aging*. Washington, DC: American Psychological Association:1996.

39. Duffy M, ed. *Handbook of Counseling and Psychotherapy with Older Adults*. New York: John Wiley & Sons; 1999.

40. Rabheru K. Special issues in the management of depression in older patients. *Can J Psychiatry*. 2004;49(3 suppl 1):41S–50S.

41. Clark WG, Vorst VR. Group therapy with chronically depressed geriatric patients. *J Psychosoc Nurs Mental Health Serv*. 1994;32: 9–13.

42. Katz IR, Beaston-Wimmer P, Parmelee P, Friedman E, Lawton MP. Failure to thrive in the elderly: exploration of the concept and delineation of psychiatric components. *J Geriatr Psychiatr Neurol*. 1993;6:161–169.

Contact Information

Alzheimer's Association
225 N. Michigan Ave., 17th Floor
Chicago, IL 60601-7633
Telephone: (800) 272–3900
Web site: www.alz.org

AARP
601 East Street NW
Washington, DC 20049
Telephone: (888) 687–2277
Fax: (202) 434–2588
Web site: http://www.aarp.org
E-mail: member@aarp.org

American Society on Aging (ASA)
833 Market Street, Suite 511
San Francisco, CA 94103-1824
Telephone: (415) 974–9600
Fax: (415) 974–0300
Web site: http://www.asaging.org
E-mail: info@asaging.org

Case Management Society of America (CMSA)
6301 Ranch Dr.
Suite 230
Little Rock, AR 72223-4623
Telephone: (501) 225–2229
Fax: (501) 221–9068
Web site: http://www.cmsa.org
E-mail: cmsa@cmsa.org

Internal Revenue Service (IRS)
1111 Constitution Avenue NW
Washington, DC 20224
Telephone: (202) 622–5000
Web site: www.irs.gov

National Academy of Elder Law Attorneys (NAELA)
1604 North Country Club Road
Tucson, AZ 85716-3102
Telephone: (520) 881–4005
Fax: (520) 325–7925
Web site: http://www.naela.org
E-mail: info@naela.com

National Association of Insurance and Financial Advisors (NAIFA)
2901 Telestar Ct.
P.O. Box 12012
Falls Church, VA 22042-1205
Telephone: 877-TO–NAIFA
Web site: www.naifa.org

National Association of Professional Geriatric Care Managers
1604 North Country Club Road
Tucson, AZ 85716-3102
Telephone: (520) 881–8008
Fax: (520) 325–7925
Web site: http://www.caremanager.org
E-mail: info@caremanager.org

National Association of Social Workers (NASW)
750 First Street NE, Suite 700
Washington, DC 20002-4241
Telephone: (202) 408-8600
Web site: http://www.socialworkers.org
E-mail: info@naswdc.org

National Council on Aging (NCOA)
1901 L Street, 4th Floor
Washington, DC 20036
Telephone: (202) 479-1200
Fax: (202) 479-0735
Web site: http://www.ncoa.org
E-mail: info@ncoa.org

National Organization for Competency Assurance (NOCA)
2025 M Street NW, Suite 800
Washington, DC 20036
Telephone: (202) 367-1165
Fax: (202) 367-2165
Web site: info@noca.org

The Gerontological Society of America (GSA)
1030 15th Street NW, Suite 250
Washington, DC 20005
Telephone: (202) 842-1275
Fax: (202) 842-1150
Web site: http://www.geron.org
E-mail: geron@geron.org

Service Corps of Retired Executives
409 3rd Street SW, 6th Floor
Washington, DC 20024
Telephone: (800) 634-0245
Fax: (202) 205-7636
Web site: http://www.score.org

Small Business Administration (SBA)
SBA Answer Desk
6302 Fairview Road
Suite 300
Charlotte, NC 28210
Telephone: (800) 827-5722
Web site: http://www.sba.gov

U.S. Chamber of Commerce
1615 H Street NW
Washington, DC 20062-2000
Telephone: (202) 659-6000, (800) 638-6582
Fax: (202) 463-3164
Web site: http://www.uschamber.com
E-mail: custvc@uschamber.com

Index